The Endocrinology of Prostate Tumours

The Endocrinology of Prostate Tumours

EDITED BY

Reza Ghanadian

Senior Lecturer, Royal Postgraduate Medical School
University of London, Hammersmith Hospital
London

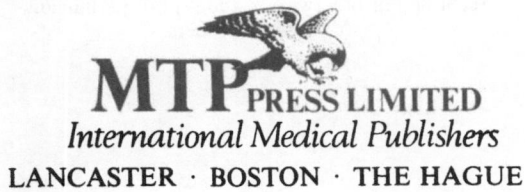

MTP PRESS LIMITED
International Medical Publishers
LANCASTER · BOSTON · THE HAGUE

Published in the UK and Europe by
MTP Press Limited
Falcon House
Lancaster, England

British Library Cataloguing in Publication Data

The Endocrinology of prostate tumours.
1. Prostate gland—Tumors
2. Endocrine therapy
I. Ghanadian, Reza
616.99'263   RC280.P7

ISBN-13: 978-94-011-7258-5

Published in the USA by
MTP Press
A division of Kluwer Boston Inc
190 Old Derby Street
Hingham, MA 02043, USA

Library of Congress Cataloging in Publication Data

Main entry under title:

The Endocrinology of prostate tumours.

Includes bibliographies and index.
1. Prostate gland—Tumors.
2. Hormones, Sex.
I. Ghanadian, Reza.
[DNLM: 1. Prostatic neoplasms—Drug therapy.
2. Prostate.
3. Hormones—Therapeutic use.
4. Hormones—Metabolism. WJ 752 E55]
RC280.P7E5 1982   616.99'263   82–17268
ISBN-13: 978-94-011-7258-5   e-ISBN-13: 978-94-011-7256-1
DOI: 10.1007/978-94-011-7256-1

Contents

Contents

Contributors

I. D. ANSELL MA, MB, B Chir, MRCPath
Consultant Histopathologist
City Hospital
University of Nottingham
Medical School
Nottingham, UK

G. AUF BSc, MSc, PhD
Research Officer
Prostate Research Laboratory
Royal Postgraduate Medical School
University of London
London, UK

L. L. BEYNON MA, MB, MChir, FRCS
Senior Registrar
Department of Surgery
Western General Hospital
Edinburgh, UK

N. J. BLACKLOCK OBE, MB, FRCS
Professor of Urology
Department of Urology
University of Manchester
    and Consultant Urological Surgeon
University Hospital of South Manchester,
Manchester, UK

G. D. CHISHOLM ChM, FRCS, FRCSE
Professor of Surgery
University of Edinburgh
Consultant Urological Surgeon
Western General Hospital
Edinburgh
    and Hon. Senior Lecturer
St. Peter's Hospital
Institute of Urology
London, UK

C. CHEN PhD
Ben May Laboratory for
Cancer Research
Department of Biochemistry
University of Chicago
Illinois, USA

R. GHANADIAN BSc, DPharm, PhD
Senior Lecturer
Prostate Research Laboratory
Department of Surgery
Royal Postgraduate Medical School
University of London
Hammersmith Hospital
London, UK

S. LIAO PhD
Professor
Ben May Laboratory for
Cancer Research
Department of Biochemistry
University of Chicago
Illinois, USA

C. M. PUAH BSc, MSc
Senior Scientific Officer
Institute of Urology and Prostate
Research Laboratory
Royal Postgraduate Medical School
University of London
London, UK

C. B. SMITH MA, MPhil
Research Assistant
Prostate Research Laboratory
Royal Postgraduate Medical School
University of London
London, UK

G. WILLIAMS MB, BS, FRCS
Consultant Urological Surgeon
Hammersmith Hospital
    and Hon. Senior Lecturer
Royal Postgraduate Medical School
University of London
London, UK

Preface

Tumours of the prostate are the commonest types of neoplasm in the male. Whilst the benign form is virtually a universal condition in the ageing male, malignant tumours rank amongst the top causes of cancer death. Despite the fact that the involvement of the testis in the growth of the prostate has been recognised for almost two centuries, it was not until the early 1940s that Charles Huggins' studies on the effect of orchidectomy and oestrogen therapy on prostatic cancer initiated endocrine manipulation in the management of this malignancy.

During the 1960s progress in the understanding of the mechanism of hormone action, achieved through advances in molecular biology and the recognition of certain aspects of hormonal control in relation to the genome, introduced a new dimension for approaching endocrine manipulation of prostàtic tumours. By the end of that decade a new scientific discipline devoted to prostate research had been born, which brought together investigators in the fields of molecular biology, biochemistry, endocrinology, immunology, urology and pathology to search for the cause and to explore methods for advancing the management of abnormal prostatic growth. Since then a wealth of scientific data has accumulated on the prostate in which endocrinology has manifested itself as the cardinal aspect to which most of the findings can be related.

During the last decade, several international scientific gatherings have attempted to assess progress and to highlight problems in prostate research, but despite all the excellent contributions which can be derived from publication of these meetings and other books, the need to bring together our current understanding of the endocrine control of the prostate and to relate it to a rationale for hormonal manipulation in patients with prostatic tumours seems long overdue. I have tried to accomplish this task, by considering the developmental and morphological background of prostatic growth in relation to the basic endocrinological environment and to follow these through to their mechanism of action at the molecular level. In addition, the current clinical status for the conservative management of prostatic tumours has been discussed and the predictive value of a number of biochemical markers with a special reference to steroid receptors have been presented. Throughout the book, attention has been directed to a critical analysis of the problem to achieve a balanced view of the current research.

It is my hope that this book will complement other contributions in this field and provide a framework from which both research scientists and urologist alike can benefit. In the compilation of this book it has not been possible to

ix

cover all the areas of research which are pertinent to the prostate, in particular some aspects of general biochemistry and immunology have been omitted in order to keep the text within the central theme of endocrinology, and inevitably other relevant contributions might have been omitted for which I take this opportunity to extend my apologies.

I have been most privileged to receive contributions from some distinguished colleagues and friends for which I am most grateful. I also wish to extend my thanks to my colleagues at the Prostate Research Laboratory, to my colleagues and the secretaries at the Urology Unit, Department of Surgery, Royal Postgraduate Medical School and last but not least to my publishers.

July 1982   *Reza Ghanadian*

1
The development and morphology of the prostate

N. J. BLACKLOCK

The prostate gland is a composite structure which includes glandular elements and a stroma of collagenous and muscle tissue. A well defined muscular layer invests the anterior and anterolateral aspects of the gland and interdigitates with the predominantly collagenous capsule enclosing it laterally and posteriorly. This muscular layer extends from the detrusor muscle above to the external sphincter below with which it is continuous. There are both involuntary and striated muscle fibres in this, the latter predominating in the lower half although there are fairly constant fasciculi of striated muscle which extend on either side up to the detrusor and trigonal regions. This muscle is presumed to be predominantly sphincteric in function. A second well defined fibromuscular structure encircles the upper half of the urethra which passes through the gland and consists entirely of involuntary muscle fibres. It is continuous with the deep trigone and internal sphincter above, lies deep to the anterior muscular investment already described and interdigitates with this at its lower termination at the level of the verumontanum. This has been designated the preprostatic sphincter by McNeal (1972) and is functional at the time of ejaculation when it closes off the upper prostatic urethra, preventing reflux of the ejaculate, but it may also have some sphincteric function in urinary continence. The glandular parenchyma lies both posterior and lateral to the urethra from which it is separated above the verumontanum

1

by the preprostatic sphincter and it lies behind the layer of striated and involuntary muscle investing the anterior aspect of the gland. Although this anterior investment of the gland is largely unaltered throughout life, the glandular parenchyma undergoes considerable change during the development, maturation and subsequent degeneration of the gland and the preprostatic sphincter is similarly involved in the degenerative process of benign prostatic hyperplasia (BPH). The morphology of the gland is therefore inconstant and dependent upon age.

Studies suggest two distinct regions in the adult gland (McNeal, 1968, 1972) and there is evidence from embryological and comparative primate studies in support of this (Glenister, 1962; Blacklock and Bouskill, 1977).

1.1   ORIGIN AND DEVELOPMENT OF THE PROSTATE

The rudimentary ducts of the prostate originate as outgrowths of epithelium from the urogenital sinus. Those which originate below the level of the Mullerian tubercle are composed of urogenital sinus endoderm and this part of the sinus later forms the lower part of the definitive prostatic urethra and penile urethra. In this respect it is solely represented in the male.

Glenister (1962) noted that the epithelium of the urogenital sinus at and above the level of the Mullerian tubercle was composite and represented the site of mingling of epithelia from the urogenital sinus, the mesonephric and paramesonephric ducts. In this respect it is distinctive and different from the lining of the rest of the sinus. This composite epithelium gives rise to the prostatic utricle and primitive ducts which extend cranially into the undifferentiated fibromuscular stroma at the base or cranial extremity of the primitive prostate. The two levels of origin of these ducts are well seen in a sagittal section of the urethra and prostate of a 125 mm fetus (Figure 1.1). The part of the sinus above the Mullerian tubercle is represented both in the male and the female and in the latter forms the greater part of the urethra. The paraurethral glands of the female are therefore homologous with the glands in the male which take origin from the urogenital sinus at and above the level of the Mullerian tubercle.

Animal studies (Franks, 1954) showed that oestrogens given to castrated guinea-pigs lead to atrophy and mucinous metaplasia of a lower group of glands but continuation of active secretion by an upper group having its origin near the Mullerian tubercle. Andrews (1951) observed in the human fetus that metaplasia and hyperplasia due to maternal oestrogenic stimulation was most marked in the epithelium of ducts originating around the colliculus and above the opening of the ejaculatory ducts. This area corresponds to that part of the urethral wall whose epithelium has a composite origin from endodermal, mesonephric and paramesonephric primordia. Huggins and Webster (1948) found that oestrogens caused greater degenerative change in the apical or lower portion of the prostate compared with the upper basal region whose ducts arise from the urethra at and above the colliculus.

Thus in the embryo there is the evidence for a dual origin of the adult prostate with different hormone sensitivity of the epithelium.

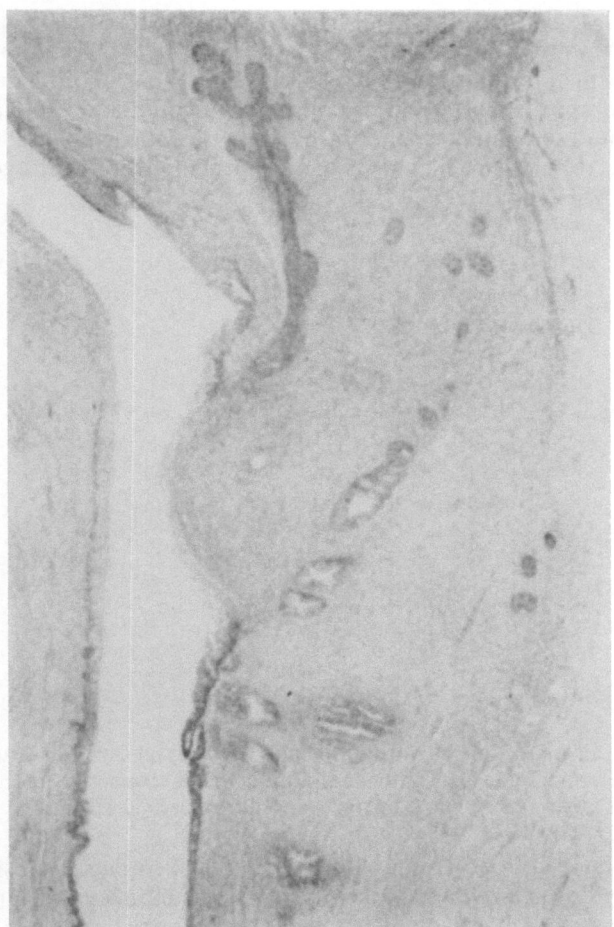

Figure 1.1 Sagittal section through prostatic urethra of 125 mm fetus showing the two levels of origin of the primitive prostatic ducts above and below the Mullerian tubercle

1.2 POSTNATAL DEVELOPMENT

When compared with the growth of the prostate gland in animals the human gland develops slowly. The primary ducts and acini formed in the embryo show little early change but there is a differentiation of the muscle fibres around the lobules of acini. Although the ducts originating from above the colliculus are slower in their appearance and development at the outset, this part of the gland (central zone, McNeal, 1972, Figure 1.4) shows duct branching and the development of new gland buds and subsequently acini within the fibromuscular stroma to a greater extent than the lower and peripheral moiety (peripheral zone, McNeal, 1972, Figure 1.4) in the prepubertal stage. The differential acinar development of the two parts of the gland is obvious in a transverse section of a 9-year-old boy (Figure 1.2). Since the epithelium of the ducts and acini of this central zone of the gland originate from the composite epithelium of both the Mullerian and Wolffian systems and urogenital sinus and responds by hyperplasia and metaplasia to maternal oestrogens, an inference is that it is less dependent upon androgen.

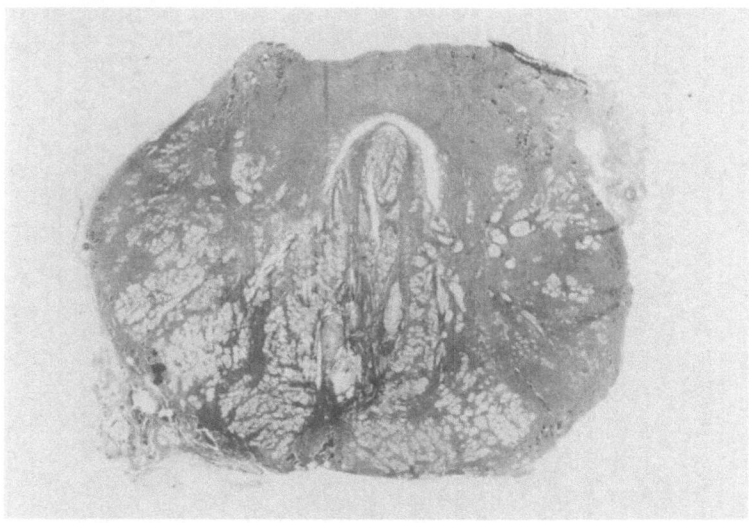

Figure 1.2   Cross-section of prostate of boy aged 9 y at level of verumontanum. Greater differentiation of acini in the central zone than in the peripheral zone laterally which is still largely represented by ducts and fibromuscular stroma

Ghanadian *et al.* (1977) found that the uptake of tritiated testosterone was significantly less in the cranial lobe of the Rhesus monkey prostate than the caudal lobe and the cranial lobe morphologically appears to be homologous with the human central zone.

With the onset of puberty there is progressive development of the fibromuscular stroma and advance of acinar development in the peripheral zone and maturation of the glandular and ductal epithelium in both parts of the gland. Gyorkey (1964) found acid phosphatase activity in epithelial cells of the central zone acini prepubertally although it was present in only some of the peripheral acinar cells.

1.3   COMPARATIVE MORPHOLOGY

The prostate of the lower orders of animals varies in its morphology and in the rodent consists of at least three distinct lobes. The animals for which most information is available are the rat and the dog which have been used extensively in research on the prostate.

The rat, representative of the rodent, has a prostate with dorsolateral, craniodorsal and ventral lobes which are clearly separate and whose fine structure and histochemistry have distinctive features. The dorsolateral lobe has distinctive properties as between its dorsal and lateral extremities; the dorsal tip does not concentrate ^{65}Zn in contrast with the epithelium of the tip of the lateral extremity. The epithelium of the midsection of this lobe has characteristics of both extremities. The ability of the lateral tip to concentrate ^{65}Zn suggests homology of this part with the caudal lobe of the baboon (Schoonees *et al.*, 1969) and the peripheral zone of the human (Kerr *et al.*, 1960). The craniodorsal lobe or coagulating gland in the rat has a flatter epithelium which contains many of the enzymes found in other lobes. This part of the rodent prostate is so called because of the property of its secretion in causing a coagulum when mixed with the secretion of the seminal vesicles.

The prostate of the non-human primate lies on the dorsal aspect of the urethra and has two discrete lobes (Blacklock and Bouskill, 1977) (Figure 1.3).

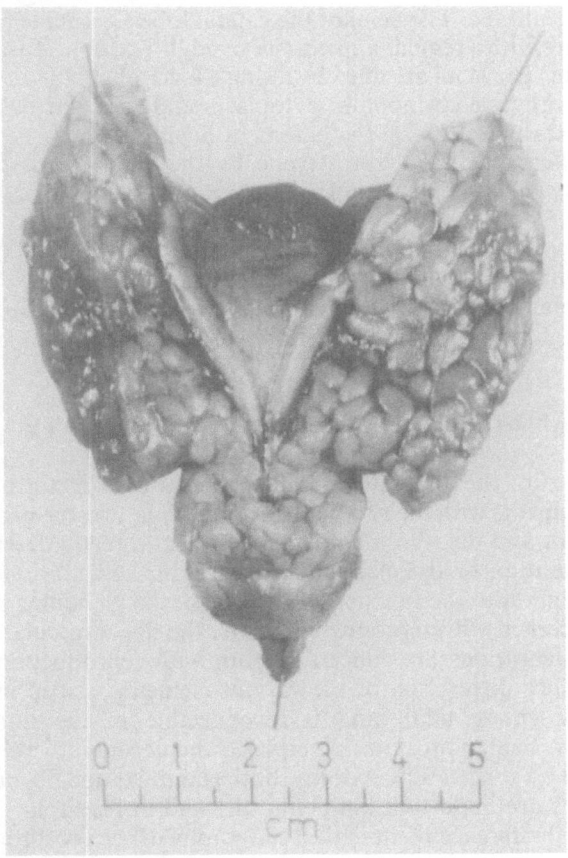

Figure 1.3 Posterior aspect of bladder, cranial and caudal prostate and seminal vesicles of Rhesus monkey. The cranial and caudal lobes of the primate are clearly recognizable

The upper, cranial lobe has a furrowed surface resembling the external appearance of the seminal vesicles. The caudal lobe has a smooth external surface. A thin capsule invests both parts of the prostate and extends on to the seminal vesicles. The caudal lobe is more closely applied to the urethra than the cranial. The terminal vas deferens and the duct of the seminal vesicles on each side pass downwards and forwards through the cranial lobe to enter the urethra. There is almost complete anatomical separation between the cranial and caudal lobes peripherally but they merge anteromedially where the ducts from the cranial lobe in company with the common ejaculatory ducts penetrate the flat upper surface of the caudal lobe to pass into the urethra.

Histologically the appearances of cranial and caudal lobes are different. The acini of the cranial lobe are large, irregular branching tubules with prominent intervening fibromuscular stroma widely separating the individual acini. The acinar epithelium is tall columnar with strongly eosinophilic cytoplasm and dense basal nuclei with their long axes at right angles to the basement membrane. The acini of the caudal lobe are smaller and consist of simple tubules with a regular appearance overall. The fibromuscular stroma is more delicate. The acini are lined by a single layer of cuboidal, low columnar epithelium with pale eosinophilic cytoplasm and vesicular basal nuclei with their long axes parallel with the basement membrane.

The uptake of tritiated testosterone by the caudal lobe of the Rhesus monkey prostate is significantly greater than the cranial lobe (Ghanadian et al., 1977).

Van Wagenen (1936) observed that the secretion from the cranial lobe of the monkey prostate gland formed a coagulum when mixed with the secretion of the seminal vesicles. In this respect it resembled the secretion of the coagulating gland of the rodent with which it may be homologous.

·1.4   THE ANATOMY OF THE HUMAN PROSTATE

Morphologically the prostate is a heterogeneous structure composed of glandular elements with their own intrinsic musculature, the prostatic portion of the urethra and the fibromuscular investment already described.

The distribution of the glandular parenchyma and fibromuscular tissue provides insight into the function of the organ; the glandular parenchyma is entirely concerned with reproduction whilst the fibromuscular tissue and its various condensations are concerned both with reproduction and urinary continence. The disposition of the various elements is seen in its definitive form in the young adult and is recognizable in the immature gland prepubertally. Benign prostatic hyperplasia and degenerative changes later in life considerably distort this anatomy, both glandular and fibromuscular, and these changes are important both clinically and in research.

The natural reference point in the topography of the prostate is the urethra which enters the prostate cranially at its base and exits on its anterior surface just above its apex caudally. During its course caudally through the gland the urethra passes in a posterior direction from the bladder neck to the level of the verumontanum where it angulates forwards to exit from the anterior surface of the gland through the external sphincter muscle. Between the internal meatus and the level of the verumontanum in the young adult the urethra is invested with a well defined fibromuscular sheath disposed in circular manner which is continuous with the deep trigone and internal sphincter above. McNeal (1972) has called this the preprostatic sphincter (Figure 1.4). It terminates abruptly at the level of the verumontanum but the fibres on its anterior aspect fan outwards at this level to interdigitate with the underside of the smooth and striated muscle sheath investing the anterior aspect of the gland. The function of the preprostatic sphincter is the closure of this part of the urethra at the time of ejaculation to prevent retrograde reflux of seminal fluid into the bladder. How much it is additionally involved in the active control of urinary continence at the bladder neck level is controversial. The prostatic part of the urethra can therefore be subdivided into an upper, 'preprostatic' segment and a lower part – the prostatic urethra proper – which extends from the upper level of the verumontanum to the point where the urethra passes through the external sphincter. This part of the prostatic urethra receives the three contributions which make up the seminal fluid – the testicular, seminal vesicular and prostatic fractions.

McNeal (1968, 1972 and 1978) has described four separate groups of glands in specific locations within the organ:-

Periurethral group
Central zone group
Peripheral zone group
Transitional zone group

The periurethral glands are the smallest component and are contained within the cylindrical sleeve of the preprostatic sphincter. They are simple straight glands whose ducts are at the most a few millimetres in length which run parallel to the urethra before opening into this upper part of the prostatic urethra. They rarely branch, have few or no acini and are invested with collagenous tissue. They are devoid of the smooth muscle investment which is so typical of the acini in other locations. This absence of specific acinar muscle and the closure by the preprostatic sphincter of this part of the urethra at the time of ejaculation suggests that they have no function in reproduction.

The central zone (Figure 1.4) comprises about 25% of the total gland complement. It is roughly triangular in the coronal section with its base forming the base of the prostate just beneath the trigone and bladder neck. Its apex is at the verumontanum and it lies on the posterior and posterolateral aspect of the preprostatic sphincter. It is traversed by the vas deferens and duct of the seminal vesicle, whose union forms the common ejaculatory duct on each side within the substance of the zone before these enter the urethra on either side of the verumontanum. The central zone therefore separates these structures from the peripheral zone which is contiguous posteriorly and laterally.

The characteristics of this zone are a prominent thick fibromuscular stroma and the complex branching of ducts and arborization of acini compared with the peripheral zone. The acini are large and angular and of irregular shape. Septa with fibromuscular core frequently traverse these. The lining epithelium

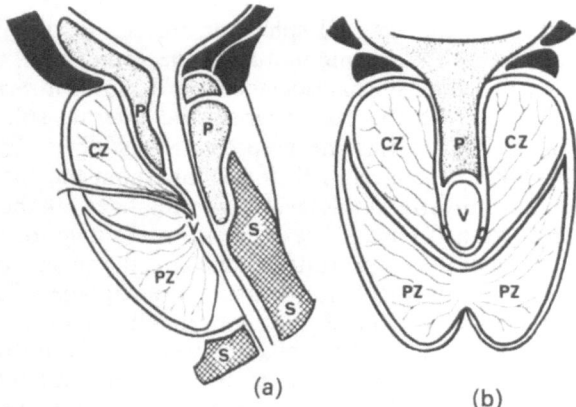

Figure 1.4   The morphology of the prostate (McNeal, 1968, 1972 and 1978) showing central zone (CZ) and peripheral zones (PZ) in diagrammatic midline sagittal section (a) and coronal section behind the urethra (b).
P – preprostatic sphincter; S – striated sphincter of the urethra and external sphincter; V – verumontanum

is compound with multiple layers of cells whose cytoplasm is opaque and vacuolated. The nuclei are large and more variable in size than those of the peripheral zone. When present corpora amylacea tend to be confined to the acini in this part of the gland (Blacklock, 1976). The central zone ducts pass downwards through the gland to exit in a restricted area of the urethra above and on each side of the verumontanum.

The peripheral zone forms the apex of the gland and encloses the lower part of the central zone in a concavity on its anterosuperior aspect. This zone comes into direct relationship with the lower prostatic urethra to which it is a posterior and lateral relation. Anterolaterally this zone is contiguous with the lower part of the anterior muscular sheath already described. A variable amount of striated muscle of the external urethral sphincter extends upwards between the urethra and the peripheral zone at the apex where there is interdigitation of glandular parenchyma and muscle. Immediately inferior to the apex is the collagenous and muscular condensation of the perineal body and posteriorly the peripheral zone of the gland is in direct relationship to the rectum with the intervention of a leaf of Denonvillier's fascia.

The peripheral zone comprises approximately 75 % of the total gland mass and is characterized by having a much finer fibromuscular stroma than the central zone. The acini are smaller, more regular in size and round. Each acinus has its own individual investment of smooth muscle as in the case of the central zone. The epithelium is simpler, consisting of columnar cells with pale cytoplasm and small dark nuclei in the basal position. The ducts of the peripheral zone pursue a long course through the gland, curving posteromedially and then forward to exit in the urethra on each side of the midline at the base of the inverted V-shaped posterior urethral fold whose apex is at the verumontanum.

The distinctive appearances of these two zones suggest that they have different functions. They have a different embryological origin, the central zone deriving from composite epithelium which includes epithelium from the urogenital sinus, Wolffian and Mullerian systems whilst the peripheral zone primordia arise entirely from urogenital sinus epithelium. The central zone primordia are also represented in the female in which they later form the paraurethral glands. The peripheral zone arises from that part of the urogenital sinus which is solely represented in the male. It is therefore also conceivable that the hormone sensitivity of the epithelium of each of these zones is different.

McNeal (1978) has described a transitional zone on each side of the urethra in the angle between the peripheral and central zones and the lower extremity of the preprostatic sphincter. Ducts from this zone enter the lateral urethral wall having passed round the lower edge of this sphincter. The duct branching of this zone is simpler than either central or peripheral zones but the acini have their individual slings of smooth muscle. The definition of this zone is difficult in view of its proximity to the fibromuscular stroma of the preprostatic sphincter which fans out through it towards the investing anterior muscular sheath. McNeal (1978) described the transition zone as a miniature model of the peripheral zone but observed that its acinar tissue is often less well developed and its stroma somewhat confused by this intermingling with the tissues of the preprostatic sphincter. The importance of the glands of this transition zone is their propensity with the periurethral glands and the stroma of the preprostatic sphincter to give origin to the changes of benign hyperplasia (BPH) (McNeal, 1978).

1.5 PATHOLOGICAL ANATOMY

The main pathological processes which involve the gland are inflammation, atrophy, hyperplasia (BPH) and carcinoma. The gland is not homogeneously involved by these and each pathology has typical location.

Both inflammation, as prostatitis, and atrophy are characteristically more common in the peripheral than the central zone. McNeal (1968) observed prostatitis significantly more frequently in the peripheral zone and in a series of 40 cases the central zone was solely involved in only two. In some there was some overlap of inflammatory change between the two zones from the main focus in the peripheral zone.

McNeal (1968) furthermore noted local atrophy to occur more commonly in the peripheral than the central zone. This was observed in comparatively young men and Moore (1936) observed this to begin in the fifth decade. Focal atrophy is accompanied by infiltration with inflammatory cells and fibrosis. It is of significance in that the changes can be quite widespread within the gland and influence the diagnosis if these areas are sampled in biopsy specimens. With advancing age a more diffuse atrophy occurs in which inflammation is absent and fibrosis less prominent. Whilst this is common in men in their eighth decade it can also occur in younger men in accompaniment of chronic debilitating diseases including malignancy.

A further change is also found characteristically in the peripheral zone. This is focal hyperplasia (McNeal, 1968, 1970). In some foci there is increased nuclear pleomorphism and hyperchromatism with cellular crowding such as to suggest uninhibited cellular growth. The nature of this focal hyperplasia is not clear but may represent the emergence of focal autonomous growth potential. This change may be a form of carcinoma *in situ* and in some cases invasive cancer has been found developing in these foci.

McNeal (1970) has also observed a further type of premalignant change in the form of the budding of new small acini on existing acini with the preservation of normal nuclear characteristics. Again this type of process suggests the re-emergence of embryonic potential and in some this change has been found to merge with areas of well differentiated carcinoma. These changes indicate alteration of the biological characteristics of the gland epithelium.

Benign prostatic hyperplasia (BPH) has its origin in the submucosal periurethral glands, the transitional zone and the fibromuscular stroma of the preprostatic sphincter (Figure 1.5). This hyperplasia involves at least three types of tissue – epithelium, muscle and collagen – the relative proportion of each varying markedly between one nodule and another even in the same patient. The location of origin of the hyperplasia anterolaterally accounts for the characteristic 'lateral lobe' intrusion seen on endoscopy. A further focus of hyperplasia is located in the midline of the urethra posteriorly just beneath the bladder neck (subcervical region). In this location the hyperplasia displaces

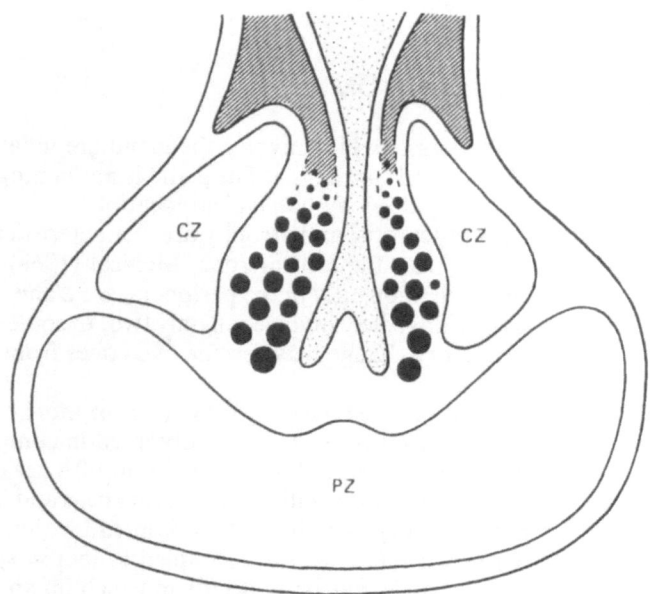

Figure 1.5 Diagrammatic vertical coronal section through prostate showing sites of origin of BPH in relation to urethra, central zone (CZ) and peripheral zones (PZ)

the internal sphincter posteriorly and as enlargement takes place projects into the bladder. Progressive enlargement of the hyperplastic process in both locations destroys the integrity of the preprostatic sphincter and compresses posteriorly the functional parenchyma of the peripheral zone. In the subcervical region the hyperplasia displaces the central zone posterolaterally and this splits into two moieties lying lateral to the hyperplasia on each side. In many sections showing hyperplastic change the peripheral zone and central zone tissue can be found uninvolved in this process although compressed and displaced.

Carcinoma of the prostate typically originates in the peripheral zone of the gland, the same location as areas of focal atrophy and hyperplasia are also found. The central zone may be involved secondarily but the frequency of carcinoma originating within this part of the gland is not known. Carcinoma may form an isolated focus or may occur diffusely as separate multiple foci within the gland. Because of its situation in the peripheral zone which is often further displaced from the urethra by accompanying hyperplastic change the urethra is only involved at a later stage of the disease, delaying symptoms and allowing extra-prostatic spread and metastases. Carcinoma *in situ* can also occur in areas of hyperplasia and the biological potential of such a tumour is probably different from tumour originating in the peripheral zone. Enucleated specimens showing invasion by carcinoma at the periphery of the nodule, however, indicate a coexisting tumour of the peripheral zone which has invaded the hyperplastic nodule as a secondary phenomenon.

1.6 CONCLUSIONS

Both the embryological and developmental history of the two zones of the prostate suggest differential function, which has not been defined, and differential hormone responsiveness. There is a requirement to define the steroid hormone receptor status of the epithelium of each of these zones and the differential histochemistry or some other marker which will allow characterization of tissue removed by biopsy.

With normal anatomy, perineal or transrectal biopsy will encounter peripheral zone tissue and, secondarily, tissue from the central zone. Where BPH is marked, however, this normal tissue may be so compressed or displaced that these biopsies return only typically hyperplastic material (Figure 1.6). Since carcinoma typically arises in the peripheral zone the type of biopsy which is most likely to succeed in providing a tissue diagnosis is either a perineal or transrectal Trucut needle biopsy. By either route it should be possible to direct the needle into the suspicious area of the gland. There is a clear case in view of the incidence of carcinoma in the older age groups for such biopsy – preferably by the perineal route – to be done at the time of transurethral resection or open enucleation of hyperplastic nodules.

From the normal and pathological anatomy and the origins and development of BPH it is clear that hyperplasia can be removed or resected from a gland without encountering hidden foci of neoplasia in the peripheral zone. Whilst enucleation will usually remove most of the BPH down to and beyond

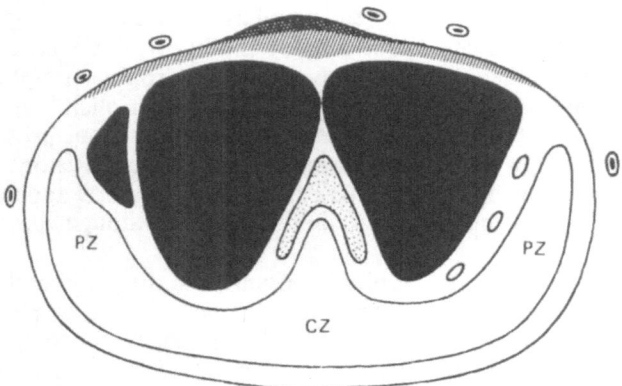

Figure 1.6 Cross-sectional diagram of prostate depicting established BPH with compression of functional prostate (CZ and PZ) posteriorly

the verumontanum, transurethral resection confines itself to removing BPH intrusion down to but not usually below the verumontanum for fear of injuring the external sphincter. Where hyperplasia extends below the veru as is quite common (Shah *et al.*, 1979) resection can only be accomplished by pushing this apical hyperplastic tissue upwards by pressure from a finger in the rectum.

It is of help to the pathologist if the resection material for histological study is selectively chosen and specifically includes the most peripheral part of the resection procedure since this is the material which is most likely to be infiltrated by carcinoma extending from the peripheral zone if this is present.

The morphological features both of the normal and pathological gland are relevant in the research context when tissue culture, cell kinetic techniques and receptor studies are contemplated. Whilst hyperplastic tissue is most often the most convenient tissue to use, the biological characteristics of the epithelium and stroma probably differ considerably from those of the tissues of the functional parenchyma – either peripheral or central zone – in view of the observed origins of hyperplasia from other tissues than these. From all the evidence – embryological, developmental and functional – it is likely that the biological characteristics of the epithelium both of the central and peripheral zones, the latter the common seat of carcinoma, are distinctive both from one another and from the epithelium of hyperplastic tissue.

1.7 REFERENCES

Andrews, G. S. (1951). The histology of the human foetal and pre-pubertal prostates. *J. Anat.*, **85,** 44
Blacklock, N. J. (1976). Surgical anatomy of the prostate. In Williams, I. D. and Chisholm, G. D. (eds.), *Scientific Foundations of Urology*, p. 113–115. (London: Heinemann)

Blacklock, N. J. and Bouskill, K. (1977). The zonal anatomy of the prostate in man and in the Rhesus monkey. *Urol. Res.*, **5**, 163

Franks, L. M. (1954). Benign nodular hyperplasia of the prostate: a review. *Ann. R. Coll. Surg. Engl.*, **14**, 92

Ghanadian, R., Smith, C. B., Chisholm, G. D. and Blacklock, N. J. (1977). Differential androgen uptake by the lobes of the Rhesus monkey prostate. *Br. J. Urol.*, **49**, 701

Glenister, T. W. (1962). The development of the utricle and of the so-called 'middle' or 'median' lobe of the human prostate. *J. Anat.*, **96**, 443

Gyorkey, F. (1964). The appearance of acid phosphatase in human prostate gland. *Lab. Invest.*, **13**, 105

Huggins, C. and Webster, W. O. (1948). Duality of the human prostate in response to oestrogens. *J. Urol.*, **59**, 258

Kerr, W. K., Keresteci, A. G. and Mayoh, H. (1960). The distribution of zinc within the human prostate. *Cancer*, **13**, 550

McNeal, J. (1968). Regional morphology and pathology of the prostate. *Am. J. Clin. Pathol.*, **49**, 347

McNeal, J. (1970). Age related changes in prostatic epithelium associated with carcinoma. In Griffiths, K. and Pierrepoint, C. G. (eds.) *Some Aspects of the Aetiology and Biochemistry of Prostatic Cancer*, pp. 23–32. (Cardiff: Alpha Omega Alpha Publishing)

McNeal, J. (1972). The prostate and prostatic urethra: A morphologic synthesis. *J. Urol.*, **107**, 1008

McNeal, J. (1978). Origin and evolution of benign prostate enlargement. *Invest. Urol.*, **15**, 340

Moore, R. A. (1936). The evolution and involution of the prostate gland. *Am. J. Pathol.*, **12**, 599

Schoonees, R., De Klerk, J. N. and Murphy, G. P. (1969). Correlation of prostatic blood flow with [65]Zinc activity in intact castrated, and testosterone treated baboons. *Invest. Urol.*, **6**, 476

Shah, P. J. R., Abrams, P. H., Feneley, R. C. L. and Green, N. A. (1979). The influence of prostatic anatomy on the differing results of prostatectomy according to the surgical approach. *Br. J. Urol.*, **51**, 549

Van Wagenen, G. (1936). The coagulating function of the cranial lobe of the prostate gland in the monkey. *Anat. Rec.*, **86**, 411

2
Histopathology of prostatic tumours

I. D. ANSELL

2.1 BENIGN PROSTATIC HYPERPLASIA (BPH)

It is probable that some degree of hyperplasia occurs in all males after the age of 40 but that in only a percentage does this give clinical symptoms. The precise aetiology of this condition is unknown but it is almost certainly the result of some form of hormonal imbalance in which androgens play a definite role since the condition is never seen in castrates (see chapter 4). The alteration of the normal architecture so produced varies considerably according to the type of tissue involved and the degree of hyperplasia present and it is important to recognize their different patterns so that they may be distinguished from the better differentiated varieties of prostatic carcinoma.

The cardinal feature of prostatic hyperplasia is nodularity and for this reason it has been suggested that nodular prostatic hypertrophy is a more appropriate term (Elbadawi, 1980). As mentioned in the previous chapter, hyperplasia occurs in the inner groups of glands and affects all the tissues that comprise the normal prostate. The first element to proliferate is thought to be the connective tissue (Cameron, 1974). In the suburethral area this is

15

perivascular in situation and produces nodules composed of vascular fibrous tissue; this particular type of nodule is only found in this situation and thus when they are seen they enable one to orientate transurethral resection chippings. Since these nodules are composed of supporting tissue only they are frequently called stromal nodules (Figure 2.1). Proliferation of periductal and intralobular connective tissue is followed by proliferation of muscular and glandular tissue and the nodules so produced are designated accordingly. Hence fibromuscular, muscular, fibroadenomatous and fibromyoepithelial nodules may be found although in practice the latter is much the most frequent.

Macroscopically, the hyperplastic gland removed suprapubically has a nodular external appearance. On bisection the nodules are either a yellowish colour, if composed predominantly of adenomatous tissue, or have a microcystic appearance exuding white milky fluid if the glandular element has undergone cystic change. Microscopically, stromal nodules are composed of circumscribed ovoid masses of stellate cells in a vascular stroma (Figure 2.1) whilst fibromuscular and muscular nodules are very reminiscent of leiomyomas. In those nodules containing glandular elements (Figures 2.2 and 2.3) the proliferation of epithelial cells first produces papillary growths into the lumen of glands but later accumulation of secretions and other factors produce cystic dilation of acini (Figure 2.4). The enlargement of the inner group of glands in BPH tends to produce atrophy and compression of the outer group of glands, which come to form a pseudocapsule to the gland

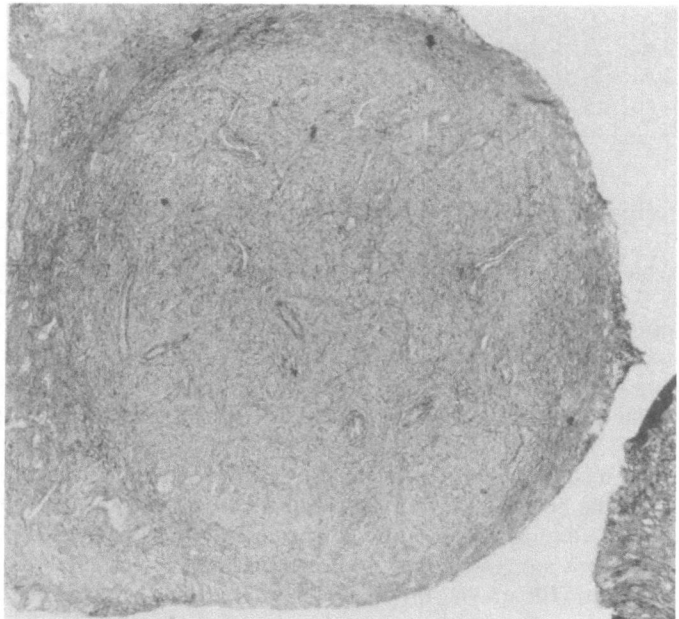

Figure 2.1   Stromal nodule in transurethral resection, a circumscribed spherical mass of vascular fibrous tissue (H & E × 35)

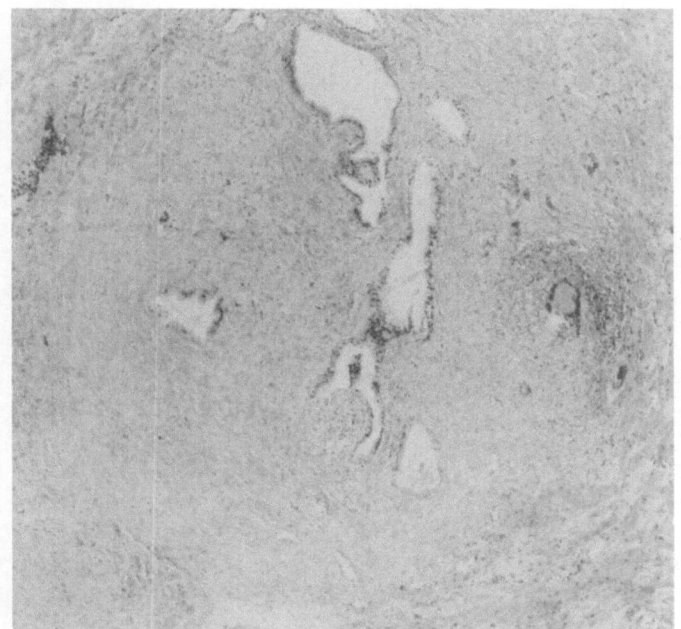

Figure 2.2 Fibroadenomatous nodule in which predominant tissue is fibrous (H & E × 40)

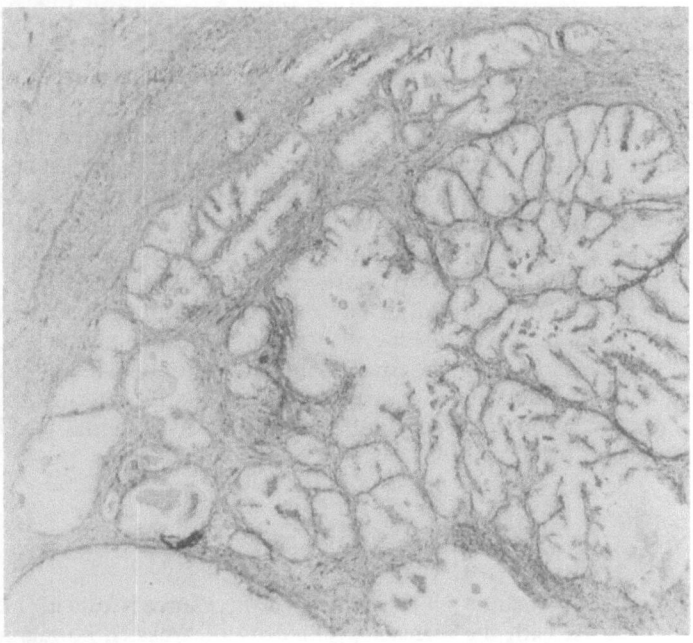

Figure 2.3 Periphery of fibromyoepithelial nodule compressing adjacent connective tissue to form a pseudocapsule (H & E × 35)

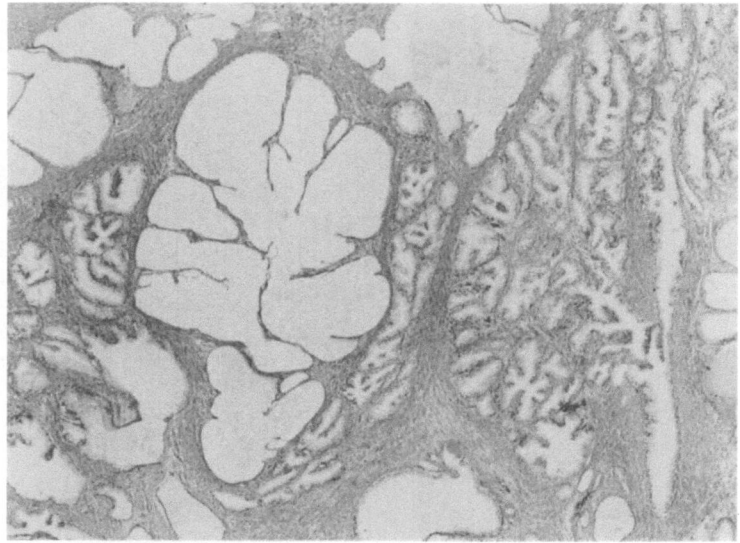

Figure 2.4 Cystic dilation of glands in centre of fibromyoepithelial nodule (H & E × 30)

which is left behind when enucleation methods of prostatectomy are employed.

Cyst formation is not the only sequel to BPH. The accumulation of secretions together with desquamation of epithelial cells is thought to be the origin of the round eosinophilic bodies called corpora amylacea often seen in acini in this condition. These are of more than histological interest in that they may undergo calcification and result in a gland that feels firm and irregular on rectal examination. The other sequel to BPH which is of clinicopathological importance is infarction. Prostatic infarcts initially have a congested haemor-rhagic appearance and often have marked squamous metaplasia of adjacent surviving epithelium (Figure 2.13). Their role in precipitating acute retention in BPH has yet to be clarified since, although it would be perfectly logical to consider that oedema of the prostate following infarction might precipitate retention, such patients have invariably undergone catheterization and/or instrumentation prior to surgery and the infarcts could equally well be the result of these procedures.

2.2 CARCINOMA OF THE PROSTATE

Carcinoma of the prostate is a tumour whose incidence rises with increasing age and therefore, with the increasing longevity of Western populations, it is becoming an increasingly important cause of cancer deaths in these societies. Indeed, it is now the second most frequent cause of cancer deaths in males in the USA and the fourth in the UK. The pathogenesis of the condition is far from understood, although the response of some tumours to changes in sex hormone levels has been known for many years. Although an increased risk of cancer in BPH has been reported (Armenian *et al.*, 1974) this association has been vigorously disputed (Byar, 1975). There are certain racial differences in the incidence of prostatic carcinoma, it being more prevalent in American blacks than whites and it is also more common in urban populations compared to rural (King *et al.*, 1963).

2.2.1 Clinical types

The accepted British clinical classification of prostatic cancer recognizes three different clinical types (Thackray, 1978): *clinical* – in which the tumour produces prostatic symptoms with or without evidence of metastatic disease, *occult* – when the only evidence of tumour is from metastases with no prostatic symptoms and *latent* – a term used to denote those cancers that come to light following the histopathological examination of tissue removed from what was initially thought to be benign prostatic hyperplasia. There is no doubt that the latter two terms may be confused and Mostofi and Price (1973) have accordingly suggested that they should be abandoned. They recommend a clinical subdivision into *clinically manifest carcinoma* and *incidental carcinoma not clinically manifest*. One must have sympathy with these views and many clinicians would now recommend abandonment of the term 'latent'. However, there still remains the problem of predicting the natural history of this group of patients and of deciding whether or not to recommend treatment. The important factors determining whether or not such tumours will metastasize appear to be *size* and *degree of differentiation*. Bauer *et al.* reported in 1960 that well differentiated small tumours seldom developed metastases and this was confirmed by Varkarakis *et al.* 10 years later. It is obviously not quite so easy to assess the size of a tumour in transurethral resection specimens but the same general principles were found to hold true in such specimens by Correa *et al.* (1974). Latent or incidental carcinoma is by definition stage A in the North American nomenclature and is subdivided by them into A1, composed of well differentiated tumour involving a quarter of the gland or less, and A2 in which most of the gland is infiltrated by more poorly differentiated tumour. Heaney *et al.* (1977) in a 10 year series of 100 patients showed that all but one cancer death occurred in patients who would fall into the A2 category. For practical purposes then, treatment should be restricted to patients in the A2 group and should be withheld from those with A1 tumours. Inevitably this staging of TUR specimens will not be wholly accurate and indeed McMillen and Wettlaufer (1976) found that 26% of patients initially staged as A1 were restaged as A2 following a repeat TUR.

2.2.2 Histopathology

The prostate gland is composed of numerous glands, or acini, which drain via a system of ducts into the prostatic urethra. These acini are lined by tall, columnar, secretory cells and have a layer of basal or reserve cells between them and the basement membrane (Mao and Angrist, 1966). The ducts are lined by more cuboidal cells but similarly have a basal layer and are often difficult to convincingly distinguish from acini. Just before reaching the prostatic urethra the ductal epithelium changes to a transitional epithelium (Lowsley and Kirwin, 1956). A fibromuscular stroma envelops the glandular system and contributes substantially to the hyperplasia seen in benign prostatic hyperplasia.

The vast majority of tumours of the prostate arise from acinar epithelium and are thus adenocarcinomas. Some carcinomas originate from ductal epithelium and only very rarely do malignant tumours (sarcomas) arise from the fibromuscular stroma. Tumours of other organs may also metastasize or spread into the prostate although, except for malignant lymphomas and direct extension of carcinoma of the bladder, this is very unusual. Carcinoma of the rectum is prevented from spreading anteriorly into the prostate by the dense Denonvillier's fascia and this is only rarely penetrated to give prostatic problems. Earlier studies which had identified that benign hyperplasia occurred in the inner (mucosal and submucosal) groups of glands and that carcinoma arose from the peripheral (main) group of glands were confirmed by the elegant studies of Franks (1954). He also showed that with increasing age these outer glands became atrophic whilst the inner group became hyperplastic. This apparent anomaly of tumours arising from atrophic glands has been discussed and illustrated by Mostofi and Price (1973), who stress that the acinar cells are dormant rather than atrophic. McNeal (1969) also showed that the majority of tumours arose at the periphery of the gland but claimed that many tumours were preceded by hyperplasia of acinar epithelium. This origin of cancer from peripheral glands explains the apparent anomaly of prostatic carcinoma occurring after prostatectomy since enucleation methods of transvesical and retropubic prostatectomy only remove the inner groups of glands, leaving the peripheral group of cancer-forming glands behind.

Retropubic prostatectomies are now performed with decreasing frequence such that the problem of macroscopic diagnosis of carcinoma of prostate is becoming of much less importance (except, perhaps, in autopsy practice). It was always recognized that such naked eye diagnosis was difficult. Features indicating the presence of tumour are firmness to palpation, an indistinct border to the area under scrutiny and often a yellow colour to the cut surface (prostatic cancer often contains appreciable quantities of fat – *vide infra*).

Histological recognition of prostatic cancer may also be difficult. The tumours are often well differentiated with abundant gland formation and, except in the more anaplastic tumours, it is uncommon to see mitoses. Diagnosis in the better differentiated tumour therefore tends to depend upon assessment of the overall architecture, which in cancer loses the organized lobular arrangement always perceptible in benign hyperplasia. Higher power examination will invariably reveal that the tumour cells have nuclei that are larger than normal, often have prominent nucleoli and that they have reduced quantities of cytoplasm. These features are not always easy to assess when viewing an individual acinus but are readily appreciated when neoplastic and non-neoplastic glands are in opposition (Figure 2.5). The 'back to back' appearance of crowded neoplastic glands is generally not so helpful in diagnosis as in the other sites (such as endometrium) but the loss of the regular whorled arrangement of smooth muscle found in the benign prostate, with replacement by obvious splitting of muscle by neoplastic glands, is often a very useful feature. The less well differentiated tumours with virtually no gland formation (Figure 2.6) present no difficulties in diagnosis although, with

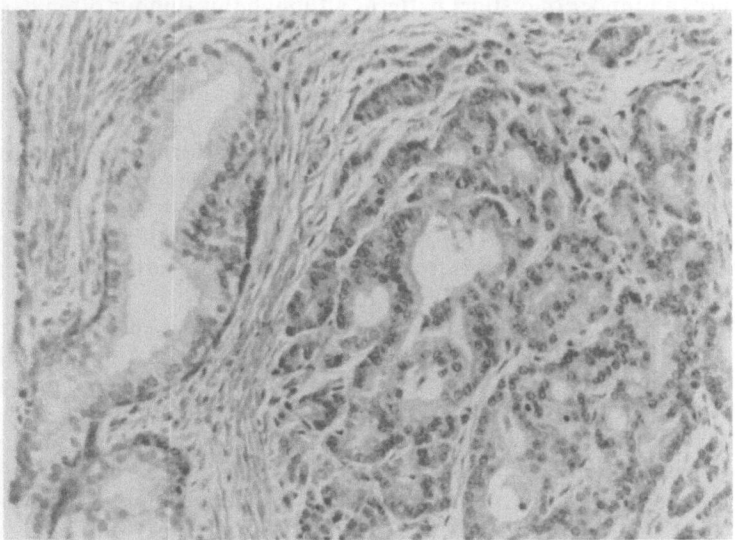

Figure 2.5 Well differentiated adenocarcinoma (right) adjacent to normal acinus (left). Tumour cells have larger, darker nuclei with more prominent nucleolus and have less cytoplasm. Glandular arrangement of tumour is also irregular. Note abundant clear apical cytoplasm of benign acinus and obvious layer of basal cells (H & E × 200)

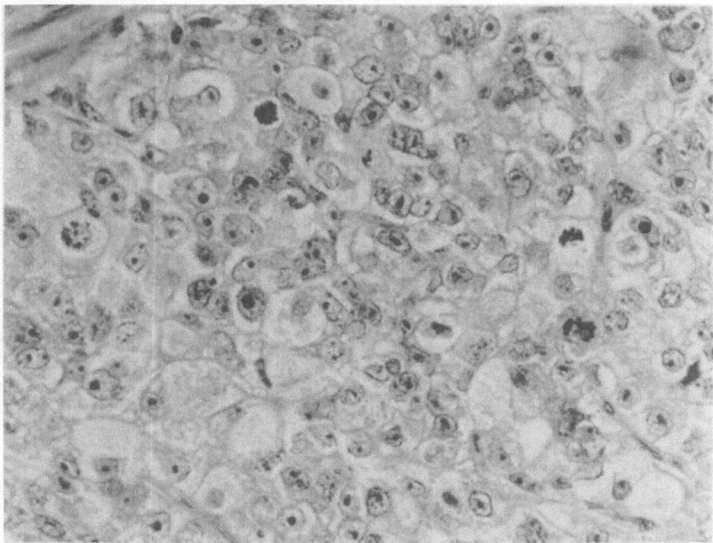

Figure 2.6 Anaplastic carcinoma of prostate showing no glandular differentiation and with numerous mitoses (H & E × 290)

these poorly differentiated tumours, distinction from anaplastic carcinoma of the bladder can be very difficult.

The variable degree of glandular differentiation in prostatic cancer produces a number of distinct patterns although this tumour often has a very variable histological appearance in different areas of the one tumour (Byar and Mostofi, 1972). Well defined glandular differentiation will give a definite *acinar* appearance which may produce discrete nodules (Figure 2.7) or may have a more infiltrative appearance (Figure 2.8).

A *cribriform* appearance (or gland within gland formation) is commonly found but is rarely the only pattern present (Figure 2.9). The most undifferentiated tumours have sheets of carcinoma cells and may be termed *medullary* (Figure 2.6). The relationship of these different patterns to prognosis and response to treatment is not clear and is discussed later when grading is considered.

Obvious infiltrative or invasive activity is, of course, definite evidence of malignancy and older articles stress the value of looking carefully for perineural invasion in order to confirm the diagnosis of carcinoma. This invasion of perineural spaces is much easier to see at the periphery of prostatectomy specimens than in the chippings obtained at transurethral resection, although it is not infrequently seen in the tissue obtained by needle biopsy. Rodin *et al.* (1967) showed that the spaces around nerves have no endothelium and therefore are not true lymphatic spaces. Somewhat surprisingly identification of this feature has no prognostic significance (Pennington *et al.*, 1967; Byar and Mostofi, 1972). Similarly the presence of striated muscle between prostatic acini does *not* imply invasion of periprostatic muscle by

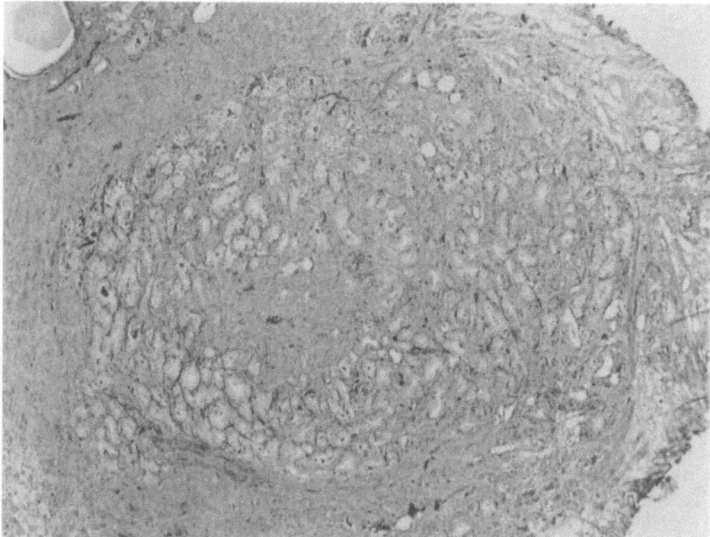

Figure 2.7 Circumscribed nodule of well differentiated prostatic carcinoma. Such isolated small well differentiated tumours have been called 'latent' carcinomas in the past (H & E × 30)

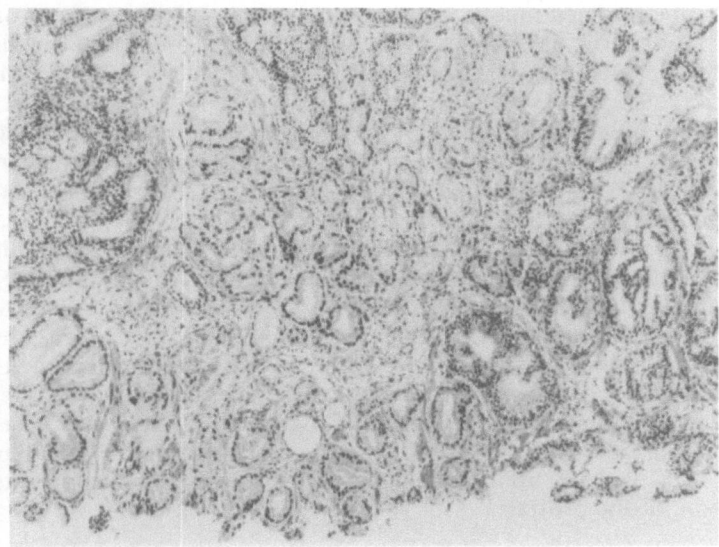

Figure 2.8 Well differentiated carcinoma of prostate (centre) in needle biopsy (H & E × 76)

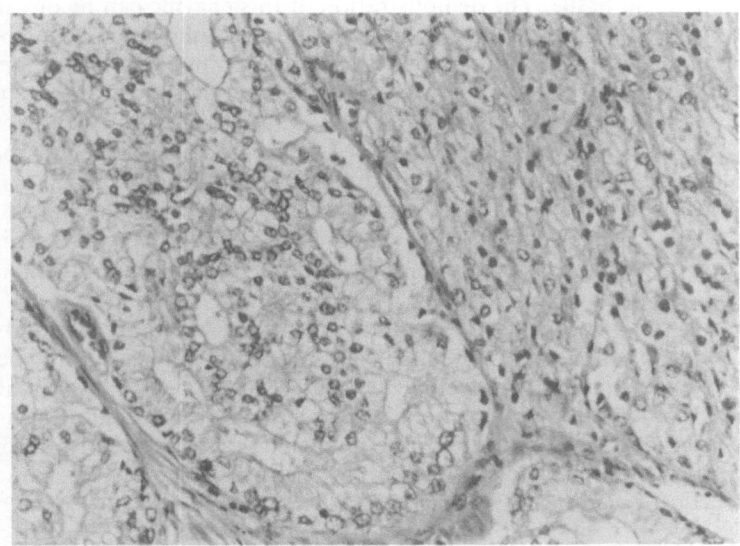

Figure 2.9 Poorly differentiated carcinoma: sheets of tumour cells on right, cribriform appearance on left (H & E × 200)

tumour since striated muscle may be seen in the normal prostate (Kost and Ewan, 1964). True vascular invasion is not often a prominent histological feature although is said, when present, to indicate a poorer outcome (Mostofi and Price, 1973).

As is so frequently the case, tumour *stage* is a much more accurate predication of prognosis than tumour *grade* and was amply illustrated in Byar and Mostofi's (1972) evaluation of a large number of radical prostatectomies in which they showed that invasion of seminal vesicle or of prostatic capsule were the most accurate unfavourable prognostic features. Their findings confirmed those of Arduino and Glucksman (1962) who showed that pelvic lymph node metastases occurred in 80 % of cases with seminal vesicle invasion but had only a 7 % incidence if there was no seminal vesicle invasion.

However, radical prostatectomy is rarely, if ever, performed in the United Kingdom and consequently histopathological assessment is never the technique employed in this country for tumour staging. Whilst pieces of seminal vesicle are occasionally seen in TUR specimens and even in needle biopsies, the urologist will rely upon radiologing techniques for staging patients with carcinoma of the prostate.

2.2.3 Histochemistry

The histochemical properties of prostatic cancer have been extensively studied and have been claimed to help in both distinguishing benign from malignant tissue and also to aid in the accurate identification of metastases. The acid phosphatase produced by carcinoma of the prostate is formaldehyde resistant (Maramba, 1965) and therefore fresh (unfixed) material is not required but only unblocked tissue. The demonstration of this enzyme can be of value in prostatic resection specimens when there is difficulty in distinguishing poorly differentiated urothelial from prostatic cancer. A number of other tumours produce acid phosphatase and so loss of activity following exposure to tartrate should be shown before suggesting that a metastasis is of prostatic origin (Scott *et al.*, 1974). The clear cytoplasm of prostatic epithelium, benign or malignant, contains neutral fat and phospholipid (Braunstein, 1964) and since this is absent in rectal and urothelial cancer (Dobrogonski and Braunstein, 1963) examination for lipid may be helpful in distinguishing prostatic cancer from these tumours, again provided that unembedded material is available.

Adenocarcinomas of prostate produce mucins to a varying degree and it has been shown that these are sulphated sialo-mucins in contrast to the neutral mucins produced in the non-neoplastic gland (Franks *et al.*, 1964; Hukill and Vidone, 1967). Although the practical application of this technique is limited by the fact that not all tumours produce mucin it is more frequently elaborated by better differentiated tumours and may be of help in distinguishing these from foci of hyperplasia (Taylor, 1979).

2.2.4 Other carcinomas

A minority of carcinomas of prostate do not originate from the periphery of the gland but arise centrally from the cells lining ducts and ductules. The cells lining these ducts are either transitional or columnar and the tumours are therefore either urothelial carcinomas or adenocarcinomas. These tumours have only gradually been recognized over the last 20 years and their classification is still somewhat contentious (Melicow and Uson, 1976; Zaloudek *et al.*, 1976). This group of central tumours more frequently present with either haematuria or prostatic obstruction and in addition may not be palpable rectally. A number of them, more especially the urothelial tumours and those with a papillary pattern, do not produce acid phosphatase, have osteolytic bone secondaries and are unresponsive to hormonal therapy. For the latter reason and because of their central location surgical extirpation is probably the treatment of choice (Catalona *et al.*, 1978).

Primary transitional cell carcinoma of the prostate was first described in 1963 (Ende *et al.*) and a large series in which the clinicopathological correlates mentioned above were described was reported by Rhamy *et al.* (1972). These tumours and squamous carcinoma arising in this area, present little in the way of diagnostic problems except for distinguishing primary tumours of the prostate from those that have spread from urethra or bladder, a task for the clinician rather than the pathologist.

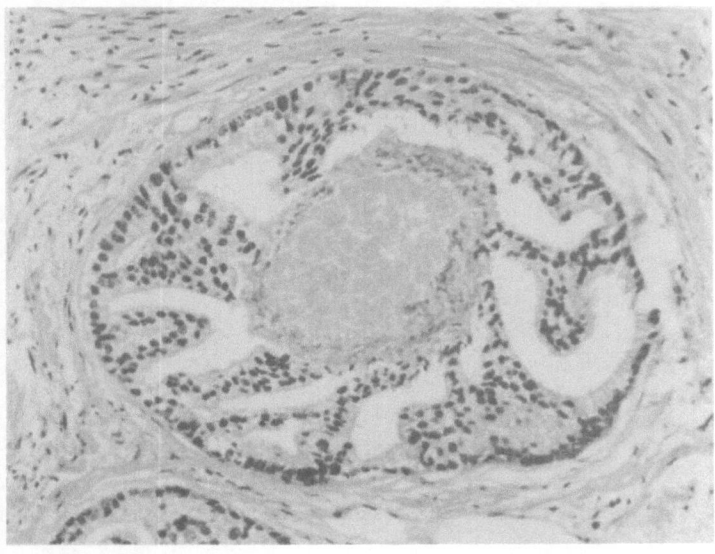

Figure 2.10 Comedo-like carcinoma with an area of central necrosis, probably arising from a prostatic duct (H & E × 190)

It is with central adenocarcinomas that problems of nomenclature and histogenesis arise. Dube *et al.* (1973) reviewed 4286 cases of carcinoma of prostate seen at the Mayo clinic and found 55 cases that they considered to be of ductal origin. 47 were thought to arise from secondary ducts and had a characteristic cribriform appearance often with much central eosinophilic necrosis to give a comedo appearance (Figure 2.10). Unlike the cribriform areas seen in more peripheral acinar carcinomas, nuclei are usually very hyperchromatic and cytoplasm is often clear or hypernephroid in appearance. However, they also described a group of mixed acinar and ductal adenocarcinomas and this reflects the difficulty of distinguishing this group of tumours, especially in TUR specimens. The eight primary duct tumours described by these workers had a definite fronded and papillary structure (Figure 2.11) and on occasions these fronds were seen projecting into the urethra at endoscopy. As with the secondary duct tumours, acid phosphatase levels were often elevated and bone metastases were frequently osteoblastic. The relationship of these tumours to those described as arising from the uterus masculinus of the verumontanum (Melicow and Tannenbaum, 1971) is arguable. Melicow and Uson (1976) argue that tumour and serum acid phosphatase levels differentiate these tumours from primary duct cancers but Zaloudek *et al.* (1976) deny this: too few cases have yet been described to resolve this argument.

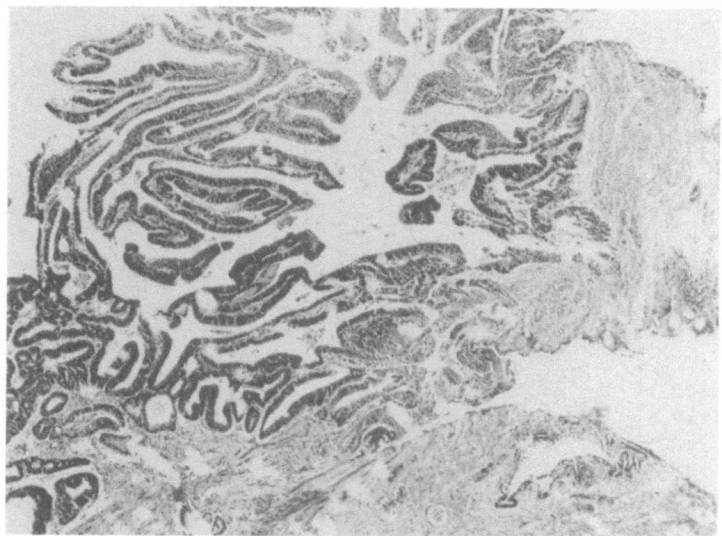

Figure 2.11   Fronded tumour of prostate considered to arise from primary ducts (H & E × 36)

Apart from the attempts at microanatomical classification of prostatic carcinoma discussed above, a number of other entities should be mentioned. Some carcinomas produce such a gross quantity of mucin that they may be properly termed 'mucoid' or 'colloid' (Figure 2.12). It is claimed that they may arise centrally and they certainly seem to have a better prognosis (Joshi *et al.*, 1967). Adenoid cystic carcinoma and adenosarcoma are mentioned by Mostofi and Price (1973) but are very infrequent.

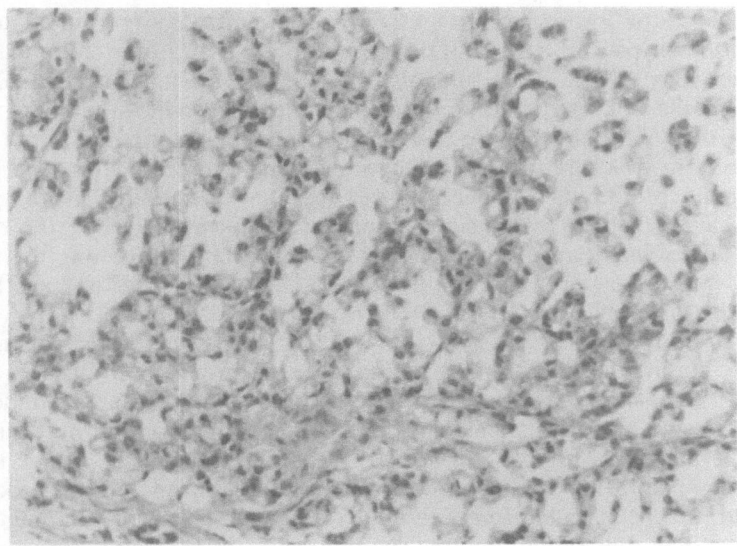

Figure 2.12 Mucoid carcinoma of prostate. Poorly formed glands and isolated tumour cells in pools of mucus (H & E × 200)

Squamous cell carcinoma of the prostate is also rare, they often arise in the ducts and may follow the squamous metaplasia that is induced by oestrogen therapy. Sarcomas of varying type are also only infrequently encountered although rhabdomyosarcoma is the commonest tumour of this organ in the first two decades of life.

2.2.5 Diagnosis

The vast majority of patients with carcinoma of the prostate present with either prostatism or with symptoms from metastatic disease. In both instances rectal examination will usually reveal a firm irregular prostate. Those patients with prostatism will require surgical resection to relieve their symptoms and the prostatic tissue so obtained should provide histological confirmation of the diagnosis. However, on occasions the diagnosis may be missed either because an inadequate resection leaves the tumour-bearing peripheral part of the gland behind or because an insufficient sample of the prostatic chippings is obtained. The latter problem can be overcome by separating the more peripheral resection specimens and only processing these histologically (O'Donoghue and Pugh, 1977). Patients with no local symptoms will require some form of biopsy procedure to obtain a tissue diagnosis of malignancy prior to the consideration of any hormonal or chemotherapeutic regime with their attendant risks and side effects.

It is particularly important to confirm the clinical diagnosis of carcinoma made by palpation of a firm nodule in the prostate since it has been shown that only about half of such nodules are in fact tumours (Hudson and Stout, 1966).

Local areas of firmness can result from such conditions as granulomatous or eosinophilic prostatitis, prostatic stones, infarcts and even some cases of benign hyperplasia. It should also not be forgotten that many Stage I carcinomas will, by definition, be impalpable on rectal examination.

There is no doubt that the easiest and most efficient method of obtaining tissue from such cases is by needle biopsy (Hendry and Williams, 1971). This procedure produces a cylinder of tissue which may be examined histologically. It has a high success rate and an acceptable incidence of side-effects (Ward *et al.*, 1980). Only very rarely is there tumour implantation along the needle track (only seven reported cases up to 1973, according to Mostofi and Price), and this theoretical objection can be safely ignored in clinical practice.

Aspiration cytology of suspicious nodules has its advocates and no one would doubt its accuracy and efficiency when performed by enthusiasts (Trott *et al.*, 1973). However, in inexperienced hands cytology is generally much less accurate and reliable than histology and therefore in most units needle biopsy will be the most suitable and accurate technique. Using the needle biopsy technique abnormal nodules felt rectally can be sampled and this procedure would thus be expected to give a higher a higher success rate in diagnosing cancer than the more random sampling that occurs with transurethral resection. In addition, it should be remembered that transurethral resection removes tissue from the central part of the gland and it is in the peripheral area that carcinoma originates and this predictable lower success rate was shown soon after the introduction of needle biopsy (Purser *et al.*, 1967).

2.2.6 Histopathological pitfalls

There are two entities which are often misdiagnosed as carcinoma, squamous metaplasia and basal cell hyperplasia. The occurrence of squamous metaplasia around areas of infarction has been known for many years (Mostofi and Morse, 1951) and is readily appreciated as such in prostatectomy specimens when the infarct is of recent origin (Figure 2.13). When the infarct heals the metaplasia may be mistaken for squamous carcinoma and this may account for the relatively high incidence of this tumour in older series (3 % in that reported by Kahler, 1939). Problems also arise in TUR chippings when infarction may not be quite so obvious as when seen in the larger prostatectomy specimens. The other entity which it is important to be aware of is basal cell hyperplasia, an uncommon finding in the nodular hyperplastic gland characterized by an apparent proliferation of small regular lobules composed predominantly of cells with oval dark-staining nuclei and only a small amount of cytoplasm (Figure 2.14). These cells are similar to the basal cells of the normal prostate and hence the terminology.

Problems in diagnosis may also occur when a patient has had oestrogen treatment prior to biopsy or prostatectomy. Fergusson and Franks (1953) described the accumulation of intracytoplasmic vacuoles that occurs following this therapy, coalescence of these vacuoles producing bloated balloon cells (Figure 2.15). The nuclei are also affected becoming first hyperchromatic and then pyknotic such that finally they may be mistaken for histiocytes or, with eventual loss of cytoplasm, even considered to be lymphocytes.

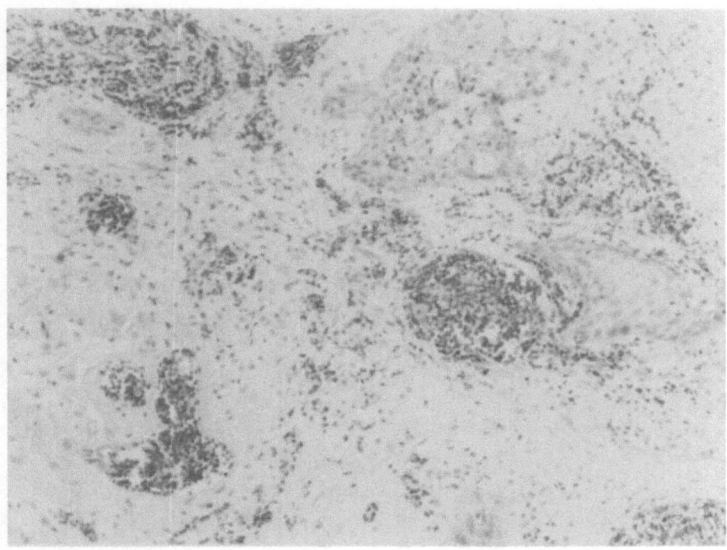

Figure 2.13 Squamous metaplasia at edge of infarct; note congested vessels and extravasated red cells (H & E × 130)

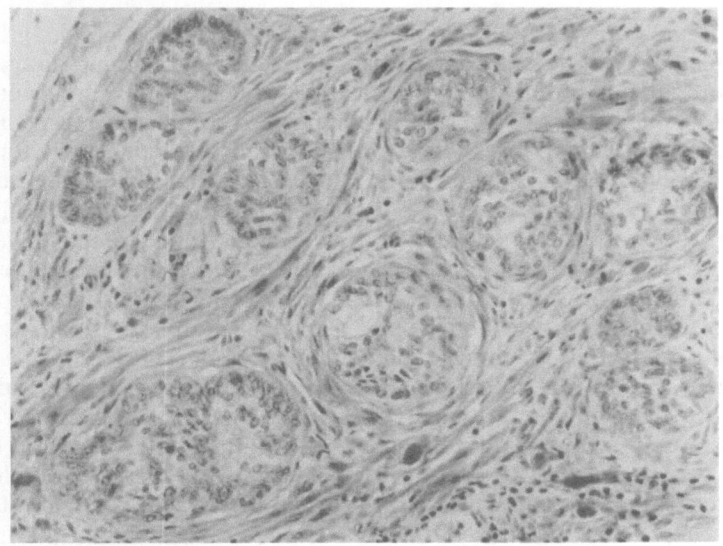

Figure 2.14 Basal cell hyperplasia – a benign condition frequently mistaken for carcinoma (H & E × 190)

2.2.7 Histological grading

The importance of the size of a prostatic carcinoma and the degree of spread (stage) in assessing prognosis has been mentioned earlier when considering

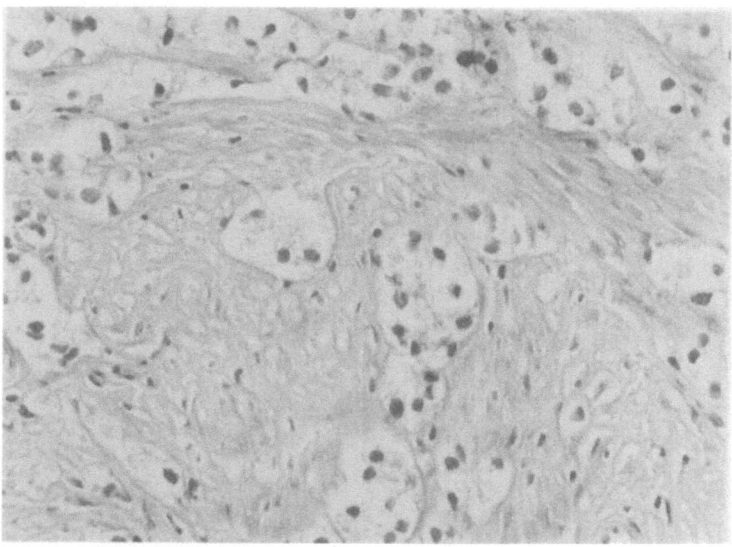

Figure 2.15 Pyknotic nuclei and clear cytoplasm of prostatic cancer following oestrogen therapy (H & E × 310)

'latent' carcinoma. It follows therefore that any investigation into the importance of histological characteristics in assessing outcome should only compare patients of comparable clinical stage. Modern staging techniques such as bone-scanning and pelvic lymphadenectomy have shown how unreliable clinical staging can be (Donohue *et al.*, 1979) and thus we should perhaps view older publications on the role of grading with some caution. Another problem with grading is the great variability in the histological appearance of prostatic cancer that may be seen in the one tumour (Byar and Mostofi, 1972). The widespread use of needle biopsy in the diagnosis of prostatic cancer has resulted in much less tissue being available for appraisal by the histopathologist, although it has been claimed that this smaller sample does not produce problems (Murphy and Whitmore, 1979).

Franks *et al.* in 1958 found no correlation between histological grade and survival, although Vickery and Kerr in 1963, when assessing radical prostatectomy specimens, found that better differentiated tumours had a better prognosis. The Veterans Administration Co-operative Urological Research Group has conducted large trials on the effectiveness of oestrogen therapy in prostatic cancer and has employed a grading technique devised by Gleason (1966). This system recognizes both a primary and secondary histological pattern to take into account the variability that may occur in the one tumour. Five patterns of varying degrees of differentiation in gland formation are recognized and are assigned numerical values. Gleason and Mellinger (1974) have shown that by combining the values obtained from this grading system with a figure derived from the clinical stage the prognosis of the patient can be accurately predicted. Workers from the Armed Forces

Institute of Pathology in Washington have criticized this system since it does not take into account the degree of anaplasia in individual cells and have devised a system in which both the degree of glandular differentiation and cellular anaplasia are assessed (Mostofi, 1975).

Other grading systems are also in use and were compared and assessed at a series of workshops in 1979 (Murphy and Whitmore). The consensus from this was that the Gleason system should be adopted, although the author has considerable doubts as to the applicability of this system to the very small samples obtained by needle biopsy. The role of grading in the management of carcinoma of the prostate is thus still actively being investigated, not only for prediction of prognosis but hopefully also in order to identify those patients who are more likely to respond to newer chemotherapeutic regimes.

2.3 REFERENCES

Arduino, L. J. and Glucksman, M. A. (1962). Lymph node metastases in early carcinoma of the prostate. *J. Urol.*, **88**, 91

Armenian, M. K., Lilienfield, A. M., Diamond, E. L. and Bross, I. D. J. (1974). Relationship between prostatic hyperplasia and cancer of the prostate. *Lancet*, **2**, 115

Bauer, W. C., McGavran, M. H. and Carlin, M. R. (1960). Unsuspected carcinoma of the prostate in suprapubic prostatectomy specimens. A clinicopathological study of 55 consecutive cases. *Cancer*, **13**, 370

Braunstein, M. (1964). Staining lipid in carcinoma of the prostate gland. *Am. J. Clin. Pathol.*, **41**, 44

Byar, D. P., Mostofi, F. K. and the Veterans Administration Co-operative Urological Research Group (1972). Carcinoma of the prostate – prognostic features in 208 radical prostatectomies. *Cancer*, **30**, 5

Byar, D. P. (1975). Benign prostatic hyperplasia and cancer of the prostate. *Lancet*, **1**, 866

Cameron, K. M. (1974). Pathology of the prostate. *Br. J. Hosp. Med.*, **11**, 348

Catalona, W. J., Kadmon, D. and Martin, S. A. (1978). Surgical considerations in the treatment of intra-ductal carcinoma of the prostate. *J. Urol.*, **120**, 259

Correa, R. J., Anderson, R. G., Gibbons, R. P. and Tate Mason, J. (1974). Latent carcinoma of the prostate – why the controversy. *J. Urol.*, **120**, 259

Dobrogonski, O. J. and Braunstein, M. (1963). Histochemical study of staining lipid, glycogen and mucins in human neoplasms. *Am. J. Clin. Pathol.*, **40**, 435

Donohue, R. E., Fauver, H. E., Whitesel, J. A. and Pfister, R. R. (1979). Staging prostatic cancer – a different distribution. *J. Urol.*, **122**, 327

Dube, V. E., Farrow, G. M. and Greene, L. F. (1973). Prostatic adenocarcinoma of ductal origin. *Cancer*, **32**, 402

Elbadawi, A. (1980). Benign proliferative lesions of the prostate gland. In Spring-Mills, E. and Hafez, E. S. E. (eds). *Male Accessory Sex Glands*. (Amsterdam: Elsevier/North Holland Biomedical Press)

Ende, N., Woods, L. P. and Shelley, M. S. (1963). Carcinoma originating in ducts surrounding the prostatic urethra. *Am. J. Clin. Pathol.*, **40**, 183

Fergusson, J. D. and Franks, L. M. (1953). The response of prostatic carcinoma to oestrogen treatment. *Br. J. Surg.*, **40**, 422

Franks, L. M. (1954). Latent carcinoma of the prostate. *J. Pathol. Bact.*, **68**, 603

Franks, L. M., Fergusson, J. D. and Murnaghan, G. E. (1958). An assessment of factors influencing survival in prostatic cancer – the absence of reliable prognostic features. *Br. J. Cancer*, **12**, 321

Franks, L. M., O'Shea, J. D. and Thompson, A. E. R. (1964). Mucin in the prostate; a histochemical study in normal glands, latent, clinical and colloid cancers. *Cancer*, **17**, 983

Gleason, D. F. (1966). Classification of prostatic carcinomas. *Cancer Chemother. Rep.*, **50**, 125

Gleason, D. F., Mellinger, G. T. and the Veterans Administration Co-operative Urological Research Group (1974). Prediction of prognosis for prostatic adenocarcinoma by combined histological grading and clinical staging. *J. Urol.*, **111**, 58

Heaney, J. A., Chang, H. C., Daly, J. J. and Prout, G. R. (1977). Prognosis of clinically undiagnosed prostatic carcinoma and the influence of endocrine therapy. *J. Urol.*, **118**, 283

Hendry, W. F. and Williams, J. P. (1971). Transrectal prostatic biopsy. *Br. Med. J.*, **4**, 595

Hudson, P. B. and Stout, A. P. (1966). Prostatic Cancer XVI. Comparison of physical examination and biopsy for detection of curable lesions. *NY. State J. Med.*, **66**, 357

Hukill, P. B. and Vidone, R. A. (1967). Histochemistry of mucus and other polysaccharides in tumours. II. Carcinoma of prostate. *Lab. Invest.*, **16**, 395

Joshi, D. P., Seery, W. H. and Neier, C. R. (1967). Mucogenic adenocarcinoma of prostate. *J. Urol.*, **98**, 241

Kahler, J. E. (1939). Carcinoma of the prostate gland – a pathological study. *J. Urol.*, **41**, 557

King, H., Diamond, H. and Lillienfield, A. M. (1963). Some epidemiological aspects of cancer of the prostate. *J. Chronic Dis.*, **16**, 117

Kost, L. V. and Ewan, G. W. (1964). Occurrence and significance of striated muscle within the prostate. *J. Urol.*, **92**, 703

Lowsley, O. S. and Kirwin, T. J. (1956). *Clinical Urology*. 3rd Edn., p. 375. (Baltimore: Williams & Wilkins)

McMillen, S. M. and Wettlaufer, J. N. (1976). The role of repeat transurethral biopsy in Stage A carcinoma of the prostate. *J. Urol.*, **116**, 759

McNeal, J. E. (1969). Origin and development of carcinoma in the prostate. *Cancer*, **23**, 24

Mao, P. and Angrist, A. (1966). The fine structure of the basal cell of human prostate. *Lab. Invest.*, **15**, 1768

Maramba, T. P. (1965). Histochemical differentiation of carcinoma of the prostate from other tumours by a modified acid phosphatase reaction. *Am. J. Clin. Path.*, **43**, 319

Melicow, M. M. and Tannenbaum, M. (1971). Endometrial carcinoma of uterus masculinus (prostatic utricle). Report of 6 cases. *J. Urol.*, **106**, 892

Melicow, M. M. and Uson, A. C. (1976). A spectrum of malignant epithelial tumours of the prostate gland. *J. Urol.*, **115**, 696

Mostofi, F. K. (1975). Grading of prostatic carcinoma. *Cancer Chemother. Rep.*, **59**, 111

Mostofi, F. K. and Morse, W. H. (1951). Epithelial metaplasia in 'prostatic infarction'. *Arch. Pathol.*, **51**, 340

Mostofi, F. K. and Price, E. B. (1973). Tumours of the male genital system. Fascicle 8 of the second *Series of Atlas of Pathology*. (Washington, DC: AFIP)

Murphy, G. P. and Whitmore, W. F. (1979). A report of the workshops of the current status of the histological grading of prostatic cancer. *Cancer*, **44**, 1490

O'Donoghue, E. P. N. and Pugh, R. C. B. (1977). Early diagnosis of prostatic cancer: the role of transurethral resection. *Br. J. Urol.*, **49,** 705

Pennington, J. W., Prentiss, R. J. and Howe, G. (1967). Radical prostatectomy for cancer – significance of perineural lymphatic invasion. *J. Urol.*, **97,** 1075

Purser, B. W., Robinson, B. C. and Mostofi, F. K. (1967). Comparison of needle biopsy and transurethral resection in the diagnosis of carcinoma of the prostate. *J. Urol.*, **98,** 244

Rhamy, R. K., Buchanan, R. D. and Spalding, J. J. (1972). Intraductal carcinoma of the prostate gland. *J. Urol.*, **97,** 457

Rodin, A. E., Larson, D. L. and Roberts, D. K. (1967). Nature of the perineural space invaded by prostatic carcinoma. *Cancer*, **20,** 1772

Scott, J., Robb-Smith, A. M. T. and Burns, I. (1974). Bilateral breast metastases from carcinoma of the prostate. *Br. J. Urol.*, **46,** 209

Taylor, N. S. (1979). Histochemistry in the early diagnosis of prostatic carcinoma. *Hum. Pathol.*, **10,** 513

Thackray, A. C. (1978). The male reproductive system. In Symmers, W. StC. (ed.) *Systemic Pathology.* Chap. 26 (London: Churchill Livingstone)

Trott, P. A., Hendry, W. F., Pugh, R. C. B. and Williams, J. P. (1973). Franzen-needle transrectal prostatic biopsy. *Lancet*, **2,** 620

Varkarakis, M., Castro, J. E. and Azzopardi, J. C. (1970). Prognosis of stage 1 carcinoma of the prostate. *Proc. R. Soc. Med.*, **63,** 91

Vickery, A. L. and Kerr, W. S. (1963). Carcinoma of the prostate treated by radical prostatectomy – a clinicopathological survey of 187 cases followed for 5 years and 148 cases followed for 10 years. *Cancer*, **16,** 1598

Ward, D. C., Taylor, M., Ansell, I. D. and Kulatilake, A. E. (1980). Transrectal needle biopsy of the prostate. Presented at the *British Association of Urological Surgeons*, June, Liverpool

Zaloudek, C., Williams, J. W. and Kempson, R. L. (1976). Endometrial adenocarcinoma of the prostate. A distinctive tumour of probable prostatic duct origin. *Cancer*, **37,** 2255

3
Hormonal environment of the normal prostate

R. GHANADIAN

The growth of the human prostate greatly depends on the supply of a number of steroids and peptide hormones. Among these hormones, the testicular androgens have been shown to play a prominent role in the differentiation and growth of this gland from the time of embryogenesis to puberty, and throughout adulthood. Orchidectomy prior to puberty appears to prevent secondary growth of the gland, which emphasizes the critical role of testicular androgens. Other sources of androgens, including the adrenal cortex and the peripheral conversion of other steroids, have been shown to be significant factors contributing to the supply of circulating androgens. Other hormones involved in the growth of the prostate, including gonadotrophins and their releasing hormones, form part of the overall complex mechanism of steroid production and exert their effect indirectly on the prostate. In addition to these peptide hormones the role of prolactin in the growth and functional activity of the prostate requires particular attention as this hormone is believed to have both direct and indirect effects on this gland. Most of these hormones are subject to various physiological variation, and age dependent changes of steroid and gonadotrophic hormones have a direct effect on the secondary growth of the normal gland which also changes with age. In this chapter, the production, secretion and circulating levels of certain hormones are discussed together with their relevance to the growth of the prostate and major emphasis directed to the factors affecting these hormones and their net effect on the growth of the gland.

3.1 TESTICULAR ANDROGENS

The recognition that testicular secretion is essential for the growth of the prostate dates from the 18th century when John Hunter (1792), demonstrated that castration causes a decrease in the size of the prostate. The isolation of the active testicular hormone, testosterone, by David et $al.$ (1935) and its subsequent characterization and quantitation by several research groups has provided the basis for the study of the role of androgenic steroids in the maintenance and the growth of the prostate. The Leydig cells of the normal testis produce almost all the androgens secreted by the testes, although it has been reported that in rats the semeniferous tubules also produce some androgens, mainly 5α-dihydrotestosterone, which has been derived from C_{19} steroids, but not from cholesterol (Dufau et $al.$, 1971). The Leydig cells produce androgenic steroids from acetate and cholesterol in response to gonadotrophin luteinizing hormone (LH) which is also known as interstitial cell stimulating hormone (ICSH). The production of LH by the pituitary is in turn controlled by hypothalamic releasing hormone (LH-RH), which is secreted into the hypothalamic portal circulation. The secretion of LH is inhibited by negative feedback from circulating testosterone.

The production of testosterone and other androgenic steroids by the testes occurs through a series of enzymatic pathways of which the Δ^4 and Δ^5 steroids provide the major pathways which are shown in Figure 3.1.

The Δ^5 pathway (Neher and Wettstein, 1960) is via 17α-hydroxy-pregnenolone, dehydroepiandrosterone and androst-5-ene-$3\beta,17\beta$-diol, whilst the Δ^4 pathway (Slaunwhite and Samuels, 1956) is via progesterone, 17α-hydroxyprogesterone and androstenedione. The interconversion between the Δ^4 and Δ^5 steroids' pathways is achieved by an isomerase enzyme. Furthermore, the 3β-hydroxysteroid dehydrogenase enzyme can alter the 3β-hydroxy group to that of a 3 ketone. As a direct result of the action of these two enzymes, the Δ^5 steroid pathway is converted to that of a Δ^4 steroid.

The other important steps in these two pathways are the hydroxylation at position 17 by the enzyme 17 hydroxylase, and the subsequent cleavage of C20 and C21 by a lyase, which results in the formation of C_{19} steroids. This pathway is completed by the formation of a 17β-hydroxy group through the effect of the enzyme 17β-hydroxy dehydrogenase. It is rather difficult to evaluate the relative importance of the Δ^5 and Δ^4 pathways, in the testis, but nevertheless, it would appear that whichever pathway is used the synthesis of androstenedione is an important intermediary step as the conversion of androstenediol to testosterone accounts for less than 1 % of testosterone biosynthesis (Chapdelaine and Lanthier, 1966).

The secretion of testosterone by the testes is 5–10 mg/day. Apart from the

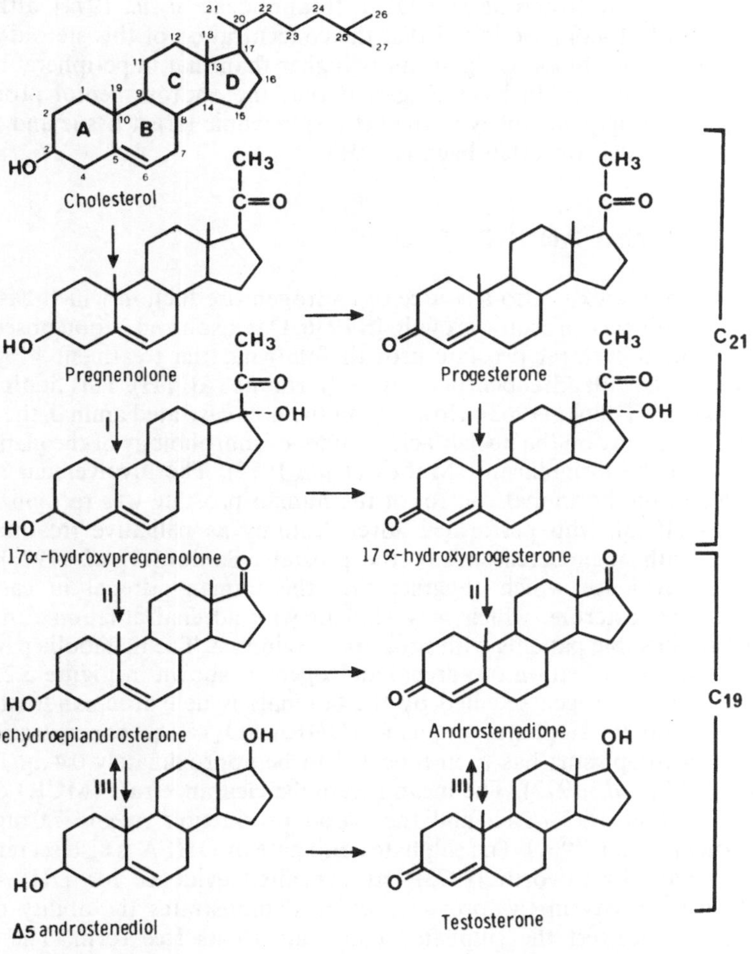

Figure 3.1 Pathways of testosterone synthesis in the testis

testosterone secretion, approximately 30% of the plasma androstenedione has a testicular origin (Vermeulen, 1979), either by direct secretion or indirectly by peripheral conversion of testosterone. The testes also produce small quantities of 5α-dihydrotestosterone (DHT) (Fiorelli *et al.*, 1976) but its exact contribution to the plasma DHT level has not been fully investigated. In addition to these androgenic steroids the testes are reported to secrete substantial amounts of dehydroepiandrosterone (DHEA) (Laatikainen *et al.*, 1971) and androstenediol (Demisch *et al.*, 1973). Finally data with regard to 5α-androstane-3α,17β-diol suggests that most of this steroid originates through the peripheral conversions of testosterone and DHT (Mahoudeau *et al.*, 1971), although Moneti *et al.* (1980) have found that the concentration of this steroid in the spermatic venous blood is significantly higher than that in peripheral blood. Morimoto *et al.* (1980) have suggested that the androstanediol produced peripherally originates solely in the extra splanchnic target tissue and that a major fraction is converted back to DHT.

3.2 ADRENAL ANDROGENS

The adrenal cortex is also a source of androgen production which has been shown to influence prostatic growth. In 1936, Davidson and Moon observed a stimulation of ventral prostate growth following the treatment of young castrated rats with adrenocorticotrophic hormone (ACTH). This finding was confirmed by Tullner (1963). However, in the non-castrated animal, the effect of adrenalectomy on the nucleic acid content or morphology of the gland was reported to be insignificant (Mobbs *et al.*, 1973). The involvement of the adrenals in the hormonal control of the human prostate was recognized by Huggins (1945), who performed adrenalectomy as palliative treatment in patients with adenocarcinoma of the prostate. Sanford *et al.* (1977) have provided evidence which suggests that the human adrenal in castrates produces testosterone which may explain why adrenal ablation can offer palliation in some patients with prostatic carcinoma. The metabolic pathway leading to the formation of adrenal androgens is shown in Figure 3.2.

The main androgen secreted by the adrenals is dehydroepiandrosterone (DHEA) and its sulphate conjugate (DHEA-SO$_4$). The concentration of DHEA in the plasma has been reported to be approximately 0.4 μg/100 ml (Rosenfield *et al.*, 1972). The mean metabolic clearance rate (MCR) of this steroid is 1640 $\pm$ 93 l/24 h and the blood production rate is 7.0 mg/24 h (Horton and Tait, 1967). The sulphate conjugate of DHEA is also secreted by the adrenals. Farnsworth (1973) has presented evidence for DHEA-SO$_4$ sulphatase activity in the prostate, which demonstrates the ability of the prostate to convert the sulphated conjugate to its free form. The mean concentration of DHEA-SO$_4$ in circulating blood is 135 μg/100 ml (37 μmol/l). The metabolic clearance rate of this steroid conjugate is 8–10 l/24 h (Sandberg *et al.*, 1964) and its production rate about 8 mg/24 h (MacDonald *et al.*, 1965).

The adrenals are also the main source of circulating androstenedione. The blood circulating level of androstenedione is reported to be 120 ng/100 ml (4.2 nmol/ml) (Baulieu and Robel, 1970). The metabolic clearance rate is 2430 $\pm$ 150 l/24 h and the production rate is 1.40 mg/24 hours (Horton and Tait, 1966). The conversion of androstenedione to testosterone as well as to oestrogens (Siiteri and MacDonald, 1973) emphasizes the importance of this androgen in relation to its contribution to the growth of the prostate. Other androgens secreted by the adrenals are androstenediol (Demisch *et al.*, 1973) and 17β-hydroxy androstenedione (Jeanloz *et al.*, 1953). The physiological significance of the latter steroid is unknown.

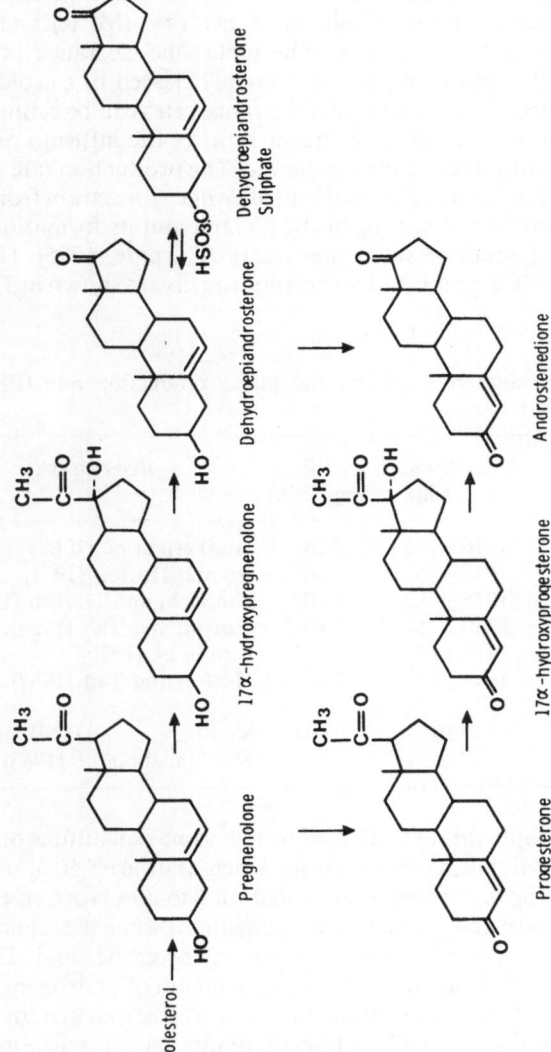

Figure 3.2 Pathway of androgens' biosynthesis in the adrenal

3.3 CIRCULATING ANDROGENS

Following the secretion of androgens by the testes and the adrenals into the general circulation, androgens are taken up by the cells, where they undergo metabolism and produce a number of metabolites, some of which escape into the circulation. The production of androgens in the blood compartment can be measured by the product of the metabolic clearance rate (MCR) and the concentration of androgen in the plasma. The metabolic clearance rate is defined as the volume of blood or plasma irreversibly cleared of steroid per unit time (Tait and Horton, 1966). Metabolic clearance rates can be estimated following a single injection of radioactive tracer or after the infusion of the tracer at a constant rate until steady state is achieved. The production rate (PR) of androgens is generally defined as the total rate of *de novo* formation from all sources and includes secretion of androgens by a gland and its formation by peripheral conversion of other secreted precursors (Gurpide, 1975). Using these criteria, values for MCR and PR of several androgens are shown in Table 3.1.

Table 3.1 Metabolic clearance rate (MCR) and blood production rate (PR) of androgens in normal men

Androgens	MCR (mean) (1/24 h)	PR (mg/24 h)	References
Testosterone	1216 ± 263	6.23	Southern *et al.* (1968)
5α-dihydrotestosterone	652 ± 35	0.302	Ito and Horton (1971)
5α-androstane-3α,17β-diol	1776 ± 492	0.208	Kinouchi and Horton (1974)
Androstenedione	2430 ± 150	1.40	Horton and Tait (1966)
Δ^5-androstene-3α,17β-diol	1311 ± 67	1.357	Bird *et al.* (1976)
Dehydroepiandrosterone	1640 ± 93	7.0	Horton and Tait (1967)
Dehydroepiandrosterone sulphate	8–10	8.0	Sandberg *et al.* (1964) and MacDonald *et al.* (1965)

In normal men the peripheral formation of testosterone constitutes only a minor fraction of the total plasma testosterone, whereas at least 50% of the plasma DHT is derived through peripheral formation (Ito and Horton, 1971; Ishimaru *et al.*, 1977) whilst the plasma androstanediol is almost exclusively formed through the peripheral conversion of testosterone and DHT (Mahoudeau *et al.*, 1971). The site of peripheral conversion of androgens and their escape into the blood have been studied by several research groups and the blood conversion ratio (CR), which is the ratio of plasma concentration of product appearing in the blood to the plasma concentration of the precursor, is reported for a number of androgens (Vermeulen, 1979). The concentration of several important circulating androgens is shown in Table 3.2.

Values in this table represent the unconjugated fraction of androgens which is the sum of unbound (free) and the protein bound steroid. The free fraction of testosterone in normal men, which is reported to be the biologically active

Table 3.2 Concentration of androgens in plasma or serum of normal men

Androgens	Mean concentrations (ng/100 ml)	(nmol/l)	Range (ng/100 ml)	References
Testosterone	512	17.75	244–986 ⎱	Lewis *et al.*
5α-dihydrotestosterone	78	2.68	42–130 ⎰	(1976)
5α-androstane-3α,17β-diol	23	0.8	12–34	Ghanadian and Puah (1980)
5α-androstane-3β, 17β-diol	61	2.08	–	Hopkinson *et al.* (1977)
Androstenedione	120	4.2	50–300	Baulieu and Robel (1970)
Dehydroepiandrosterone	400	13.9	350–700	Rosenfield *et al.* (1972)
Dehydroepiandrosterone sulphate	100700	2870	32000–206000	Plager (1966)
Androstenediol	108	3.7	63–207	Bird *et al.* (1976)
Androsterone	27	0.9	12–47	Hammond *et al.* (1977b)

fraction, constitutes only 2 % of unconjugated testosterone. The other 98 % are bound to plasma proteins. Vermeulen (1977) reported that the binding distribution of testosterone for protein binding component was as follows: sex hormone binding globulin, SHBG, (56 %), albumin (40 %) and transcortin or corticosteroid binding globulin, CBG (2 %). The corresponding values at 4 °C were reported to be 43 %, 29 % and 26 % respectively (Baulieu and Robel, 1970). Corticosteroid binding globulin which is a low capacity α-globulin, displays a low binding affinity for testosterone at 37 °C, whereas it binds up to 26 % at 4 °C. On the other hand SHBG possesses a high affinity but low capacity for testosterone and other 17β-hydroxy androgens. The binding capacity of SHBG is reported to be $3–5 \times 10^{-8}$ mol/l in adult men (Vermeulen, 1979). Albumin has a high capacity but low affinity for testosterone. It is generally accepted that a steroid hormone bound non-covalently to a serum protein is biologically inactive and this has been found for CBG and serum albumin (Westphal, 1980). Androstenedione and DHEA are almost exclusively bound to albumin.

The importance of these protein binding components in blood is not only that they transport steroids from the biosynthesis site to the target cell, but also act as a buffering factor (Daughaday, 1959; Burton and Westphal, 1972). Furthermore, Burke and Anderson (1972) have suggested a special role for SHBG in oestrogen–androgen balance. A change in the concentration of the binding proteins in the blood could result in changes in the unbound steroid fraction.

Circulating androgens are subjected to a number of variations. It has been reported that both the testes and the adrenal cortex show secretory episodes. For testes, the frequency of these episodes is about 1–2 pulses in 6 hours, resulting in transitory spikes of testosterone levels. (Naftolin *et al.*, 1973). On the other hand, both androstenedione and DHEA are secreted synchronously with the secretion of cortisol which results in a pulsatile variation (Rosenfield *et al.*, 1971). In addition, circulating androgens such as testosterone (Resko and Eik-Nes, 1966; Faiman and Winter, 1971; Rose *et al.*, 1972), androstenedione (Vermeulen and Verdonck, 1976a) and DHEA (Vermeulen and Verdonck 1976b) have shown diurnal variation with the highest levels between 4.00 and 8.00 hours and lowest between 22.00 and 24.00 hours.

Apart from the above mentioned variations in the content of circulating androgens, there is now ample evidence in support of age associated changes of these steroids. Despite the controversy as to the decline of androgen with age during the 1960s (Kent and Acone, 1966; Gandy and Peterson, 1968; Frick and Kincle, 1969), most if not all of the studies during the 1970s have demonstrated changes of androgens with age. Vermeulen *et al.*, 1972, Pirke and Doerr, 1973, Sterns *et al.*, 1974, Ghanadian, 1976 and Lewis *et al.*, 1976 have all demonstrated that circulating testosterone decreases with age and that the decline is more significant from the sixth to eighth decades of life. There is a wide range of individual variation, and some individuals of 60–80 years age have testosterone levels well within the younger age group of 20–40 years. However, analysis of the results as a group demonstrates a statistically significant decline with age (Table 3.3).

Table 3.3 Age related changes of testosterone, 5α-dihydrotestosterone, 5α-androstane-3α, 17β-diol and androstenedione in normal men. Values are Mean ± SEM expressed in ng/100 ml serum*. The number of estimations are shown in parenthesis

Androgens	Age groups (years)		
	20–40	40–60	60–80
Testosterone	559 ± 25 (19)	491 ± 25 (20)	475 ± 28 (18)
5α-dihydrotestosterone	84 ± 4 (21)	79 ± 3 (19)	67 ± 3 (18)
5α-androstane-3α, 17β-diol	25 ± 1 (22)	25 ± 0.9 (20)	18 ± 0.7 (18)
Androstenedione	164 ± 10 (21)	129 ± 11 (11)	77 ± 13 (10)

* Conversion factor for 1 ng/100 ml to 1 nmol/1 is as follows: Testosterone 34.67; 5α-dihydrotestosterone 34.43; 5α-androstane-3α, 17β-diol 34.19; androstenedione 34.91. (Data from author's laboratory)

These studies have also been extended to DHT (Lewis *et al.*, 1976; Ghanadian and Puah, 1981a) and 5α-androstane-3α, 17β-diol (Ghanadian and Puah, 1981b) and decline of these androgens with age has also been demonstrated (Table 3.3). Pirke *et al.* (1977) have reported a decline for several testosterone precursors with age in normal men. These include: dehydroepiandrosterone, pregnenolone, androstenediol, 17α-hydroxyprogesterone and androstenedione. However, Vermeulen and Verdonck (1976a) did not observe changes of androstenedione with age. In a recent laboratory study (Ghanadian and Puah, unpublished) we have clearly demonstrated a decline in the content of circulating androstenedione with age (Table 3.3). In parallel with the decrease of androgens with age, SHBG is shown to increase with age and consequently the level of free testosterone declines with age (Vermeulen et al., 1972; Pirke and Doerr, 1973). Based on the fact that gonadotrophic secretion increases with age (Isurugi et al., 1974; Sterns et al., 1974), it appears that the decrease in testicular androgen production is caused by processes within the testes (Baker et al., 1976). Pirke et al. (1980) have suggested that these age-dependent changes are caused by an impaired oxygen supply to the ageing testes. The age associated changes of androgens are not confined to man. A number of androgens including testosterone and 5α-dihydrotestosterone have been shown to decline with age in experimental animals (Ghanadian et al., 1975).

The age related changes of steroids and, in particular, androgens are of paramount importance, as the secondary growth of the prostate leading to the development of benign and malignant tumours of the gland is commonly encountered in men after the fifth decade of life. The decline in the content of the androgens testosterone, 5α-dihydrotesterone and 5α-androstane-3α, 17β-diol together with the increase in the level of the principle oestrogen in man, oestradiol-17β, as well as SHBG which leads to an androgen–oestrogen imbalance, should be taken as an important consideration in the aetiology of prostatic tumours.

3.4 OESTROGENS

The possibility that oestrogens are involved in the development of prostatic tumours has been the subject of much study. The main source of plasma oestrogens in normal men (> 75 %) is derived from the peripheral conversion of androstenedione and testosterone. The sites where oestrogen production does occur have not been determined. However, it has been suggested that adipose tissues may be involved (MacDonald, 1976). Testicular secretion accounts for 25 % of the oestradiol-17β production (Kelch et al., 1972) but less than 5 % of oestrone production (Weinstein et al., 1974). The formation of C18 steroids (oestrone and oestradiol) from C19 steroids (androstenedione and testosterone) involves the loss of the methyl groups at C-10 and one each of the hydrogens from C_1 and C_2. This is achieved by the formation of 19 hydroxy androgens and subsequent aromatization of the A ring (Figure 3.3).

The production rate of oestradiol-17β, in normal men is 30–65 μg/24 h (Ridgway et al., 1975). It has been estimated that, based on a daily production of 7.0 mg of testosterone in man, 0.35 % was converted directly to oestradiol and accounted for 25 μg/day of oestradiol-17β production. Together with the interconversion of oestrone and oestradiol this results in a total peripheral production of approximately 40 μg oestradiol-17β/day, whereas, of the daily production of 2.5 mg androstenedione, 1.7 % was converted to oestrone, producing 42 μg/day (Siiteri and MacDonald, 1973). The plasma concentration of oestradiol in normal men aged between 22 and 61 years is reported to

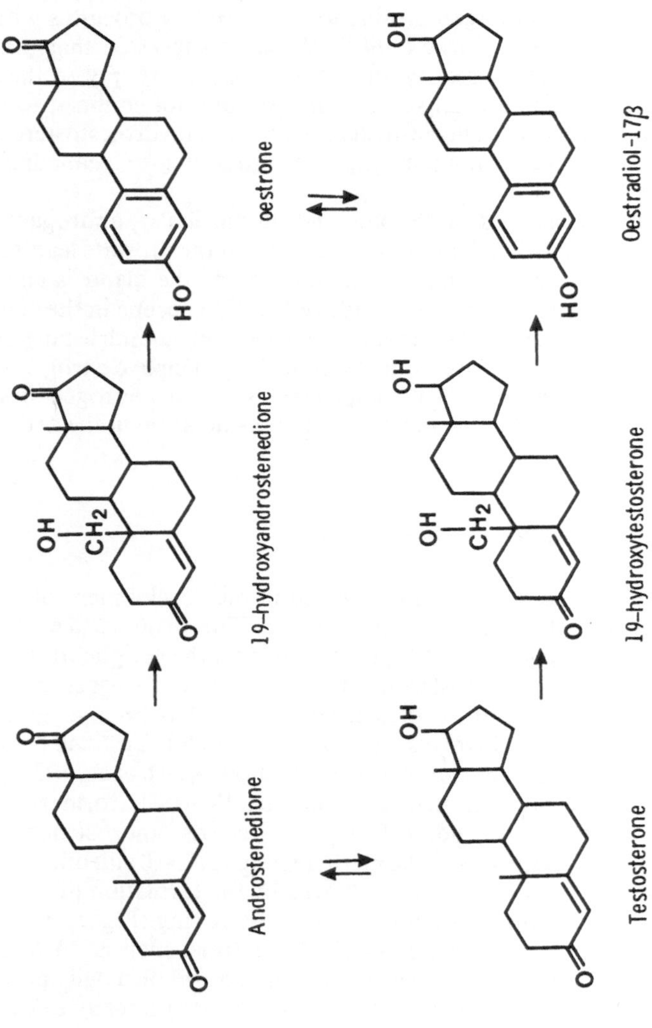

Figure 3.3 Pathway for the formation of oestrogens from androgens

vary between 1.07 and 2.70 with a mean of 1.66 ng/100 ml (60.9 pmol/l). This concentration has been shown to increase with age (Pirke and Doerr, 1973). In normal men aged between 67 and 90 years values for the concentration of oestradiol range between 1.59 and 4.13 with a mean of 2.56 ng/100 ml (93.9 pmol/l). For plasma oestrone similar changes with age have been reported. In two groups of normal subjects of 22–61 and 67–90 years the mean plasma oestrone is reported to be 2.81 ng/100 ml (103.9 pmol/l) and 3.41 ng/100 ml (126.1 pmol/l) respectively (Doerr, 1976). The metabolic clearance rate (MCR) for oestradiol-17β and oestrone in normal men is reported to be 1890 $\pm$ 100 and 2570 $\pm$ 160 l/24 h respectively (Longcope et al., 1968). Changes in the concentration of oestrogens with age are reported to be associated with peripheral conversion of androgens to oestrogens rather than production by the testes. Mannelli et al. (1979) have studied the changes in the concentration of testosterone, androstenedione and oestradiol-17β, in spermatic venous blood with increasing age. In 25 subjects aged 20–70 years undergoing a hernia operation there was a significant reduction in the concentration of both androgrens but not oestradiol-17β with age in the spermatic venous blood. They concluded that in old age the increase of oestradiol-17β in systemic blood is not due to an increased secretion of this steroid by the human testis, but it may be due to an increase in the peripheral conversion of aromatizable androgen and to the reduction of the metabolic clearance rate of this oestrogen.

3.5 PROGESTERONE AND 17α-HYDROXYPROGESTERONE

The significance of other steroids, and in particular progesterone, lies partly in that these compounds may be intermediary precursors in androgen and oestrogen synthesis. Most of the progesterone in normal men originates in the adrenal cortex, since the content of progesterone significantly increases after the administration of ACTH and markedly declines after the administration of dexamethasone (Vermeulen and Verdonck, 1976a). In addition, these authors have reported that the administration of human chorionic gonadotrophins (hCG) does not significantly alter the level of progesterone in either castrated or normal men. However, the presence of progesterone has also been reported in the testes. Hammond et al. (1977b) have measured the concentration of progesterone in human spermatic venous blood and found a mean value of 10.2 mg/ml (32.4 nmol/l). The concentration of circulating progesterone in normal men is reported to vary between 0.02 and 0.57 ng/ml (0.06–1.8 nmol/l) (Strott et al., 1969; Vermeulen and Verdonck, 1976a; Hammond et al., 1977b). The blood production rate of progesterone is reported to be approximately 0.3 mg/24 h (1.0 μmol/24 h) and the metabolic clearance rate about 2000 l/24 h (Strott et al., 1969).

Another important precursor of the androgrens is 17α-hydroxy-progesterone. Unlike progesterone this steroid is reported to have a testicular origin (Strott et al., 1969; Vermeulen and Verdonck, 1969a). Steward-Bentley and Horton (1971) and Pirke et al. (1977) have found that the testicular contribution accounts for approximately 75 % of the peripheral 17α-hydroxyprogesterone level. The mean concentration of this steroid in human spermatic venous blood is reported to be approximately 90 ng/ml (Pirke et al., 1980). However, the level of circulating 17α-hydroxyprogesterone is reported to vary between 0.34 and 2.2 ng/ml (Hammond et al., 1977b; Vermeulen and Verdonck, 1976a). A significant decline in the level of 17α-hydroxy-progesterone with age has been reported by Vermeulen and Verdonck (1976a) and Pirke et al. (1977). With regard to the changes of progesterone with age limited data is available. Vermeulen and Verdonck (1976a) did not detect any changes with age for this steroid, when they compared men aged less than 50 years with those who were over 50 years of age. It is interesting that, whilst Pirke et al. (1980) observed a reduction in testosterone, progesterone and 17α-hydroxyprogesterone in the testicular tissue and spermatic vein of elderly men, the relative concentration of progesterone and its hydroxylated derivative increase in relation to testosterone.

3.6 GONADOTROPHINS

The effect of gonadotrophins on the prostate is indirect, acting through the regulation of testicular secretion. The hypothalamic pituitary gonadal system which is involved in a feedback control mechanism plays an extremely important role in regulating the supply of androgens and thus influencing the growth and functional activity of the prostate.

The two pituitary gonadotrophins, follicle stimulating hormone (FSH) and luteinizing hormone (LH; also referred to as interstitial cell stimulating hormone, ICSH) are glycopeptides which are named as a result of their functions in the female, but are produced in both sexes. They are synthesized in the anterior pituitary gland, circulate in the blood and thus reach the gland where they exert their effects. Their main effect on the prostate is indirectly through the regulation of testicular secretion. The secretion of gonadotrophins is an episodic process. Pulses of LH occur every 2−4 hours with the peak concentration being two or three times the mean value (Nankin and Troen, 1971; Bayer et al., 1972). Fluctuations in FSH also occur, but they are less pronounced. The metabolic clearance rate of LH is significantly higher than that of FSH. Serum gonadotrophins rise progressively after the age of 40−50 y (Isurugi et al., 1974; Baier et al., 1974; Hammond et al., 1977a) and correspond with the fall of testosterone and dihydrotestosterone.

There is good evidence for a negative feedback control of testosterone on gonadotrophins. Testosterone exerts an inhibitory effect on the secretion of gonadotrophins, the effect being preferentially towards LH (Franchimont et al., 1975). Suppression of testosterone by orchidectomy has produced a significant rise in LH and FSH (Walsh et al., 1973). Apart from testosterone, which is considered to be the primary inhibitor of LH secretion, a number of other androgens such as DHT and 5α-androstane-3α, 17β-diol as well as oestrogens at certain doses (Steward-Bentley et al., 1974; Franchimont et al., 1975) have been shown to inhibit gonadotrophin secretion. Oestradiol is reported to be a stronger inhibitor of LH and FSH than testosterone (Swerdloff and Walsh, 1973).

Gonadotrophins are controlled by the hypothalamus through the gonado-trophin releasing hormone (Gn-RH) which is generally known as luteinizing hormone releasing hormone (LH-RH), also referred to as LH-RH/FSH-RH. However, no separate FSH-RH has been identified (Schally et al., 1979). The secretion of LH-RH is in part under the influence of the central nervous system (CNS). LH-RH is a decapeptide (Nair and Schally, 1972) which is produced in the hypothalamus and transported to the pituitary gland by a short portal venous system.

Both natural and synthetic LH-RH are capable of releasing LH and FSH. The response of the pituitary to LH-RH is also influenced by the presence of gonadal steroids. Testosterone has inhibitory effects on LH and FSH secretion after LH-RH administration (Wollesen et al., 1974), whilst orchidectomy or hypogonadism cause augmented responses (Marshall, 1975). Changes in the binding of testosterone to sex hormone binding globulin (SHBG) are reported to be important, since it is only the unbound circulating testosterone which exerts the control on gonadotrophins release (Anderson, 1974). It has been suggested that in addition to the aforementioned effect of oestradiol in the feedback control of gonadotrophins, local aromatization of testosterone or other androgen precursors to oestradiol may occur in the hypothalamus. This local metabolic conversion would inhibit LH-RH production (Naftolin et al., 1971). There is also the possibility for other mechanisms, since androgens, such as dihydrotestosterone, that cannot be converted to oestradiol, are potent inhibitors of LH and FSH (Naftolin and Feder, 1973; Steward-Bentley et al., 1974).

There is as yet no firm evidence for the existence of a separated FSH-RH (Schally et al., 1979). An alternative mechanism for the control of FSH has been suggested by postulating the existence of a non-steroidal substance 'inhibin' secreted by sertoli cells, which acts in the feedback mechanism of FSH. Support for the existence of such a feedback mechanism and a separate tubular factor is based on the observation of an increase in FSH concentration where there is extensive tubular damage (Franchimont et al., 1972). However, both a tubular inhibitor factor and gonadal steroids are thought to be important in maintaining the normal serum FSH.

3.7 PROLACTIN

Prolactin was identified as a lactogenic hormone by Striker and Gueter in 1928, but the isolation and purification of human prolactin from the pituitary gland was first reported by Lewis et al. (1971). Evidence for the existence of a relationship between pituitary prolactin and prostate was originally presented using experimental animals. Huggins and Russell (1946) found a more profound atrophy of the dog prostate following the removal of the pituitary than after simple castration. Grayhack et al. (1955) reported that in castrated and hypophysectomized rat, administration of testosterone alone was not capable of restoring normal prostatic weight unless it was given with a supplement of commercial luteotrophins. Lawrence and Launda (1965) found a fall in prostatic uptake of labelled testosterone following hypophysectomy.

The synergism between testosterone and prolactin has been further investigated (Chase et al., 1957; Grayhack and Lebowitz, 1967; Hafiez et al., 1972) and a similar relationship has also been reported between adrenal androgens and prolactin (Tullner, 1963). In contrast to these findings, Thomas et al. (1976) found that prolactin reduces the formation of tritiated dihydrotestosterone, indicating that it exerts an inhibitory effect upon prostatic 5α-reductase. In 1965 Asano found that the pituitary prolactin content and release increased not only following castration, but also after total prostatectomy in the rat. These studies have provided some experimental evidence for a direct effect of prolactin on the prostate. Furthermore, the presence of specific prolactin binding sites has been reported in the rat ventral prostate (Kledzik et al., 1976; Aragona and Friesen, 1975). Rubens et al. (1976) have reported that in normal adult men prolactin may increase testosterone secretion and Farnsworth (1972) has suggested that prolactin accentuates the effect of androgens of both testicular and adrenal origin on the prostate. The plasma concentration of prolactin has been estimated in normal men. The mean concentration of this hormone in normal men is reported to be 6.0 ± 0.3 ng/ml (Franks, 1979). Studies on the 24 hour pattern of plasma prolactin suggest that this hormone is released in a pulsatile fashion, but these pulses are not large except during sleep, when a significant increase has been observed (Nokin et al., 1972).

3.8   STEROIDS IN NORMAL HUMAN PROSTATE

The finding that prostatic tissues are able to take up testosterone and subsequently metabolize and retain its active metabolite has prompted much interest in the quantitation of endogenous steroids and in particular androgens in this gland. In line with other investigations in the human prostate, the shortage of normal prostate for research purposes compared to tumours, has been a hindrance to progress in the elucidation of the hormonal control of the normal prostate. In a classical study, Siiteri and Wilson (1970) demonstrated higher levels of DHT compared to testosterone and androstenedione in the normal gland. There were also differences in the levels of these hormones, and in particular DHT, when they compared normal prostate with benign prostatic tumours. The importance attached to this original investigation was that it has not only demonstrated the accumulation of DHT in this gland, but also, differences in the hormonal profile of the tissue with that of the circulating blood. In this study, the mean concentrations of androstenedione, testosterone and DHT in normal prostate measured by a double isotope derivative technique were 0.09, 0.09 and 0.13 μg/100 g tissue respectively. These values were obtained from the prostates of 15 subjects with a mean age of 33 ± 4 years. The mean weight of the prostate from this group was 18 ± 2 g which is within the normal weight of the gland. The regional studies on only three normal prostates revealed that the DHT content was 2 to 3 fold greater in the periurethral region, when compared to the outer region of the gland. Geller et al. (1976) have measured the concentration of DHT and 5α-androstane-3α, 17β-diol by radioimmunoassay and have found the concentration of these two steroids in the prostate of subjects not older than 45 years to be 2.1 ng/g and 10.2 ng/g tissue respectively. These authors did not study the regional content of these androgens. A similar study reported by Krieg *et al.* (1979) who measured the content of testosterone, 5α-dihydrotestosterone and 5α-androstane-3α,17β-diol in normal subjects aged 19–43 years, found the mean ± SD concentrations of these steroids to be 0.2, 1.6 and 1.7 ng/g tissue respectively. Hammond (1978) has measured several steroids including testosterone, androstenedione, 5α-androstane-3α,17β-diol, androsterone, progesterone and 17α-hydroxyprogesterone. In this study no significant differences in the tissue concentration of these steroids in the periurethral compared to the outer region of the gland was observed. This is in contrast to the previous report by Siiteri and Wilson (1970) who found regional differences for the distribution of DHT. However, when the levels of these steroids in the prostate derived from different age groups were compared (Hammond, 1978), certain differences were observed. Apart from 5α-androstane-3α, 17β-diol, the level of which tended to increase after 6 days of age, the concentrations of all steroids were lower in the infant and pubertal prostates. The high concentration of progesterone and 17α-hydroxyprogesterone in the prostate of the newborn is attributed to exposure of the fetus to circulating maternal hormones. It is interesting to note that in this study, despite the high concentrations of progesterone and its hydroxylated derivative which could reduce the activity of 5α-reductase, when present in pharmacological doses, the level of both DHT and other 5α-reduced metabolites is reported to be high. However, based on the limited numbers of prostates reported by Hammond (1978), no apparent explanation can be given for this high concentration of DHT and androstanediol in the prostate of this age group. Other important observations by this author were the significant correlation between the combined concentration of testosterone and androstenedione and the combined concentration of 5α-androstane-3α,17β-diol and androsterone in the normal gland. The author has concluded that in the normal prostate the latter two androgens are major metabolites of testosterone and androstenedione via the formation of DHT and 5α-androstanedione (see Figure 6.2, Chapter 6). There is no information on the concentration of oestradiol-17β, in the normal prostate. However, the levels of this oestrogen in the benign and malignant tumours of the prostate has been reported by Ghanadian and Puah (1980). The concentration of steroids in the normal prostate is summarized in Table 3.4.

3.9 CONCLUSIONS

The normal prostate is dependent upon a number of steroid and peptide hormones for its growth and functional activity. Androgens are the most important hormones, without which the gland ceases to grow and undergoes atrophy. The main source of androgens is derived from the testis, which is capable of synthesizing these compounds from cholesterol through two major pathways, namely the Δ^4 and Δ^5 pathways. The major androgen which originates in the testes is testosterone, although it does secrete androstenedione, dehydroepiandrosterone and a number of other androgens to a much

Table 3.4 The concentration of endogenous steroids in normal human prostates

Steroids	Mean ± SEM (ng/g wet tissue)	No. of prostates	Age (years)	References
Testosterone	0.90 ± 0.30	15	15–66	Siiteri & Wilson (1970)
	0.25 ± 0.04	18	20–75	Hammond (1978)
5α-dihydrotestosterone	1.30 ± 0.50	15	15–66	Siiteri & Wilson (1970)
(DHT)	1.20 ± 0.14	18	20–75	Hammond (1978)
	2.10 ± 0.32	6	< 50	Geller et al. (1976)
5α-androstane-3α,17β-diol	10.2 ± 2.4	6	< 50	Geller et al. (1976)
(3α-diol)	4.32 ± 0.49	18	20–75	Hammond (1978)
Androstenedione	0.9 ± 0.40	15	15–65	Siiteri & Wilson (1970)
	0.13 ± 0.03	18	20–75	Hammond (1978)
5α-androstane-3,17-dione	1.13 ± 0.30	18	20–75	Hammond (1978)
Androsterone	4.15 ± 1.07	18	20–75	Hammond (1978)
Progesterone	0.39 ± 0.07	18	20–75	Hammond (1978)
17α-hydroxyprogesterone	0.42 ± 0.06	18	20–75	Hammond (1978)

lesser extent. Another source of androgens is the adrenal cortex which contributes largely towards the levels of androstenedione, dehydroepiandrosterone and its sulphate conjugate as well as a number of other androgens to a lesser degree. Apart from these two major sources of androgen production, some circulating androgens came from the peripheral conversion of other steroids. Circulating androgens in men are present in either conjugated or unconjugated form. The latter consists of the fraction bound to the blood proteins and the free fraction. In the case of testosterone the free fraction accounts for approximately 2% of the unconjugated fraction. Thus the majority of circulating androgens are bound to plasma proteins. These proteins and in particular SHBG, are involved in the transport and buffering of hormones. They also appear to play an important role in oestrogen–androgen balance. The circulating androgens are subject to a number of variations mainly diurnal and pulsatile. Another factor which significantly influences the level of circulating androgens is the age-dependency of these steroids, there being a general concensus of opinion supporting the decline of androgens, notably testosterone, 5α-dihydrotestosterone, 5α-androstane-3α,17β-diol as well as the precursors of testosterone, with increasing age. These changes become more pronounced after the 5th decade of life and are commonly associated with the ageing testis.

Another important class of steroids which is thought to be involved in the maintenance and growth of the prostate are the oestrogens and especially oestradiol-17β. The main source of this oestrogen in normal men is through peripheral conversion, although the testicular contribution is important. The concentration of this oestrogen is also subject to a number of variations. However, unlike the androgens this steroid is shown to increase with age in normal men, possibly due to peripheral aromatization of androgens rather than an increased testicular secretion. This imbalance between circulating androgens and oestrogens could influence the hormonal control of the prostate and may play a role in the secondary growth of this gland. With regard to other classes of steroid hormones and, in particular, progesterone, little is known on the role of these steroids in the growth of the prostate. However, the importance of progesterone and 17α-hydroxyprogesterone, appears to be related to the fact that these steroids are precursors of androgens and oestrogens. The role of gonadotrophic hormones LH and FSH in the hormonal control of the prostate is indirect through the regulation of gonadal steroids. The secretion of gonadotrophins is an episodic process, and is accompanied by an age-dependent change. Both LH and FSH rise progressively after the 5th decade of life and this rise corresponds to the fall of testosterone and DHT. These polypeptides are synthesized in the anterior pituitary, and are in turn controlled by the hypothalamus, through the gonadotrophin releasing hormones, the latter being in part under the influence of the central nervous system. Another important peptide hormone, which is shown to influence the growth of the prostate both directly and indirectly, is prolactin. This hormone is capable of increasing testosterone secretion and enhancing the effect of androgens of both testicular and adrenal origin.

The current available data on the mode of entry, accumulation and release of hormones in the normal prostate is limited. However, a number of research groups have estimated the concentration of several steroids including testosterone, 5α-dihydrotestosterone, 5α-androstane-3α,17β-diol, androstanedione, androstenedione, 5α-androstane, 3,17-dione, androsterone, dehydroepiandrosterone, progesterone and 17α-hydroxyprogesterone in the normal prostate. Some of these steroids are reported to have a differential regional distribution and also show age associated changes. It is suggested that in the normal gland 5α-androstane-3α,17β-diol and androsterone are the major metabolites of testosterone and androstenedione via the formation of DHT and 5α-androstane-3α,17β-diol, but this requires further experimental support.

It would appear from our present knowledge on the hormonal environment of the normal prostate, that despite the importance of the androgens in the control and development of this gland, a rather complicated multifactor mechanism is involved, which requires further elucidation.

3.10 REFERENCES

Anderson, D. C. (1974). Sex hormone-binding globulin. *Clin. Endocrinol.*, **3**, 69

Aragona, C. and Friesen, H. G. (1975). Specific prolactin binding sites in the prostate and testis of rats. *Endocrinology*, **97**, 677

Asano, M. (1965). Basic experimental studies of the pituitary prolactin–prostate interrelationships. *J. Urol.*, **93**, 87

Baier, H., Biro, G. and Weinges, K. F. (1974). Serum levels of FSH, LH and testosterone in human males. *Horm. Metab. Res.*, **6**, 514

Baker, H. W. G., Burger, H. G., De Kretser, D. M., Hudson, B., O'Connor, S., Wang, C., Mirovics, A., Court, J., Dunlop, M. and Rennie, G. C. (1976). Changes in the pituitary-testicular system with age. *Clin. Endocrinol.*, **5**, 349

Baulieu, E. E. and Robel, P. (1970). Catabolism of testosterone and androstenedione. In Eik-Nes, K. (ed.). *The Androgens of the Testis*, pp. 49–71. (New York, London: Marcel Dekker. Inc.)

Bayer, R. M., Parlow, A. F., Hellman, L., Kapen, S. and Weitzman, E. (1972). Twenty-four hour pattern of luteinizing hormone secretion in normal men with sleep stage recording. *J. Clin. Endocrinol. Metab.*, **35**, 73

Bird, E. C., Morrow, L., Fukumoto, Y., Marcellus, S. and Clark, A. F. (1976). Δ5 Androstenediol: kinetics of metabolism and binding to plasma proteins in normal men and women. *J. Clin. Endocrinol.*, **43**, 1317

Burke, C. W. and Anderson, D. C. (1972). Sex-hormone globulin is an oestrogen amplifier. *Nature (London)*, **240**, 38

Burton, R. M. and Westphal, U. (1972). Steroid hormone-binding proteins in blood plasma. *Metabolism*, **21**, 253

Chapdelaine, A. and Lanthier, A. (1966). *In vivo* metabolism of androgens. In *2nd International Congress on Hormonal Steroids*, p. 281. (Amsterdam: Excerpta Medica)

Chase, M. D., Geschwind, I. I. and Bern, H. A. (1957). Synergistic role of prolactin in response of male accessories to androgen. *Proc. Soc. Exp. Med.*, **96**, 480

Daughaday, W. H. (1959). Steroid protein interaction. *Physiol. Rev.*, **39**, 885

David, K., Dingemanse, E., Freud, J. and Laquer, E. (1935). Uber Krystallinisches mannliches hormon aus hoden (testosteron), Wirksamer als aus harn oder aus cholesterin bereittes androsteron. *Hoppe-Syel. Z. Physiol. Chem. Phys.*, **233**, 281

Davidson, C. S. and Moon, H. D. (1936). Effect of adrenotropic extracts on accessory reproductive organs of castrate rats. *Proc. Soc. Exp. Biol. Med.*, **35**, 281

Demisch, K., Magnet, W., Naubauer, M. and Schoffling, K. (1973). Studies about unconjugated androstanediol in human peripheral plasma. *J. Clin. Endocrinol. Metab.*, **37**, 129

Doerr, P. (1976). Radioimmunoassay of oestrone in plasma. *Acta Endocrinol.*, **81**, 655

Dufau, M. L., de Krester, D. M. and Hudson, B. (1971). Steroid metabolism by isolated rat seminiferous tubules in tissue culture. *Endocrinology*, **88**, 825

Faiman, C. and Winter, J. S. A. (1971). Diurnal cycles in plasma FSH, testosterone and cortisol in men. *J. Clin. Endocrinol.*, **33**, 186

Farnsworth, W. E. (1972). Prolactin and the prostate. In Boynes, A. R. and Griffiths, K. (eds.) *Prolactin and Carcinogenesis*. pp. 217–8. (Cardiff: Alpha Omega Alpha Publishing)

Farnsworth, W. E. (1973). Human prostatic dehydroepiandrosterone sulfate sulfatase. *Steroids*, **21**, 647

Fiorelli, G., Borrelli, D., Forti, G., Gonnelli, P., Pazzagli, M. and Serio, M. (1976). Simultaneous determination of androstenedione, testosterone and 5α-dihydrotestosterone in human spermatic and peripheral venous plasma. *J. Steroid Biochem.*, **7**, 113

Franchimont, P., Chari, S. and Demoulin, A. (1975). Hypothalamus–pituitary–testis interaction. *J. Reprod. Fertil.*, **44**, 335

Franchimont, P., Millet, D., Vendrely, E., Letawe, J., Legros, J. J. and Netter, A. (1972). Relationship between spermatogenesis and serum gonadotrophin levels in azoospermia and oligospermia. *J. Clin. Endocrinol. Metab.*, **34**, 1003

Franks, S. (1979). Prolactin. In Gray, C. H. and James, V. H. T. (eds.) *Hormones in Blood.*, 3rd Edn., pp. 279–331. (London, New York: Academic Press)

Frick, J. and Kincle, F. A. (1969). The measurement of testosterone by competitive protein binding assay. *Steroids*, **13**, 495

Gandy, H. M. and Peterson, R. E. (1968). Measurement of testosterone and 17-ketosteroids in plasma by the double isotope dilution derivative techniques. *J. Clin. Endocrinol.*, **27**, 949

Geller, G., Albert, J., Lopez, D., Geller, S. and Niwayama, A. (1976). Comparison of androgen metabolites in benign prostate hypertrophy (BPH) and normal prostate. *J. Clin. Endocrinol. Metab.*, **43**, 686

Ghanadian, R. (1976). Endocrine control of the prostate: mechanism of action of androgens. In Williams, D. I. and Chisholm, G. D. (eds.) *Scientific Foundation of Urology.* pp. 138–146. (London: Heinemann)

Ghanadian, R., Lewis, J. G. and Chisholm, G. D. (1975). Serum testosterone and dihydrotestosterone changes with age in rat. *Steroids*, **25**, 753

Ghanadian, R. and Puah, C. M. (1980). Relationship between oestradiol-17β, testosterone, dihydrotestosterone and 5α-androstane-3α,17β-diol in human benign hypertrophy and carcinoma of the prostate. *J. Endocrinol.*, **88**, 255

Ghanadian, R. and Puah, C. M. (1981a). Age related changes of serum 5α-androstane-3α,17β-diol in normal men. *Gerontology*, **27**, 281

Ghanadian, R. and Puah, C. M. (1981b). Changes of androgens in normal men. *Age Ageing*, **10**, 204

Grayhack, J. T., Bunce, P. L., Kearn, J. W. and Scott, W. W. (1955). Influence of pituitary on prostatic response to androgen in the rat. *Bull. Johns Hopkins Hosp.*, **96**, 154

Grayhack, J. T. and Lebowitz, J. M. (1967). Effect of prolactin on citric acid of lateral lobe of prostate of Sprague-Dawley rat. *Invest. Urol.*, **5**, 87

Gurpide, E. (1975). *Tracer Methods in Hormone Research.* (Heidelberg and New York: Springer Verlag)

Hafiez, A. A., Lloyd, C. W. and Bartke, A. (1972). The role of prolactin in the regulation of testis function: the effects of prolactin and luteinizing hormone on the plasma level of testosterone and androstenedione in hypophysectomized rats. *J. Endocrinol.*, **52**, 327

Hammond, G. L. (1978). Endogenous steroid levels in the human prostate from birth to old age: a comparison of normal and diseased tissues. *J. Endocrinol.*, **78**, 7

Hammond, G. L., Kontturi, M., Maattala, M., Puukka, M. and Vihko, R. (1977a). Serum FSH, LH and prolactin in normal males and patients with prostatic disease. *Clin. Endocrinol.*, **7**, 129

Hammond, G. L., Roukoneu, A., Konttuir, M., Koskela, E. and Vihko, R. (1977b). The simultaneous radioimmunoassay of seven steroids in human spermatic and peripheral venous blood. *J. Clin. Endocrinol. Metab.*, **45**, 16

Hopkinson, C. R. R., Park, B. K., Johnson, M. W., Stram, G., Steinbach, K. and Hirschauser, C. (1977). Concentration of unconjugated 5α-androstane-3β, 17β-diol in human peripheral plasma as measured by radioimmunoassay. *J. Steroid Biochem.*, **8**, 1253

Horton, R. and Tait, J. E. (1966). Androstenedione production and inter-conversion rates measured in peripheral blood and studies on the possible state of its conversion to testosterone. *J. Clin. Invest.*, **45**, 301

Horton, R. and Tait, J. F. (1967). *In vivo* conversion of dehydroepiandrosterone to plasma androstenedione and testosterone in man. *J. Clin. Endocrinol. Metab.*, **27**, 79

Huggins, C. (1945). The physiology of the prostate gland. *Physiol. Rev.*, **25**, 281

Huggins, C. and Russell, P. S. (1946). Quantitative effects of hypophysectomy of testis and prostate of dogs. *Endocrinology*, **39**, 1

Hunter, J. (1792). *Observation on Certain Parts of Animal Oeconomy.* 2nd Edn., p. 44. (London: Bibliotheca Oesteriana)

Ishimaru, T., Pages, L. and Horton, R. (1977). Altered metabolism of androgens in elderly men with benign prostatic hyperplasia. *J. Clin. Endocrinol. Metab.*, **45**, 695

Isurugi, K., Fukutani, K., Takayasu, H., Wakabayashi, K. and Tamaoki, B. I. (1974).

Age related changes in serum luteinizing hormone (LH) and follicle stimulating hormone (FSH) levels in normal men. *J. Clin. Endocrinol. Metab.*, **39**, 955

Ito, T. and Horton, R. (1971). The source of plasma dihydrotestosterone in man. *J. Clin. Invest.*, **50**, 1261

Jeanloz, R. W., Levy, H., Jacobson, R. P., Hechter, O., Schenker, V. and Pincus, G. (1953). Chemical transformations of steroids by adrenal perfusion. *J. Biol. Chem.*, **203**, 453

Kelch, R. P., Jenner, M. R., Weinstein, R., Kaplan, S. L. and Grunbach, M. M. (1972). Estradiol and testosterone secretion by human, simian and canine testes, in males with hypogonadism and in male pseudohermaphrodites with the feminizing testes syndrome. *J. Clin. Invest.*, **51**, 824

Kent, J. R. and Acone, A. B. (1966). Plasma testosterone levels and ageing in males. *International Congress Series*, Vol. **101**, p. 31. (Amsterdam: Excerpta Medica)

Kinouchi, T. and Horton, R. (1974). 3α-androstanediol kinetics in man. *J. Clin. Invest.*, **54**, 646

Kledzik, G. S., Marshall, S., Campbell, G. A. and Gelato, M. (1976). Effects of castration, testosterone, oestradiol and prolactin on specific prolactin-binding activity in ventral prostate of male rats. *Endocrinology*, **98**, 373

Krieg, M., Bartsch, W., Janssen, W. and Voigt, K. D. (1979). A comparative study of binding, metabolism and androgen levels of androgens in normal hyperplastic and carcinomatous human prostate. *J. Steroid Biochem.*, **11**, 615

Laatikainen, T., Laitmen, E. A. and Vihko, R. (1971). Secretion of free and sulphate-conjugated neutral steroids by the human testis. Effect of administration of human chorionic gonadotrophin. *J. Clin. Endocrinol. Metab.*, **32**, 59

Lawrence, A. M. and Launda, R. L. (1965). Impaired ventral prostate affinity for testosterone in hypophysectomized rats. *Endocrinology*, **77**, 1119

Lewis, J. G., Ghanadian, R. and Chisholm, G. D. (1976). Serum 5α-dihydrotestosterone and testosterone changes with age in man. *Acta Endocrinol.*, **82**, 444

Lewis, U. J., Singh, R. N. P. and Seavey, B. K. (1971). Human prolactin: isolation and some properties. *Biochem. Biophys Res. Commun.*, **44**, 1169

Longcope, C., Layne, D. S. and Tait, J. F. (1968). Metabolic clearance rates and interconversions of estrone and 17β-estradiol in normal males and females. *J. Clin. Invest.*, **47**, 93

MacDonald, P. C. (1976). Origin of estrogen in men. In Grayhack, J. J., Wilson, J. D. and Scherhenske, M. J. (eds.) *Benign Prostatic Hyperplasia*. pp. 191–2. (Washington: US Govt. Printing Office)

MacDonald, P. C., Chapdelaine, A., Gonzales, O., Gurpide, E., Van de Wide R. L. and Liebeiman, S. (1965). Studies on the secretion and interconversion of the androgens. III. Results obtained after the injection of several radioactive C_{19} steroids single or as mixtures. *J. Clin. Endocrinol. Metab.*, **25**, 1557

Mahoudeau, J. A., Bardin, C. W. and Lipsett, M. B. (1971). The metabolic clearance rate and origin of plasma dihydrotestosterone in man and its conversion to the 5α-androstanediols. *J. Clin. Invest.*, **50**, 1338

Mannelli, M., Borrelli, D., Gonnelli, P., Fiorelli, G., Forti, G. and Serio, M. (1979). 17β-oestradiol concentration in spermatic venous blood with increasing age. *Int. J. Androl.*, **2**, 131

Marshall, J. C. (1975). Investigative procedures. *J. Clin. Endocrinol. Metab.*, **4**, 545

Mobbs, B. G., Johnson, I. E. and Connolly, J. G. (1973). Influence of the adrenal gland on prostatic activity in adult rats. *J. Endocrinol.*, **59**, 335

Moneti, G., Pazzagli, M., Fiorelli, G. and Serio, M. (1980). Measurement of 5α-androstane-3α,17β-diol in human spermatic venous plasma by mass-fragmentography. *J. Steroid Biochem.*, **13**, 623

Morimoto, I., Edmiston, A. and Horton, R. (1980). Origin of androstanediol (3α-diol) and its glucoronide (G) in man. Proceedings *62nd Annual meeting, The Endocrine Society*, pp. 258, Washington.

Naftolin, F. and Feder, H. H. (1973). Suppression of luteinizing hormone secretion in male rats by 5α-androstan-17-ol-3-one (dihydrotestosterone) propionate. *J. Endocrinol.*, **56**, 155

Naftolin, F., Gudd, J. H. and Yen, S. S. C. (1973). Pulsatile patterns of gonadotrophins and testosterone in man: the effects of clomiphene with and without testosterone. *J. Clin. Endocrinol. Metab.*, **36**, 285

Naftolin, F., Ryan, K.J. and Petro, Z. (1971). Aromatization of androstenedione by the diencephalon. *J. Clin. Endocrinol. Metab.*, **33**, 368

Nair, R. M. G. and Schally, A. V. (1972). Structure of hypothalamic peptide possessing gonadotrophin-releasing activity. *Int. J. Pept. Protein Res.*, **4**, 421

Nankin, H. R. and Troen, P. (1971). Repepitive luteinizing hormone elevations in serum of normal men. *J. Clin. Endocrinol. Metab.*, **33**, 558

Neher, R. and Wettstein, A. (1960). Occurrence and Δ⁵-3α, hydroxysteroid in adrenal and testicular tissue, *Acta Endocrinol.*, **35**, 1

Nokin, J., Vekemans, M., L'Hermite, M. and Robyn, C. (1972). Circadian periodicity of serum prolactin concentration in man. *Br. Med. J.*, **3**, 561

Pirke, K. M. and Doerr, P. (1973). Age related changes and inter-relationship between plasma testosterone, oestradiol and testosterone-binding globulin in normal adult males. *Acta Endocrinol.*, **74**, 792

Pirke, K. M., Doerr, P., Sintermann, R. and Vogt, H. J. (1977). Age dependence of testosterone precursors in plasma of normal adult males. *Acta Endocrinol.*, **86**, 415

Pirke, K. M., Sintermann, R. and Vogt, H. J. (1980). Testosterone and testosterone precursors in the spermatic vein and in the testicular tissue of old men. *Gerontology.*, **26**, 221

Plager, J. E. (1966). Extraction and purification of steroid conjugates with ion exchange resins: measurement of androsterone sulfate and dehydroepiandrosterone sulfate in plasma. *J. Clin. Endocrinol. Metab.*, **26**, 1275

Resko, J. A. and Eik-Nes, K. B. (1966). Diurnal testosterone levels in peripheral plasma of human male subjects. *J. Clin. Endocrinol.*, **26**, 573

Ridgway, E. C., Longcope, C. and Maloof, F.'(1975). Metabolic clearance and blood production rates of estradiol in hyperthyroidism. *J. Clin. Endocrinol. Metab.*, **41**, 491

Rose, R. M., Dreuz, K. E., Holaday, J. W., Sulak, K. J. and Johnson, C. E. (1972). Diurnal variation of plasma testosterone and cortisol. *J. Endocrinol.*, **54**, 177

Rosenfield, R. S., Hellman, L. and Gallagher, T. F. (1972). Metabolism and interconversion of dehydroiosoandrosterone and dehydroisoandrosterone sulfate. *J. Clin. Endocrinol. Metab.*, **35**, 187

Rosenfield, R. S., Hellman, L., Roffwaig, H., Weitzmann, E. D., Fukushima, D. K. and Gallagher, T. F. (1971). Dehydroisoandrosterone is secreted episodically and synchronously with cortisol by normal men. *J. Clin. Endocrinol. Metab.*, **33**, 87

Rubens, R. T., Poland, R. E. and Tower, B. B. (1976). Prolactin related testosterone secretion in normal adult men. *J. Clin. Endocrinol. Metab.*, **42**, 112

Sandberg, E., Gurpide, E. and Lieberman, S. (1964). Quantitive studies on the metabolism of dehydroisoandrosterone sulfate. *Biochemistry*, **3**, 1256

Sanford, E. J., Paulson, D. F., Rohner, T. J., Drago, J. R., Santen, R. J. and Bardin, C. W. (1977). The effects of castration on adrenal testosterone secretion in man with prostatic carcinoma. *J. Urol.*, **118**, 1019

Schally, A. V., Coy, D. H., Meyers, C. A. and Kastin, A. J. (1979). Hypothalamic peptide hormones: basic and clinical studies. In Choh Hao Li (ed). *Hormonal Proteins and Peptides*. pp. 1–54. (London, New York: Academic Press)

Siiteri, P. K. and MacDonald, P. C. (1973). Role of extra glandular estrogen in human endocrinology. In Greep, R. O. and Astwood, E. B. (eds.) *Handbook of Physiology.* Vol. II, pp. 615–629. (Baltimore: Williams & Wilkins)

Siiteri, P. K. and Wilson, J. D. (1970). Dihydrotestosterone in prostatic hypertrophy. 1. The formation and content of dihydrotestosterone in the hypertrophic prostate of man. *J. Clin. Invest.*, **49**, 1737

Slaunwhite, W. R. and Samuels, L. T. (1956). Progesterone as a precursor of testicular androgens. *J. Biol. Chem.*, **220**, 341

Southern, A. L., Gordon, G. G. and Tochimoto, S. (1968). Further study of factors affecting the metabolic clearance rate of testosterone in man. *J. Clin. Endocrinol. Metab.*, **28**, 1105

Sterns, E. L., MacDonnell, J. A., Kaufman, B. J., Padua, R., Lucman, T. S., Winter, J. S. D. and Faiman, C. (1974). Declining testicular function with age. *Am. J. Med.*, **57**, 761

Steward-Bentley, M. and Horton, R. (1971). 17α-hydroxyprogesterone in human plasma. *J. Clin. Endocrinol. Metab.*, **33**, 542

Steward-Bentley, M., Odell, W. and Horton, R. (1974). The feedback control of luteinizing hormone in normal adult men. *J. Clin. Endocrinol. Metab.*, **38**, 545

Striker, S. and Grueter, F. (1928). Action de l'hypophyse sur la montee laiteuse. *C.R. Soc. Biol.*, **99**, 1978

Strott, C. A., Yoshimi, T. and Lipsett, M. B. (1969). Plasma progesterone and 17-hydroxyprogesterone in normal men and children with congenital adrenal hyperplasia. *J. Clin. Invest.*, **48**, 930

Swerdloff, R. S. and Walsh, P. C. (1973). Testosterone and estradiol suppression of LH and FSH in adult male rats. Duration of castration, duration of treatment and combined treatment. *Acta Endocrinol.*, **73**, 11

Tait, J. F. and Horton, R. (1966). The *in vivo* estimation of blood production and inter-conversion rates of androstenedione and testosterone and the calculation of their secretion rates. In Pincus, G., Nakao, T., and Tait, J. F. (eds.) *Steroid Dynamics.* pp. 393–427. (New York and London: Academic Press)

Thomas, J. A., Mawhinney, M. G. and Lloyd, J. W. (1976). Some actions of proluctin on the metabolism of ³H testosteronè in prostate glands of the rat and dog *in vitro*. In Goland, M. (ed.) *Normal and Abnormal Growth of the Prostate.* pp. 534–540. (Springfield: Charles Thomas)

Tullner, W.W. (1963). Hormonal factors in the adrenal dependent growth of the rat ventral prostate. In *Biology of the prostate and related tissue, Nat. Cancer Instit. Monogr.*, **12**, 211

Vermeulen, A. (1977). Transport and distribution of androgens at different ages. In Martini and Motta, M. (eds). *Androgens and Antiandrogens* pp. 53–65. (New York: Raven Press)

Vermeulen, A. (1979). The androgens. In Gray, C. H. and James, V. H. T. (eds.) *Hormones in Blood.* Vol. 3, pp. 355–416, 3rd Edn. (London, New York: Academic Press)

Vermeulen, A., Rubens, R. and Verdonck, L. (1972). Testosterone secretion and metabolism in male senescence. *J. Clin. Endocrinol.*, **34**, 730

Vermeulen, A. and Verdonck, L. (1976a). Radioimmunoassay of 17β-hydroxy-5α-androstan-3-one, 4-androstene-3, 17-dione dehydroepiandrosterone, 17-hydroxy-progesterone and progesterone and its application to the human male plasma. *J. Steroid Biochem.*, **7**, 1

Vermeulen, A. and Verdonck, L. (1976b). Plasma androgen levels during the menstrual cycle. *Am J. Obstet. Gynecol.*, **125**, 491

Walsh, P. C., Swerdloff, R. S. and Odell, W. D. (1973). Feedback control of FSH in the male: role of estrogen. *Acta Endocrinol.*, **74**, 449

Weinstein, R. L., Kelch, R. P., Jenner, M. R., Kaplan, S. L. and Grumbach, M. M.

(1974). Secretion of unconjugated androgens and estrogen by the normal and abnormal human testis before and after human chorionic gonadotrophin. *J. Clin. Invest.*, **53**, 1

Westphal, U. (1980). How are steroid transported in the blood before they enter target cells? In Wittliff, J. L. and Dapunt, O. (eds.) *Steroid Receptors and Hormone-dependent Neoplasia.* pp. 1–17. (New York: Masson publishing)

Wollesen, F., Swerdloff, R. S., Peterson, M. and Odell, W. D. (1974). Testosterone (T) modulation of pituitary response to LHR. Differential effects of luteinizing hormones (LH) and follicle stimulating hormone (FSH). *J. Clin. Invest.*, **53**, 85a

4

Hormonal control and rationale for endocrine therapy of prostatic tumours

R. GHANADIAN

Hormone therapy is recognized as an important form of treatment for prostatic tumours. In practice this treatment has generally been confined to the malignant tumours, although a limited number of clinical trials have also been performed in patients with benign prostatic hypertrophy. Huggins and Hodges (1941) were the first to introduce endocrine therapy for prostatic carcinoma. In principle the therapy is aimed at depleting or minimizing the action of those steroids or peptide hormones which are essential for the growth of the prostatic epithelium. It is thought that the major effect of steroids in prostatic carcinogenesis is to stimulate the development and maintenance of prostatic epithelium so that sufficient number of cells are present in which malignant changes can occur (Franks, 1973). In the case of benign hypertrophy of the prostate, a wealth of evidence in favour of the hormonal dependency of this tumour has been obtained. The tumour has been shown to grow in an androgen supplemented media (Ghanadian *et al.*, 1975) and the tumour has been induced in the dog by androgen metabolites alone or in combination with oestrogens (Walsh and Wilson, 1976; DeKlerk *et al.*, 1979).

A number of clinical studies have attempted to evaluate the efficacy of endocrine therapy in the management of prostatic cancer (see Catalona and Scott, 1978). Whilst some of these studies have concluded that endocrine therapy in any form can prolong patient survival, others have not supported this conclusion (Nesib and Baum, 1950; Barnes and Ninan, 1972; Byar, 1972; Blackard, 1975). In this chapter, the hormonal control of both benign and malignant tumours of the prostate together with the rationale for endocrine therapy is discussed. Further information on the endocrine therapy of prostatic tumours can be obtained from chapters 9, 10 and 11.

4.1 CIRCULATING HORMONES

4.1.1 Circulating hormones in patients with benign prostatic hypertrophy (BPH)

Although the assessment of circulating hormones in patients with BPH has been performed by a number of research groups for many years, it is only recently that the measurement of some of these hormones has been accurately undertaken with the view to making a valid comparison between age-matched subjects. At least two major factors are critical in these studies. Firstly, the availability of a highly sensitive and reliable method for the measurement of the hormone is essential. This makes it possible to detect any difference in the concentration of circulating hormones between patients with BPH and control subjects. Secondly, the establishment of a firm criterion of normal subjects is also essential. As the incidence of BPH in elderly men is high, the use of the term 'normal' may not be fully justified, since the evaluation of prostatic status in the 'normal' subject cannot be undertaken by histological means, but only through clinical examination, such as rectal palpation and the absence of urinary obstruction in elderly patients. Consequently the term normal has been given to those elderly men who, despite the presence or absence of some adenomatous tissues, fulfil the clinical criteria of rectal palpation and lack of urinary obstruction. It is therefore quite clear that because of the existence of some ambiguities within the 'normal' group the selection procedure, which is subjective, may result in considerable differences between one centre and another. In addition to this, the diversity of patients with benign prostatic hypertrophy in terms of the size and the type of the tumours is another important consideration in these studies.

Several research groups have measured the concentration of steroids and peptide hormones in patients with BPH. In a number of independent studies the level of testosterone in these patients has been compared with the age-matched normal controls and no significant difference has been observed (Chisholm and Ghanadian, 1976; Vermeulen and De Sy, 1976; Harper et al., 1976; Ghanadian et al., 1977a; Hammond et al., 1978; Bartsch et al., 1979). There is a wide range of variation in the level of testosterone both in BPH and age-matched controls (Table 4.1).

More attention has been focused on the level of the main 5α-reduced metabolite of testosterone, i.e. 5α-dihydrotestosterone (DHT) in patients with BPH and its comparison to control subjects. This stems from the original observation that DHT is the main androgen in this tumour (Siiteri and Wilson, 1970). Data on the concentration of circulating DHT in patients with BPH has been controversial. This is partly because of the low blood level of this steroid which requires a sensitive and reliable technique, capable of measuring this steroid with great accuracy. In a preliminary report, Mahoudeau et al. (1974) reported that the level of DHT in venous blood draining from an enlarged prostate is higher than in the peripheral blood, but the mean value for peripheral DHT in the BPH group did not differ from that of the age-matched control. Subsequently, Horton et al., (1975) found a significantly higher concentration of DHT in patients with BPH aged 60–90 years compared with a group of normal men aged 20–40 years. More substantial evidence for the elevated level of DHT in patients with BPH compared to normal subjects has been provided by Vermeulen and De Sy (1976), Ghanadian et al. (1977a), Hammond et al. (1978). Despite individual variations of this steroid, the overall results indicate a statistically significant difference between the two groups (Table 4.1). However, Bartsch et al. (1979) found no difference between the concentration of DHT in patients with BPH and normal subjects. Studies on the elevated level of DHT do not provide sufficient evidence as to the origin of the increase in patients with BPH, although it has been suggested that some contribution may be made by the enlarged prostate. In addition to the increased level of DHT in patients with BPH, the ratio of DHT to its main precursor, testosterone, has been found to change significantly in these patients. Ghanadian et al. (1977a) reported the ratio of T/DHT in patients with BPH and normal age-matched controls to be 5.50 ± 0.3 and 7.1 ± 0.3 respectively. This difference was found to be statistically significant. Similar findings have been reported by Vermeulen and De Sy (1976).

Another important androgen is 5α-androstane-3α,17β-diol, which is the major metabolite of DHT. Changes of this androgen in patients with BPH have recently been investigated in our laboratory. We have found significant increases in the level of 5α-androstane-3α,17β-diol in the circulating blood of patients with BPH, when compared with age-matched normals (Ghanadian et

Table 4.1 The comparison between the concentrations of circulating hormones in patients with benign prostatic hypertrophy (BPH) and age-matched normal subjects. Figures in brackets denote number of estimations

Hormones	Normal	BPH	Age (years)	Significance	Reference
Testosterone* (ng/100 ml)	475±28 (24)	438±27 (25)	60-80	NS**	I
	366 (15)	379 (18)	60-70	NS	II
	640 (35)	590±40 (41)	50-80	NS	III
5α-Dihydrotestosterone (ng/100 ml)	67±3 (24)	81±4 (25)	60-80	$p < 0.02$	I
	41 (36)	61 (27)	60-80	$p < 0.025$	II
	52±6 (13)	56±6 (16)	56-65	NS	IV
5α-Androstane-3α,17β-diol (ng/100 ml)	20±1 (24)	24±1 (32)	51-84	$p < 0.05$	V
	11±1 (13)	14±1 (16)	56-55	NS	IV
Androstenedione (ng/100 ml)	56±6 (32)	59±6 (27)	50-80	NS	III
	104 (41)	92 (20)	60-80	NS	II
Dehydroepiandrosterone (ng/100 ml)	157 (26)	164 (17)	60-80	NS	II
Oestradiol-17β (ng/100 ml)	4±0.1 (34)	4±0.2 (41)	50-80	NS	III
	2.1 (30)	2.5 (24)	60-80	NS	II
17α-Hydroxyprogesterone (ng/100 ml)	89 (20)	107 (14)	60-80	NS	II
Sex hormone binding globulin nmol/l	35.6±4 (13)	28 ±9 (16)	56-65	NS	IV
LH (mIU/ml)	7±1.4 (35)	11.1±1.5 (41)	50-80	NS	III
FSH (mIU/ml) (μg/l)	14±4.2 (31)	6.6±1.4 (37)	50-80	NS	III
	4.1±0.7 (13)	3.7±0.6 (16)	56-65	NS	IV
Prolactin (m amp/ml) (ng/ml)	16.4±4 (35)	9.5±1.4 (41)	50-80	NS	III
	9.8±1.6 (19)	10.4±1.3 (32)	62√/69***	NS	VI

* Conversion factor for 1 ng/100 ml to 1 nmol is as follows; Testosterone 34.67; 5α-dihydrotestosterone 34.43; 5α-androstane-3α, 17β-diol 34.19; androstenedione 34.91; oestradiol-17β 36.71; 17α-hydroxyprogesterone 30.26; dehydroepiandrosterone 34.67.

** NS = Not significant.

*** Mean age for normal $\sqrt{BPH}$

References are: I. Ghanadian et al. (1977a); II. Vermeulen and De Sy (1976); III. Harper et al. (1976); IV. Bartsch et al. (1979); V. Ghanadian et al. (1981a); VI. Jacobi et al. (1980b). For further information consult the text. References without proper age-matched control are excluded.

al., 1981b). However, Bartsch *et al.* (1979) did not find differences between the concentration of this steroid in the circulating blood of normal and BPH subjects. The increased level of 5α-androstane-3α,17β-diol in the circulating blood of patients with BPH (Ghanadian *et al.*, 1981b) corresponds to a similar increase of its precursor, i.e. 5α-dihydrotestosterone (Ghanadian *et al.*, 1977a). However, neither 5α-androstane-3α,17β-diol nor 5α-dihydrotestosterone measurement in the circulation is capable of discriminating between normal and BPH subjects. This is due to the individual variation of steroid values between the two groups. The overall difference in the steroid level between the two groups is only obtained when a large number of subjects is investigated.

Other androgens including androstenedione, androsterone and dehydro-epiandrosterone have been measured in the circulating blood of patients with BPH and compared with the age-matched normal (Vermeulen and De Sy, 1976; Harper *et al.*, 1976; Hammond *et al.*, 1978). None of these steroids have shown any significant differences between the blood concentration in the two groups. This suggests that there is no alteration in the production and metabolism of these three androgens in patients with BPH.

In addition to the above mentioned androgens, three groups have studied the circulating level of oestradiol-17β, in patients with BPH and in age-matched control subjects and have found no significant differences between the levels within these two groups (Harper *et al.*, 1976; Hammond *et al.*, 1978; Bartsch et al., 1979). The precursors of testosterone, i.e. progesterone, 17α-hydroxyprogesterone and pregnenolone have also been estimated in the circulating blood of patients with BPH. No significant differences between the levels of either progesterone or pregnenolone in the circulating blood of these two groups have been observed (Vermeulen and De Sy, 1976; Hammond *et al.*, 1978). However, the available data on the circulating 17α-hydroxy-progesterone is controversial. Whilst Hammond *et al.* (1978) have detected a significantly higher level of this steroid in patients with BPH, Vermeulen and De Sy (1976) found no difference in the two groups.

Based on these observations and, in particular, reports on the precursors of testosterone in patients with BPH, it appears that the significant changes which have been detected in the concentration of androgens in the circulating blood are those related to the 5α-reductase and 3α-hydroxysteroid oxidore-ductase in these patients. The activities of these enzymes in the prostate are well established (see chapter 6). However, evidence for the differential activities of these enzymes in non-prostatic sites in patients with BPH are required, if a conclusion is to be drawn on the true origin of the elevated DHT and 5α-androstane-3α,17β-diol in these patients.

Information concerning the concentration of binding proteins and, in particular, sex hormone binding globulin (SHBG) in patients with BPH is limited. Bartsch *et al.* (1977) have compared the binding capacity of SHBG in the circulating blood of patients with BPH and age-matched controls and found no difference between the two groups.

The concentrations of the gonadotrophic hormones, LH and FSH, have also been estimated in patients with BPH (Harper *et al.*, 1976; Hammond *et al.*, 1978; Bartsch *et al.*, 1979). When comparing the levels of gonadotrophins in circulating blood between BPH and age-matched normals, no significant differences were observed for FSH by all these investigators (Table 4.1). However, Hammond *et al.* (1978) found a significant reduction in the level of LH in patients with BPH when compared to normal subjects, which corresponds to the increased level of DHT and 5α-androstane-3α,17β-diol and suggests a negative feedback of testosterone metabolites on pituitary LH secretion. However, whether the increased level in testosterone metabolites originates from the enlarged prostate and is thus suggestive of a direct link between the prostate and pituitary requires further clarification.

When the level of circulating prolactin in patients with BPH was measured and compared with normal subjects, in most studies no significant differences were observed (Harper *et al.*, 1976; Hammond *et al.*, 1978; Bartsch *et al.*, 1979; Jacobi *et al.*, 1980b). However, some investigators have found a higher level of prolactin in patients with prostatic carcinoma (Ca) than the control subjects (Giuliani *et al.*, 1979). Farnsworth (1972) demonstrated a synergestic effect between prolactin and androgens and recently Farnsworth *et al.* (1981) have measured the incorporation of labelled testosterone into minced BPH tissues obtained from subjects with high serum prolactin (40 ± 6.7 ng/ml) and found the uptake to be more than twice that of tissues, originating from patients with low serum prolactin (6.5 ± 1.9 ng/ml). In view of these findings and the previous studies on experimental animals, a reappraisal of the significance of the role of serum prolactin in relation to endocrine therapy is essential.

4.1.2 Circulating hormones in patients with prostatic carcinoma (Ca)

Parallel studies to those described for BPH have been carried out on the circulating level of hormones in patients with Ca prostate. The levels of testosterone in these patients have been measured by a number of investigations (Robinson and Thomas, 1971; Harper *et al.*, 1976; Bartsch *et al.*, 1977; Hammond *et al.*, 1978; Ghanadian *et al.*, 1979b; Jacobi *et al.*, 1980a). Some of these workers have compared their findings with those of circulating testosterone in normal men. Robinson and Thomas (1971) found no difference between the levels of plasma testosterone in patients with Ca prostate and those of normal subjects aged from 20 to 78 years. Similarly, Harper *et al.* (1976) and Bartsch *et al.* (1977) found no difference in the level of circulating testosterone in patients with Ca prostate and age-matched controls. However, Ghanadian *et al.* (1979b) found elevated levels of testosterone in patients with Ca prostate and statistical analysis of their results showed significant differences in the level of this androgen in these patients when compared to the normal groups (Table 4.2).

It is interesting to consider these changes in relation to other findings related to androgen metabolism within the prostate (Chapter 6). Whilst the metabolic pathway of androgens in BPH tissues is predominantly a reductive one, leading to 5α-dihydrotestosterone and androstanediols formation, in the malignant prostate an oxidative pathway is operative. The interconversion of testosterone and androstenedione in the malignant tissue could lead to a higher concentration of testosterone in this tissue. The increased level of testosterone in the circulating blood of patients with Ca prostate may originate

Table 4.2 The comparison between the concentrations of circulating hormones in patients with prostatic carcinoma (Ca) and age-matched normal subjects. Figures in brackets denote number of estimations

Hormones	Normal	Ca	Age (years)	Significance	References
Testosterone (ng/100 ml)	607±235 (13)	603±347 (13)	>50	NS***	I*
	640±50 (35)	545±46 (33)	55–83	NS	II
	521 (29)	473 (34)	50–85	NS	III
	483±22 (42)	604±53 (33)	50–85	$p < 0.01$	IV
	361±145 (19)	438±174 (41)	67√69**	NS	V
5α-Dihydrotestosterone (ng/100 ml)	466 (29)	37.7 (33)	50–85	NS	III
	70.6±2.6 (42)	59.8±2.6 (33)	50–85	NS	IV
	36±7 (19)	42 ±14 (41)	67√69**	NS	V
5α-Androstane-3α,17β-diol (ng/100 ml)	29.5±9.3 (19)	15.1±5.3 (41)	67√69**	$p < 0.0001$	V
	20±0.8 (24)	15.3±1.0 (32)	50–85	$p < 0.005$	VI
Androstenedione (ng/100 ml)	56±6 (32)	70±11 (23)	50–85	NS	II
Oestradiol-17β (ng/100 ml)	4±0.1 (34)	3.9 ±0.2 (30)	50–85	NS	II
	2.4 (29)	1.9 (32)	50–85	NS	III
Sex hormone binding globulin (nmol/l)	3.6 (29)	4 (32)	50–85	NS	III
	≃2.6 (19)	≃4 (64)	67√69**	$p < 0.01$	V
LH (mIU/ml)	7±1.4 (35)	8.2±1.6 (33)	50–85	NS	II
FSH (mIU/ml)	14±4.2 (31)	6.9±2.5 (31)	50–85	NS	II
Prolactin (m amp/ml)	16.4±4 (35)	19±3.5 (32)	50–85	NS	II
ng/ml	7 (29)	7 (34)	50–85	NS	III
ng/ml	9.8±1.6 (19)	9.9±0.5 (73)	62√67**	NS	VII

I. Robinson and Thomas (1971)* This reference gives a value of 364±135 ng/100 ml for nine patients with metastasis; II. Harper *et al.* (1976); III. Bartsch *et al.* (1977); IV. Ghanadian *et al.* (1979b); V. Jacobi *et al.* (1980a); VI. Ghanadian *et al.* (1981b); VII. Jacobi *et al.* (1980a).

** Mean age for normal √ Ca

***NS = Not significant

from some prostatic contribution of testosterone to the general circulation. However, this suggestion requires further experimental support.

The concentration of DHT has also been measured in patients with Ca prostate (Table 4.2) (Bartsch et al., 1977; Hammond, 1978; Ghanadian et al., 1979b; Jacobi et al., 1980a). No significant difference in the level of DHT in patients with Ca prostate with that of age-matched controls has been found. However, Jacobi et al., (1980a) have reported that total androgens in patients with Ca prostate is significantly higher than that of the control group. Ghanadian et al. (1979b) have studied the ratio of testosterone to DHT in patients with Ca prostate and found that this ratio is approximately twice that of normal subjects. This striking difference in testosterone–DHT ratio could discriminate in most cases patients with Ca prostate from the normal subjects and is a better marker than either the individual testosterone or DHT measurement in these patients.

The concentration of 5α-androstane-$3\alpha,17\beta$-diol has also been measured in patients with carcinoma of the prostate (Jacobi et al., 1980a; Ghanadian et al., 1981b). Both studies have demonstrated a significant reduction in the level of circulating 5α-androstane-$3\alpha,17\beta$-diol in patients with Ca prostate compared to age-matched controls (Table 4.2). Although this finding is in keeping with the previous suggestion that in patients with Ca prostate the reductive pathway is reduced and the predominant pathway is an oxidative one, the circulating DHT in Ca patients did not appear to be altered. Thus the tissue concentration is not always reflected in the circulating hormone levels. Further studies are required in order to clarify the cause of the reduced circulating 5α-androstane-$3\alpha,17\beta$-diol in patients with Ca prostate.

Apart from testosterone and its 5α-reduced metabolites, the concentrations of androstenedione and androsterone have been measured in patients with Ca prostate and compared with age-matched controls (Harper et al., 1976; Hammond et al., 1978). These studies indicate that there is no significant difference in the levels of these two steroids in the two groups of subjects.

In addition to androgens the precursors of these steroids including progesterone, 17α-hydroxy progesterone and pregnenolone have been estimated in patients with Ca prostate, and have been found to have similar levels to those in age-matched controls (Hammond et al., 1978).

The concentrations of oestradiol-17β and oestrone in the circulating blood of patients with Ca prostate have been measured and the values compared with those of age-matched controls (Harper et al., 1976; Bartsch et al., 1977; Hammond et al., 1978). No significant differences have been found in the levels of either of these two oestrogens between the two groups of subjects. Data reported by these investigators for oestrogens in patients with Ca prostate clearly indicate that in this disease, as in BPH, oestrogens are of no value in distinguishing patients with these two types of tumours from normal subjects.

The concentration of sex binding proteins (SHBG) in circulating blood of patients with Ca prostate has also been compared with that of the age-matched normals (Bartsch et al., 1977; Jacobi et al., 1980a). Whilst the latter authors have found elevated levels of SHBG binding capacity in patients with Ca prostate compared to normal subjects, the former authors found no difference in the binding capacity of this protein in these two groups. An increased level of

SHBG would suggest that the free forms of steroids such as testosterone, DHT and oestradiol which exhibit a high affinity for this binding protein would be significantly reduced, this being important since the free steroids are suggested to be the biologically active fraction (Anderson, 1974).

Changes of the gonadotrophins, LH and FSH, in patients with Ca prostate have also been investigated and compared with age-matched normals (Harper *et al.*, 1976; Hammond *et al.*, 1977). Whilst Hammond *et al.* (1977) have demonstrated a reduction in the level of LH in patients with Ca prostate compared to normal subjects, Harper *et al.* (1976) found no difference in the level of this gonadotrophin in these two groups. However, neither team of investigators found any significant difference in the level of FSH between the two groups. The fall of LH reported by Hammond *et al.* (1977) corresponds to the increased circulating level of testosterone in patients with Ca prostate (Ghanadian *et al.*, 1979b) and are related to each other by a negative feedback mechanism at the pituitary.

There is no unanimity on the concentration of circulating prolactin in patients with Ca prostate and age-matched controls. Whilst Harper *et al.* (1976), Bartsch *et al.* (1977), Hammond *et al.* (1977), Jacobi *et al.* (1980b) have found no difference in the circulating level of this hormone in the two groups, Giuliani *et al.* (1979) have reported that both the serum prolactin as well as prolactin reserve, elicited by TRH stimulation in patients with Ca prostate, is significantly higher than in the age-matched control group. Despite the controversy in the circulating level of prolactin in the two groups of subjects and the subsequent utilization of this hormone for discriminating patients with Ca prostate from the normal subjects, this hormone appears to play an important role in patients with Ca prostate.

The available data on circulating steroids and peptide hormones in patients with Ca prostate and age-matched control subjects, suggest that, in general, measurements of these hormones have only a limited potential as tumour markers. The measurement of testosterone and DHT when expressed as a ratio of the two steroids could offer some diagnostic value in discriminating the malignant from the normal (Ghanadian *et al.*, 1979b). However, this parameter is also subject to certain variations and could not be considered as an absolute discriminant.

4.1.3 Comparison between circulating hormones in patients with BPH and Ca

The belief that both benign hypertrophy and malignant prostates are in some way related and to a certain extent under a hormonal influence has prompted the question, whether or not the hormonal profiles in patients with these tumours differ significantly and can thereby be utilized as a discriminant. In the previous section changes of certain circulating hormones were found to be associated with patients with malignant prostates, when compared with the normal subjects of the same group. With the exception of the ratio of testosterone to DHT there is little value in the measurement of circulating hormones in order to distinguish the normal subject from the patient with Ca prostate. A similar situation exists for the comparative study between age-matched normal subjects and patients with BPH. However, it is valuable to investigate the possibility of differences between the hormonal status of the two tumour groups in order that they may be differentiated at an early stage and so assist rapid clinical management which is of particular importance when considering the malignant gland.

There have been a number of reports concerning comparative studies of circulating hormones in patients with Ca or BPH. There is no single hormone measurement which has been shown to discriminate between the two types of tumours. Despite the higher concentration of 5α-androstane-$3\alpha,17\beta$-diol (Ghanadian et al., 1981b) and the lower concentration of prolactin (Harper et al., 1976) in patients with BPH compared to those of patients with Ca, neither of these two hormones can be utilized to differentiate between the two types of patients. Regarding prolactin, however, two other groups of workers (Hammond et al., 1977 and Jacobi et al., 1980b) have reported that there is no difference in the circulating level of this hormone in the two types of disease. Other circulating hormones including testosterone, DHT, androsterone and androstenedione, pregnenolone, progesterone, 17α-hydroxyprogesterone, oestradiol, LH and FSH have been measured and compared in patients with Ca and BPH by a number of research laboratories (Harper et al., 1976; Hammond et al., 1977; Jacobi et al., 1980a).

In addition to the comparison of circulating hormones in the two types of diseased prostate, the concentration of several hormones in circulating blood of patients during different stages of the malignancy has been measured by the British Prostate Group (1979). In this study, testosterone, oestradiol, LH, FSH, prolactin and growth hormone were measured in groups of patients with prostatic carcinoma at stages T_0, T_1, T_2, T_3, and T_4. No systematic change in the group means of any of these hormones was associated with the progression of the disease from the T_0 to the T_4 stage. The growth hormone (GH) measurement was shown to be able to distinguish the combined intraprostatic $(T_0 + T_1 + T_2)$ from the combined extraprostatic $(T_3 + T_4)$ tumour category in patients without clinically evident metastases. This study also showed that the mean growth hormone values were significantly higher in patients with metastases than those without. Furthermore, the mean for testosterone was significantly higher in patients without metastases compared to those with metastases. This multicentre investigation which involved 197 patients has suggested that the clinical stage of patients with Ca prostate may, in some cases, be accompanied by differences in their endocrine status. However, apart from growth hormone and to some extent testosterone, none of the hormones measured appears to be of any value in discriminating the various stages of the tumour.

4.2. THE EFFECT OF ENDOCRINE TREATMENT ON CIRCULATING HORMONES IN Ca PATIENTS

Since the pioneering work of Huggins et al. (1941), on the treatment of carcinoma of the prostate, using the synthetic oestrogen, diethylstilboestrol, a number of research groups have attempted to evaluate the hormonal changes in these patients following treatment. In addition to oestrogen therapy of patients with carcinoma of the prostate a number of other endocrine therapies have been used for the treatment of these patients. The majority of these therapeutic regimes have been aimed at suppressing androgens in these patients, either at their source of production such as the testes, the adrenal, or peripheral conversion, as well as their regulatory centres in the pituitary and the hypothalamus or within the prostate.

4.2.1 Suppression of testicular androgens

As the testes are the main source of androgen production in man, most therapeutic regimes have been aimed at reducing the levels of testicular androgens preferably to that obtained in the castrated male. The most widely used drug for this purpose has been diethylstilboestrol (DES). A number of investigators have monitored changes of testosterone and some of its metabolites following the treatment of patients with DES, and in most studies circulating testosterone has been shown to decline significantly (Shearer *et al.*, 1973; Harper *et al.*, 1976; Ghanadian *et al.*, 1979a). The use of 3 mg of DES per day can reduce the level of testosterone to approximately that of the castrate male (Table 4.3). The mean percentage for suppression of serum testosterone in 48 patients receiving 3 mg DES per day was 96.8 % and the corresponding value in 11 orchiectomized patients was 98.2 % (Ghanadian *et al.*, 1979a). Basically, similar results have been reported by Robinson and Thomas (1971), Shearer *et al.* (1973) and Harper *et al.* (1976). Other androgens including 5α-dihydrotestosterone (Ghanadian *et al.*, 1979a) and androstenedione (Harper *et al.*, 1976) have also been measured following treatment with DES. Whilst DHT was reduced by 85 % the level of androstenedione remained unchanged. The latter androgen is mainly of adrenal origin and therefore implies that the main effect of DES is on the

Table 4.3 The effects of endocrine therapy on serum testosterone and 5α-dihydrotestosterone in patients with carcinoma of the prostate. Values are Mean ± SEM. Figures in brackets denote number of patients

Treatment	Testosterone (ng/100 ml)	% Suppression Mean	Dihydrotestosterone (ng/100 ml) Mean ± SEM	% Suppression Mean
Untreated	645 ± 43 (33)	—	60 ± 6 (33)	—
Deep X-ray	460 ± 75 (8)	23.8	50 ± 9 (8)	16.0
Cyproterone acetate	137 ± 27 (20)	77.3**	17 ± 6 (20)	72.3**
Diethylstilboestrol	19 ± 3.5 (48)	96.8**†	9 ± 3 (48)	84.9**
Primary estracyt	28 ± 9 (7)	95.4**	17 ± 4 (7)	70.9*
Primary orchidectomy	11 ± 6 (11)	98.2**†	3 ± 2 (11)	95.1**
Secondary orchidectomy	10 ± 5 (19)	98.3**†	9 ± 3 (19)	84.9**

Patients received the following treatments: cyproterone acetate, 100 mg b.d.; diethylstilboestrol, 1 mg t.d.s.; estracyt, 280 mg t.d.s.
Statistical significance: compared to deep X-ray *$p < 0.01$, **$p < 0.001$; compared to cyproterone acetate †$p < 0.001$.
Data from Ghanadian *et al.* (1979a)

production of testicular androgens. Both LH and FSH have also been reported to be reduced significantly following treatment with DES (Harper *et al.*, 1976). In addition to these effects a direct effect of oestrogenic compounds on testosterone formation by the human testis has also been reported by Yamihara and Troen (1972) and Dorner *et al.* (1975). The net effect of DES on testosterone production and secretion resembles that of castration. Thus DES treatment can be considered a form of chemical castration.

A number of other oestrogenic compounds, including diethylstilboestrol diphosphate (Honvan), chlortrianisene (TACE), ethinyloestradiol, poly-oestradiol phosphate (Estradurin), estramustine phosphate (Estracyt), have been used in the treatment of Ca prostate and have been found to suppress circulating testosterone. However, the effectiveness of these compounds varies considerably. Shearer *et al.* (1973) reported that TACE has no measurable effect on plasma testosterone, whereas, Honvan, Premarin and ethyloestradiol are equally as effective as DES in suppressing plasma testosterone. Similarly Estracyt has proved to be as effective as DES in suppressing circulating testosterone (Ghanadian *et al.*, 1979a). Other effects of some of the oestrogens include the inhibition of enzymes such as 5α-reductase (Shimazaki *et al.*, 1965; Farnsworth 1969; Jenkins and McCaffery, 1974). However, diethylstilboestrol has shown to be ineffective in suppressing binding of androgen to the specific receptor proteins in the rat ventral prostate (Ghanadian *et al.*, 1977b; Smith *et al.*, 1978), although in the castrated dog DES has been reported to decrease prostatic secretion (Huggins and Clark, 1940).

Other synthetic compounds which have been widely utilized for suppressing circulating androgens are the antiandrogens. The most commonly used compound of this type is cyproterone acetate ($1,2\alpha$-methylene-6-chloro-17α-acetoxypregna-4,6-diene-3,20-dione) which has been shown to suppress circulating androgen but to a significantly smaller extent than that of either DES or Estracyt (Ghanadian *et al.*, 1979a). This inhibitory effect of cyproterone acetate on circulating androgens has been shown to be through inhibition of LH release. However, this compound also exerts an inhibitory effect at the cellular level.

Megestrol acetate is another progestational antiandrogenic compound which has been shown to be an effective drug for the initial therapy of stage D prostatic cancer (Johnson *et al.*, 1975; Geller *et al.*, 1978b). The mode of action of this compound is thought to be twofold: firstly, a suppression of circulating testosterone through the inhibition of gonadotrophin release and, secondly, blocking of the intracellular effects of androgens including the binding of DHT to its cytoplasmic receptor protein as well as the inhibition of 5α-reductase (Geller *et al.*, 1976a). However, this compound does not provide a sustained inhibition of plasma testosterone and it has therefore been suggested that a combination of small doses of DES with this drug could result in a more effective medical castration (Geller *et al.*, 1981).

Another important endocrine manipulation in patients with Ca prostate is bilateral orchidectomy. The testes are the major source of testosterone as well as several other androgens in man (see chapter 3). In a number of studies, the level of testosterone has been measured following orchidectomy (Bartsch *et al.*, 1977; Bracci *et al.*, 1977; Ghanadian *et al.*, 1979a; Leinonen *et al.*, 1979). All these studies have shown that orchidectomy is the most effective means by which the level of testosterone may be reduced. Ghanadian *et al.* (1979a) and Leinonen *et al.* (1979) have demonstrated that orchidectomy also suppresses DHT effectively. It has been shown that plasma testosterone decreases significantly after orchidectomy and remains reasonably low for up to 5 years (Bracci *et al.*, 1977). However, the urinary excretion of total 17 ketosteroids, which include those androgens of testicular origin, substantially decreases following orchidectomy, but eventually exceeds the precastrate levels in nine out of ten Ca patients (Scott and Vermeulen, 1942). This suggests enhanced adrenal production of steroids after orchidectomy. Indeed, Bracci *et al.* (1977) have reported a progressive increase in cortisol levels up to 5 years following orchidectomy, which emphasizes the importance of measuring adrenal steroids following endocrine manipulation in patients with Ca prostate.

4.2.2 Suppression of adrenal and pituitary

The rationale behind adrenalectomy is to remove another main source of androgens. Several adrenal steroids including dehydroepiandrosterone and androstenedione can influence prostatic growth, although the potency of these steroids is much less than that of testosterone. Additionally androstenedione can be converted to testosterone and therefore the elimination of these androgens is considered to be beneficial for some patients with Ca prostate. Reynoso and Murphy (1972) have demonstrated an increase in circulating LH and FSH following adrenalectomy and have suggested that this form of surgery decreases the feedback suppression of gonadotrophins. The lack of suppressive effect of adrenalectomy on the measured testosterone level has been attributed to inaccurate assessment of this androgen at low concentrations. In another study, Bhanalaph *et al.* (1974) also found no difference in circulating testosterone levels before and after bilateral adrenalectomy. Renswick and Grayhack (1975) reported that, despite some improvement in a number of patients who have undergone adrenalectomy, the mean survival rate did not exceed 8 months after the operation.

The removal of the pituitary has been shown to be effective as an endocrine therapy in Ca patients. In this case, hypophysectomy produces both testicular and adrenal inhibition by removing the source of gonadotrophins and adrenocorticotrophin. Robinson and Thomas (1971) and Shearer *et al.* (1973) have found that, following hypophysectomy, circulating testosterone has significantly declined to that of the castrate. However, it has been reported that the total removal of the anterior pituitary is difficult to accomplish, thus a return of androgen production is to be expected if removal is inadequate (Holland and Grayhack, 1976). Hendry (1974) and Fitzpatrick *et al.* (1980) have emphasized the importance of hypophysectomy in the management of prostatic cancer. The latter authors have treated 55 patients with diffuse pain due to bone metastases from prostatic carcinoma by pituitary ablation (53 with intrasellar yttrium 90, and 2 with intrapituitary alcohol instillation). These authors have concluded that ablation of the pituitary with radioactive yttrium has an important place in the treatment of advanced carcinoma of the prostate, as it is a relatively simple and short surgical procedure which produced significant relief of pain in 80 % of patients in their series. In addition to the suppressive effects of hypophysectomy on circulating androgens, this operation eliminates the source of growth hormone and prolactin. The latter has been shown to influence prostatic growth in experimental animals and man. Farnsworth *et al.* (1981) have demonstrated the synergistic effects of prolactin on the uptake and metabolism of androgens. These authors have concluded that the best management of prostatic cancer should include depletion of prolactin as well as androgens. Prolactin can be suppressed by chemical means using bromocriptine; CB 154 (Coune and Smith, 1975).

4.2.3 Suppression of androgens within the prostate

In addition to the suppression of androgens and other circulating hormones responsible for the growth of the prostate, by surgical and chemical means, the effects of hormones may be significantly reduced by using drugs capable of interfering at the cellular level. An example of this is the use of antiandrogens capable of blocking the effects of testosterone and its active metabolite, DHT, in the prostate by interfering with the binding of androgens to their receptors. Despite the available data on the effect of antiandrogens on the circulating levels of androgens, information about the effect of these drugs on the human prostate is limited. The inhibitory effects of a number of these compounds, such as cyproterone acetate, chlormadinone acetate and flutamide, have been studied on the prostate of experimental animals (Ghanadian *et al.*, 1977b; Smith *et al.*, 1978). The mechanism of action of steroids and the inhibitory effects of the drugs at the cellular level is discussed in chapters 7, 8 and 9.

4.3 SUPPRESSIVE EFFECTS OF SURGERY ON CIRCULATING HORMONES

It has been demonstrated that surgical stress may influence circulating steroids and peptide hormones. Serum prolactin, growth hormones, (Noel *et al.*, 1972), testosterone and LH (Aono *et al.*, 1972) have been reported to change significantly during surgery. In a study involving 28 BPH patients undergoing retropubic prostatectomy, the suppressive effects of surgical stress on circulating androgens during and after prostatectomy was investigated by Ghanadian *et al.* (1981c). After operation the concentration of both testosterone and 5α-dihydrotestosterone declined and reached minimal levels 2 days after surgery. One month postoperatively testosterone had recovered to its preoperative value, whilst the recovery of DHT to its preoperative level required a minimum period of 2 months. This study indicated that any interpretation of hormone levels following surgery requires careful attention.

4.4 CONCENTRATIONS OF ENDOGENOUS STEROIDS IN PROSTATIC TUMOURS

4.4.1 Endogenous steroids in benign hypertrophied prostate

Although circulating androgens provide useful information on the function of endocrine organs and could be used in some cases for assessing patients with prostatic disease, this information does not reflect the hormonal status of the prostate gland. The measurement of hormones within the gland could provide a more accurate account of the hormonal environment of the prostate. Several research groups have measured the content of endogenous steroids in BPH tissues. The first report on the concentration of testosterone DHT and androstenedione came from Siiteri and Wilson (1970). In this original work, they found that the concentration of DHT in this tissue is significantly higher than either testosterone or androstenedione. Furthermore, these authors reported that DHT content in BPH tissues is significantly higher than that in the normal gland. This important observation led a number of other research workers to study the differential hormonal status of benign hypertrophied and normal prostates. Geller *et al.* (1976b) confirmed the original observation by Siiteri and Wilson that the tissue content of DHT is higher in BPH when compared with normal tissues. Additionally, these authors measured 5α-androstane-3α,17β-diol which is an important metabolite of DHT. In contrast to DHT, this steroid was found to be significantly lower in BPH than normal tissues. Apart from these three important androgens, a number of other steroids have been measured in the prostate. Hammond (1978) has also measured 5α-androstane-3α, 17-dione, androsterone, progesterone and 17α-hydroxyprogesterone. Values for the concentrations of several steroids in BPH tissue are shown in Table 4.4.

In addition to androgens and progestogens, the concentration of oestradiol-17β, the main oestrogen in man, has been evaluated by Ghanadian and Puah (1981b). These authors have studied the association between oestradiol-17β, and stromal and epithelial cells of BPH tissues and found that this oestrogen is mainly associated with the stromal elements (Puah and Ghanadian, 1981). Other investigators including Habib *et al.* (1976), Krieg *et al.* (1979) and Bruchovsky *et al.* (1980) have measured testosterone, DHT and androstanediol and have basically confirmed the findings of the earlier research groups. There are two aspects of these findings to be considered. Firstly, when the plasma concentration of steroids is expressed in terms of molarity and has been compared with the tissue concentration which is expressed in terms mmol or pmol per wet weight, testosterone has been found to be higher in the plasma, whilst the concentration of DHT, 5α-androstane-3α, 17β-diol and oestradiol are higher in BPH tissues (Figure 4.1). Secondly, negative correlations have been observed between the levels of oestradiol and DHT as well as oestradiol and 5α-androstane-3α,17α-diol.

4.4.2 Endogenous steroids in malignant prostate

The initial encouraging findings of the steroid contents in BPH tissues has also been extended to malignant tissues. The purposes of these measurements have

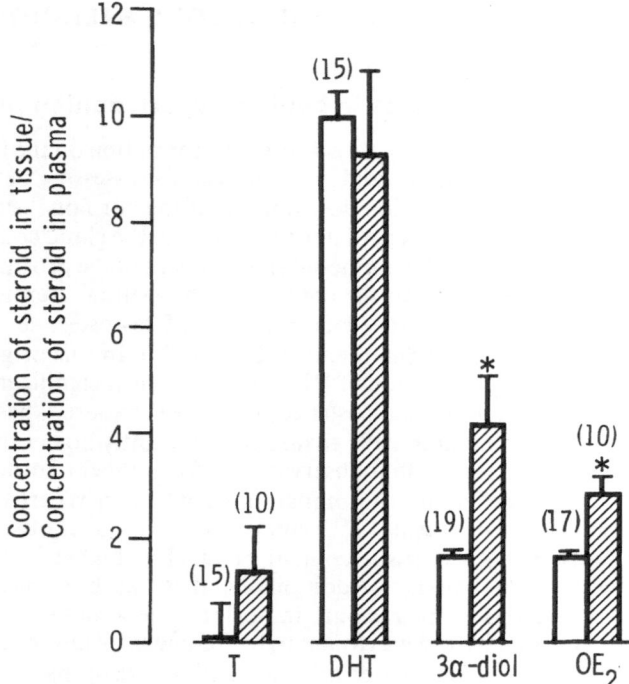

Figure 4.1 Ratio of concentration of steroids in prostatic tissues (nmol/kg) to concentration of steroids in plasma (nmol/l) for patients with benign prostatic hypertrophy (open bars) and carcinoma of the prostate (hatched bars). Height represents mean values and vertical bars represent 1 SEM.
* significant ($p < 0.001$) difference between means of groups of patients (t-test). T, testosterone; DHT, 5α-dihydrotestosterone; 3α-diol, 5α-androstane-3α, 17β-diol; OE₂, oestradiol-17β

been to study differences between the steroid profiles of the benign and malignant prostates and to investigate if this could be used as a criterion to predict the response of the tumour to hormonal manipulation. In a number of studies the concentration of testosterone, DHT, 5α-androstane-3α,17β-diol, androstanedione, oestradiol-17β, and progesterone has been measured in malignant tissues with different histological grading in most cases. However, a limited number of tissues have been investigated. Despite these shortcomings it is possible to compare the hormonal profile of malignant tumours with that of benign tissues and highlight certain differences (Table 4.4).

In general the concentration of testosterone and androstenedione is higher in cancer tissues, whereas DHT is significantly lower (Habib et al., 1976; Geller et al., 1978a; Krieg et al., 1979; Ghanadian and Puah, 1981b; Puah and Ghanadian, unpublished). Also, concentrations of 5α-androstane-3α,17β-diol and oestradiol are significantly higher in malignant prostate compared to BPH (Ghanadian and Puah, 1981b). With the exception of 5α-androstane-

Table 4.4 Concentrations of endogeneous steroids in prostatic tissues obtained from patients with benign prostatic hypertrophy (BPH) and carcinoma of the prostate (Ca). Figures in brackets denote number of estimations

	BPH	Ca	Age (years)	Significance (value for p)	References
Testosterone (ng/g tissue)	0.9 ± 0.2 (10)	—	64–94	—	Siiteri & Wilson (1970)
	0.4 ± 0.02 (24)	2.1 ± 0.3 (14)	41–89	< 0.001	Ghanadian & Puah (1981).
	0.3 ± 0.1 (11)	1.2 ± 0.8 (7)	—	< 0.002	(Krieg et al. 1979)
5α-Dihydrotestosterone (ng/g tissue)	6.0 ± 1.0 (10)	—	64–94	—	Siiteri & Wilson (1970)
	5.0 (17)	3.2 (17)	—	< 0.01	Geller et al. (1978a)
	7.5 ± 0.3 (24)	3.6 ± 0.5 (14)	41–89	< 0.001	Ghanadian & Puah (1981b)
(pmol/mg DNA)	9.3 ± 1.2 (8)	8.5 ± 1.5 (6)	53–90	NS	Bruchovsky et al. (1980).
5α-Androstane-3α,17β-diol (ng/g tissue)	0.6 ± 0.7 (14)	1.6 ± 0.6 (7)	—	< 0.05	Krieg et al. (1979)
	0.4 ± 0.03 (24)	0.6 ± 0.09 (12)	41–89	< 0.05	Ghanadian & Puah (1981b)
Androstenedione (ng/g tissue)	0.4 ± 0.3 (10)	—	64–94	—	Siiteri & Wilson (1970)
	0.7 ± 0.05 (27)	1.5 ± 0.2 (15)	48–94	< 0.001	Puah & Ghanadian (unpublished findings)
Oestradiol-17β (pg/g tissue)	62.3 ± 2.0 (22)	103.6 ± 5.3 (16)	41–89	< 0.001	Ghanadian & Puah (1980)

NS = Not significant

$3\alpha, 17\beta$-diol the findings on the tissue content of androgens are in keeping with the data obtained from the metabolism of testosterone by benign and malignant (Ghanadian *et al.*, 1981a). In these studies the percentage of recovered androstenedione is significantly higher in cancer, whilst DHT is higher in BPH. The lower level of endogenous 5α-androstane-3α, 17β-diol in BPH compared to Ca tissue (Krieg *et al.*, 1979; Ghanadian and Puah, 1981b) may be due to differences in enzyme activities between *in vitro* and *in vivo* conditions.

When the levels of circulating steroids in Ca patients were compared to the tissue content of their respective steroids, certain differences were observed. With the exception of testosterone, the concentration of DHT 5α-androstane-3α, 17β-diol and oestradiol-17β was higher in the tissue (Ghanadian and Puah, 1981b). This finding is similar to that reported for patients with BPH and clearly indicates that the endogenous tissue content of steroids in either BPH or Ca prostates is independent of circulating steroids. This is not surprising, as the prostate is able to take up steroids and in particular androgens and has the ability to metabolize and retain the active metabolites.

4.4.3 Effects of endocrine therapy on endogenous steroids in malignant prostate

It is generally accepted that a great percentage of patients with Ca prostate, especially in stages C or D, are responsive to endocrine therapy (Franks, 1974). However, no clear criteria, either to predict the response to endocrine manipulation prior to the treatment or to evaluate the hormonal changes of the tumour during treatment, have yet been established. Indeed, the measurement of circulating hormones can only monitor the hormonal changes outside the prostate gland. An appropriate approach to predict the response, and also to evaluate the effectiveness of different endocrine modalities would be to investigate the endocrine status of the tumour itself. It has been suggested that this can be achieved either by measuring the tumour concentration of active androgens or evaluating the steroid receptors and, in particular, androgen receptors in the tumour (see chapter 9). Geller *et al.* (1978a) have measured DHT content of the tissues from treated and untreated patients with carcinoma of the prostate. In this study, these authors found that in three out of four oestrogen treated patients, DHT levels were similar to untreated cancer patients. Furthermore, of six patients treated with combined castration and oestrogen or castration alone, two had a DHT concentration in the tissue similar to that of untreated patients. They concluded that either oestrogen treatment in these cases does not provide a complete suppression of testosterone metabolites or significant conversion of adrenal androgens to DHT occurs within the prostate. In a subsequent study, Geller *et al.* (1979) reported that in those patients with a tissue concentration of DHT greater than 2 ng/g tissue 11 out of 12 patients responded to treatment with DES, Megestrol acetate, or castration. They concluded that this measurement could provide a better tumour marker than histological grading. A combined measurement of androgens and Zn has also been reported to be of some value as an index for the onset of neoplasia in the prostate (Habib *et al.*, 1979). There is little or no additional data on the predictive role of tissue measurement of either DHT or any of the other steroids and the results are still far from being conclusive.

4.5 AETIOLOGICAL FACTORS INVOLVED IN THE DEVELOPMENT OF BPH

Benign prostatic hypertrophy is associated with elderly men. From a few grams at birth, the prostate undergoes androgen induced growth and reaches a weight of about 20 g by the age of 20 years and remains stable in both weight and histological appearance for another 25 years. A second growth of the gland usually commences during the 5th decade of life, which results in a mean weight about 60 g by the age of 70 (Swyer, 1944). In a study of 206 consecutive autopsies carried out on men over 40 years of age, the incidence of BPH is reported to be about 80% (Harbitz and Haugen, 1972). Although clinical evidence supporting a direct relationship between established BPH and testicular function is not conclusive (White, 1895; Deming and Wolf, 1939; Huggins and Stevens, 1940; Wendel *et al.*, 1972) most accept that the disease does not occur in men castrated during puberty and that the prostatic epithelium is under the influence of the testes. In addition, the concentration of DHT in this tumour is increased and the periurethral region of the normal gland, which is thought to be the site for the development of this tumour, has a 2–3 fold greater concentration of DHT than the outer region of the prostate (Siiteri and Wilson, 1970). Support for the hormone dependency of BPH in man has also come from experiments on the dog prostate. This animal shares with man the common phenomenon of developing prostatic hyperplasia with age. Castration is also reported to prevent the development of the disease in dog (Huggins, 1947). In earlier studies Zuckerman and Groome (1937) suggested that a combination of androgens and oestrogens might play a role in the development of prostatic hyperplasia in the dog. Walsh and Wilson (1976) were able to induce canine prostatic hyperplasia in castrated animals by the administration of 5α-androstane-$3\alpha,17\beta$-diol and the growth rate of the induced tumour was enhanced when a combination of this androgen metabolite and oestradiol-17β, was used. In a comprehensive study, DeKlerk *et al.* (1979) have carefully examined the conditions for the induction of canine prostatic hyperplasia and compared the results with spontaneous tumours of the prostate in this animal. In young dogs with intact testes prostatic hyperplasia was shown to be induced by the administration of either DHT or 5α-androstane-$3\alpha,17\beta$-diol alone or with either of these steroids in combination with oestradiol. When the animals were castrated the induction of tumours required a combination of oestradiol with either of these two testosterone metabolites. Testosterone or oestradiol alone could not induce this tumour in either the intact or castrate dog. This study has clearly demonstrated that glandular hyperplasia in the dog can be induced experimentally and that the development of the tumour requires both active androgens and oestradiol. Moore *et al.* (1974) have measured the content of androgens in canine prostatic tumours induced with 5α-androstane-3α, 17β-diol and have found a higher concentration of DHT instead of 5α-androstane-3α, 17β-diol. Similarly, in naturally occurring canine prostatic hyperplasia the tissue concentration of DHT was four times higher than in the normal gland (Lloyd et al., 1975). This would indicate that the accumulation of DHT may be causal in the development of benign hyperplasia in this animal. In a parallel study, Lloyd et al. (1975) have observed that both oestradiol and oestrone were higher in plasma and prostatic tissues of dogs with prostatic hyperplasia compared with the normal animals. The relationship between oestrogen and androgens has also been studied in the dog prostate (Moore et al., 1979). These investigators found a twofold enhancement in the cytoplasmic DHT receptors in the experimentally induced prostatic tumours following the administration of oestradiol and concluded that oestradiol regulates cytoplasmic androgen receptors in the dog prostate. Although the mechanism of this enhancement is not quite clear, there is evidence for the presence of a functional oestrogen receptor in the prostate of this animal (Dube et al., 1979). It is therefore possible that the mechanism of androgen receptor enhancement may be mediated through the oestrogen receptors. Shain and Boesel (1978) have shown that BPH tumours in dog contain significantly higher levels of androgen receptors than the normal gland.

Since the type of direct cause and effect studies which have been carried out in the dog cannot be performed in man, the elucidation of aetiological factors in man requires different experimental designs. Studies on the relationship between the endogenous steroids in human BPH tissues have revealed a negative relationship between either DHT or 5α-androstane-3α, 17β-diol and oestradiol, whereas no significant relationship could be observed between oestradiol and testosterone (Ghanadian and Puah, 1981b). This indicates that an oestrogen–androgen balance may play some role in the development of this tumour. The presence of both androgen and oestrogen receptors in human BPH is now well established (chapter 8). When the concentration of endogenous steroids or their receptors was correlated to different cell types of human BPH, as assessed by morphometric analysis, it was found that oestradiol and its receptor correlated significantly with the stroma (unpublished results). An association between oestrogen receptors and stromal elements has also been reported by Bashirelahi et al. (1980). Furthermore, we have observed significant correlations between the ratios of either 5α-androstane-3α, 17β-diol to oestradiol or androgen receptors to oestradiol receptors with the glandular elements. These studies suggest that oestradiol is somehow involved with stromal growth and thus the development of BPH. The association between oestrogens and stromal growth has been well documented in a number of experimental animals (Mawhinney and Neubauer, 1979). Moreover, in patients with BPH a significant correlation between the percentage of stroma in BPH tissues with either plasma oestradiol or total urinary oestrogen excretion but not testosterone has also been reported (Seppelt, 1978).

Based on the available data on the development of BPH in the dog and the findings in human BPH, at least two mechanisms may be envisaged for the development of this tumour in man. Firstly, it is possible that the increased level of oestradiol in elderly men (Pirke and Doerr, 1973) together with the decline in circulating androgens (Lewis *et al.*, 1976; Ghanadian and Puah, 1981b) may change the oestrogen–androgen balance. This imbalance in favour of oestrogen may induce androgen receptor which could ultimately potentiate hypertrophic growth by amplifying the androgenic stimulus. Support for this oestrogen-mediated androgen growth hypothesis comes from two lines of research. The first evidence is derived from the experiments on the dog in which oestradiol has been shown to enhance androgen receptors (Moore *et al.*, 1979). The second supportive evidence comes from our findings of a significant relationship between the total (cytoplasmic and nuclear) DHT binding sites and the total oestradiol binding sites (unpublished results).

Secondly, it is also possible that the increased oestradiol in elderly men may directly stimulate stromal elements through the oestrogen receptor. Evidence in support of this comes from the direct finding of an association between oestrogen receptors and the percentage of the stroma in human BPH (unpublished results). In addition, oestrogen is known to stimulate fibromuscular growth in a number of male accessory sexual organs (Mawhinney and Neubauer, 1979). The oestrogen enhanced stromal elements may then interact with epithelial cells, thus leading to the secondary growth of the gland. The dependence of epithelial growth on the mesenchyme (stroma) has been documented (Cunha and Lung, 1979). The common factor in both schemes is the role of oestradiol through its receptor, either in mediating androgenic action or by direct stimulation of the stroma and the subsequent interaction between stromal and epithelial elements.

4.6   AETIOLOGICAL FACTORS INVOLVED IN THE DEVELOPMENT OF MALIGNANT PROSTATE

Carcinoma of the prostate is basically associated with age and although cases of this disease have been reported in children and adolescents (Chiu and Weher, 1974) the incidence is rare before the age of 50 (Moore, 1935). A number of factors such as race and environment may be involved, e.g. low incidence of the tumour in orientals or a high incidence in environments where workers are exposed to high levels of cadmium (Kipling and Waterhouse, 1967). However, the role of hormones appears to be an important consideration in evaluating the factors influencing the development of this tumour. Earlier observations that the disease does not occur in eunuchs (Moore, 1947) and that suppression of circulating androgens could induce regression of tumour (Huggins and Hodges, 1941) have provided supportive evidence that the disease is associated with hormones and, in particular, testicular androgens. The association between the development of this tumour and BPH is not established.

Although a relationship between the incidence of the two diseases has been reported by Armenian *et al.* (1974), this has not been supported by others (Mostofi and Price, 1973; Greenwald, 1974). Studies on the hormonal environment of the malignant prostate have shown certain differences between this tumour and BPH. Steroid profiles in the tissue are significantly different to those for BPH. A higher concentration of testosterone (Habib *et al.*, 1976, Ghanadian and Puah, 1981b) and androstenedione (unpublished results) and a lower concentration of DHT (Ghanadian and Puah, 1981b) are reported for malignant tissue compared to BPH. This steroid profile is also consistent with the metabolic pathway of androgens in these two tumours (Ghanadian *et al.*, 1981a). Whilst the predominant metabolic pathway of testosterone in the cancer tissue is oxidative, that of BPH is mainly reductive. The presence of androgen (Ghanadian and Auf, 1980) and oestrogen (Bashirelahi *et al.*, 1980) receptors has also been established in this tumour, which indicates that in a large proportion of these malignant tumours a hormone-receptor mechanism is in operation and that this system may be utilized in the prediction of response to endocrine therapy (see Chapter 9). However, the link between any of the above-mentioned factors with the pathogenesis of the disease remains unclear.

4.7 CONCLUSIONS

Although endocrine therapy has long been advocated for patients with prostatic tumours, a number of important aspects of the physiological basis for this type of treatment are not understood. An important factor has been the role of circulating hormones, some with low concentration, but possessing high potency. The measurement of these hormones has revealed certain differences in patients with benign and malignant prostatic tumours when compared with age-matched normals. However, limited diagnostic value has been achieved from the measurement of hormones in individual patients, although statistically significant differences in circulating hormone profiles of a number of steroids have been obtained. The importance of hormone measurements and particularly those of testosterone, dihydrotestosterone and LH is to monitor changes which occur following hormonal manipulation. The effectiveness of the various regimes and their comparative suppression of these hormones have been reviewed. Hormone measurement within the prostate may be utilized for differentiation between benign and malignant tumours. Whilst DHT concentration is higher in BPH, testosterone is comparatively higher in Ca prostate. This differential hormonal profile can also be monitored by metabolism studies. Studies on the effects of endocrine therapy on the concentration of steroids in the prostate are limited. It has been suggested that the evaluation of clinical response may be achieved by the measurement of the tissue DHT. Hormone therapy has mainly been applied to malignant tumours whilst surgery has been the predominant approach for the treatment of benign prostatic hypertrophy. The findings on the hormonal status of patients with BPH and Ca prostates have been discussed in relation to the pathogenesis of these diseases. Several factors give prominence to the role of hormones and, in particular, androgens and oestrogens in the development of BPH and experimental evidence has supported the concept that hormones are major factors in the development of this disease. In this chapter two explanations which have certain factors in common have been presented for the development of BPH. However, these explanations cannot be readily extended to the neoplastic prostate and a more comprehensive study of the latter with particular reference to the biochemical events at the cellular level is required.

4.8 REFERENCES

Anderson, D. C. (1974). Sex hormone binding globulin. *Clin. Endocrinol.*, **3**, 69

Aono, T., Kurachi, K., Mizutani, S., Hamanaka, Y., Uozami, T., Nakasama, A., Koshiyama, K. and Matsumoto, K. (1972). Influence of major surgical stress on plasma level of testosterone luteinizing hormone and follicle stimulating hormones in male patients. *J. Clin. Endocrinol. Metab.*, **35**, 535

Armenian, H. K., Libienfeld, A. M., Diamond, E. L. and Bross, I. D. J. (1974). Relation between benign prostatic hyperplasia and cancer of the prostate: a prospective and retrospective study. *Lancet*, **2**, 115

Barnes, R. W. and Ninan, C. A. (1972). Carcinoma of the prostate: biopsy and conservative therapy. *J. Urol.*, **108**, 897

Bartsch, W., Becker, H., Pinkenburg, F. A. and Krierg, M. (1979). Hormone blood levels and their inter-relationships in normal men and men with benign prostatic hyperplasia. *Acta Endocrinol.*, **90**, 727

Bartsch, W., Horst, H. J., Becker, H. and Nehse, G. (1977). Sex hormone binding globulin binding capacity, testosterone, 5α-dihydrotestosterone, oestradiol and prolactin in plasma of patients with prostatic carcinoma under various types of hormonal treatment. *Acta Endocrinol.*, **85**, 650

Bashirelahi, N., Young, J. D., Sidh, S. M. and Sanefuji, H. (1980). Androgen, oestrogen and progestogen and their distribution in epithelial and stromal cells of human prostate. In Schroder, F. H. and deVoogt, H. J. (eds.) *Steroid Receptors, Metabolism and Prostatic Cancer.* pp. 240–256. (Amsterdam: Excerpta Medica)

Bhanalaph, T., Varkarakis, M. S. and Murphy, G. P. (1974). Current status of bilateral adrenalectomy for advanced prostatic carcinoma. *Ann. Surg.*, **179**, 17

Blackard, C. E. (1975). The Veteran Administration Co-operative Urological Research Groups studies of carcinoma of the prostate: a review. *Cancer Chemother. Rep.*, **59**, 225

Bracci, U., Di Silverio, F., Sciarra, F., Sorcini, G., Piro, C. and Santoro (1977). Hormonal pattern in prostatic carcinoma following orchidectomy: 5 year follow-up. *Br. J. Urol.*, **49**, 161

British Prostate Study Group (1979). Evaluation of plasma hormone concentrations in relation to clinical staging in patients with prostatic cancer. *Br. J. Urol.*, **51**, 382

Bruchovsky, N., Rennie, P. S. and Wilkin, R. P. (1980). New aspects of androgen action in prostatic cells: stromal localization of 5α-reductase, nuclear abundance of androstanolone and binding of receptor to linker deoxyribonucleic acid. In Schroder, F. H. and de Voogt, H. J. (eds.) *Steroid Receptors, Metabolism and Prostatic Cancer.* pp. 57–75. (Amsterdam: Excerpta Medica).

Byar, D. P. and the Veterans Administration Co-operative Urological Research Group (1972). Survival of patients with incidentally found microscopic cancer of the prostate: results of a clinical trial of conservative treatment. *J. Urol.*, **108**, 908

Catalona, W. J. and Scott, W. W. (1978). Carcinoma of the prostate: a review. *J. Urol.*, **119**, 1

Chisholm, G. D. and Ghanadian, R. (1976). Comparison between the changes in serum 5α-dihydrotestosterone and testosterone in normal men and patients with benign prostatic hypertrophy. In *5th International Congress of Endocrinology*, p. 186. (Hamburg: Bruhlsche Universitäts Druckerei)

Chiu, C. L. and Weher, D. L. (1974). Prostatic carcinoma in young adults. *J. Am. Med. Assoc.*, **230**, 724

Coune, A. and Smith, p. (1975). Clinical trial of 2-bromo-α-ergocryptine (NSC-169774) in human prostatic cancer. *Cancer Chemother. Rep.*, **59**, 209

Cunha, G. R. and Lung, B. (1979). The importance of stroma in morphogenesis and functional activity of urogenital epithelium. *In Vitro*, **15**, 50

DeKlerk, D. P., Coffey, D. S., Ewing, L. L., McDermott, I. R., Reiner, W. G., Robinson, C. H., Scott, W. W., Strandberg, J. D., Talalay, P., Walsh, P. C., Wheaton, L. G. and Zirkin, B. P. (1979). Comparison of spontaneous and experimentally induced canine prostatic hyperplasia. *J. Clin. Invest.*, **64**, 842

Deming, C. L. and Wolf, J. S. (1939). The anatomical origin of benign prostatic enlargement. *J. Urol.* **42**, 566

Dorner G., Stahl, F., Rohde, W. and Schnorr, D. (1975). An apparently direct inhibitory effect of oestrogen on the human testis. *Endokrinologie*, **66**, 221

Dube, J. Y., Lesage, R. and Tremblay, R. R. (1979). Estradiol and progesterone receptors in dog prostate cytosol. *J. Steroid Biochem.*, **10**, 459

Farnsworth, W. E. (1969). A direct effect of oestrogens on prostatic metabolism of testosterone. *J. Invest. Urol.*, **6**, 423

Farnsworth, W.E. (1972). Prolactin and the prostate. In Boyns, A. R. and Griffiths, K. (eds.) *Prolactin and Carcinogenesis*, pp. 217–228. (Cardiff: Alpha Omega Alpha Publishing)

Farnsworth, W. E., Slaunwhite, Jr., W. R., Sharma, M., Oseko, F., Brown, J. R., Gonder, M. J. and Cartagena, R. (1981). Interaction of prolactin and testosterone in the human prostate. *Urol. Res.*, **9**, 79

Fitzpatrick, J. M., Gardiner, R. A., Williams, J. P., Riddle, P. R. and O'Donoghue, E. P. N. (1980). Pituitary ablation in the relief of pain in advanced prostatic carcinoma. *Br. J. Urol.*, **52**, 301

Franks, L. M. (1973). Aetiology, epidemiology and pathology of prostatic cancer. *Cancer*, **32**, 1092

Franks, L. M. (1974). Biology of the prostate and its tumours. In Castro, J. E. (ed.). *The Treatment of Prostatic Hypertrophy and Neoplasia*. pp. 1–26. (Lancaster: MTP)

Geller, J., Albert, J., Geller, S., Lopez, D., Carter, T. and Yen, S. (1976a). Effect of megestrol acetate (Megace) on steroid metabolism and steroid–protein binding in the human prostate. *J. Clin. Endocrinol. Metab.*, **43**, 1000

Geller, J., Albert, J., Loza, D., Geller, S. and Niwayama, G. (1976b). Comparison of androgen metabolites in benign prostatic hypertrophy (BPH) and normal prostates. *J. Clin. Endocrinol. Metab.*, **43**, 686

Geller, J., Albert, J., Loza, D., Geller, S., Stoeltzing, W. and De La Vega, D. (1978a). DHT concentrations in human prostate cancer tissue. *J. Clin. Endocrinol. Metab.*, **46**, 440

Geller, J., Albert, J., Nachtsheim, D., Loza, D. and Lippman, S. (1979). Steroid levels in cancer of the prostate-markers of tumour differentiation and adequacy of anti-androgen therapy. In Murphy, G. P. and Sandberg, A. A. (eds.) *Prog. Clin. Biol. Res.*, Vol. 33, pp. 103–111. (New York: Alan R. Liss Inc.)

Geller, J., Albert, J. and Yen, S. S. C. (1978b). Treatment of advanced cancer of the prostate with megestrol acetate. *J. Urol.*, **12**, 537

Geller, J., Albert, J., Yen, S. S. C., Geller, S. and Loza, D. (1981). Medical castration with megstrol acetate and minidose of diethylstilboestrol. *J. Urol. Suppl.*, **17**, 27

Ghanadian, R. and Auf, G. (1980). Receptor proteins for androgens in benign prostatic hypertrophy and carcinoma of the prostate. In Schroder, F. H. and de Voogt, H. J. (eds.) *Steroid Receptors, Metabolism and Prostatic Cancer.* pp. 110– 125. (Amsterdam: Excerpta Medica)

Ghanadian, R., Chisholm, G. D. and Ansell, I. D. (1975). 5α-dihydrotestosterone stimulation of human prostate in organ culture. *J. Endocrinol.*, **65**, 253

Ghanadian, R., Lewis, J. G., Chisholm, G. D. and O'Donoghue, E. P. N. (1977a). Serum dihydrotestosterone in patients with benign prostatic hypertrophy. *Br. J. Urol.*, **49**, 541

Ghanadian, R., Masters, J. R. W. and Smith, C. B. (1981a). Altered androgen metabolism in carcinoma of the prostate. *Eur. Urol.*, **7**, 169

Ghanadian, R., O'Donoghue, E. P. N. and Puah, C. M. (1979a). Changes in dihydrotestosterone and testosterone following endocrine manipulation in carcinoma of the prostate. *Cancer Treat. Rep.*, **63**, 1192

Ghanadian, R. and Puah, C. M. (1981a). Age related changes of serum 5α-androstane-3α,17β-diol. *Gerontology*, **27**, 281

Ghanadian, R. and Puah, C. M. (1981b). Relationships between oestradiol-17β, testosterone, dihydrotestosterone and 5α-androstane-3α,17β-diol in human benign hypertrophy and carcinoma of the prostate. *J. Endocrinol.*, **88**, 255

Ghanadian, R., Puah, C. M. and O'Donoghue, E. P. N. (1979b). Serum testosterone and dihydrotestosterone in carcinoma of the prostate. *Br. J. Cancer*, **39**, 696

Ghanadian, R., Puah, C. M. and Williams, G. (1981b). Serum 5α-androstane-3α, 17β-diol in patients with prostatic tumours. *Br. J. Cancer*, **44**, 308

Ghanadian, R., Puah, C. M., Williams, G., Shah, P. J. R. and McWhinney, N. (1981c). Suppressive effects of surgical stress on circulating androgens during and after prostatectomy. *Br. J. Urol.*, **53**, 147

Ghanadian, R., Smith, C. B., Williams, G. and Chisholm, G. D. (1977b). The effect of anti-androgens and stilboestrol on the cytosol receptor in rat prostate. *Br. J. Urol.*, **49**, 695

Giuliani, L., Pescatore, D., Mastorana, G., Gilberti, C., Barreca, T. and Roland, E. (1979). Increased serum prolactin pituitary reserve in patients with prostatic neoplasia. *Br. J. Urol.*, **51**, 390

Greenwald, P., Kirnuis, V., Polan, A. K. and Dick, V. S. (1974). Cancer of the prostate among men with benign prostatic hyperplasia. *J. Natl. Cancer. Inst.*, **53**, 335

Habib, F. K., Lee, I. R., Stitch, S. R. and Smith, P. H. (1976). Androgen levels in the plasma and prostatic tissues of patients with benign hypertrophy and carcinoma of the prostate. *J. Endocrinol.*, **71**, 99

Habib, F. K., Mason, M. K., Smith, P. H. and Stitch, S. R. (1979). Cancer of the prostate: early diagnosis by zinc and hormone analysis? *Br. J. Cancer*, **39**, 700

Hammond, G. L., Kontturi, P., Maattala, M., Puukka, M. and Vihko, R. (1977). Serum FSH, LH and prolactin in normal males and patients with prostatic diseases. *Clin. Endocrinol.*, **7**, 129

Hammond, G. L., Kontturi, M., Vihko, P. and Vihko, R. (1978). Serum steroids in normal males and patients with prostatic diseases. *Clin. Endocrinol.*, **9**, 113

Harbitz, T. B. and Haugen, O. A. (1972). Histology of the prostate in elderly men. *Acta Pathol. Microbiol. Scand. (A)*, **80**, 756

Harper, M. E., Peeling, W. B., Cowley, T., Brownsey, B. G., Phillips, M. E. A., Groom, G., Fahmy, D. R. and Griffiths, K. (1976). Plasma steroid and protein hormone concentrations in patients with prostatic carcinoma before and during oestrogen therapy. *Acta Endocrinol.*, **81**, 409

Hendry, W. F. (1974). Adrenalectomy and hypophysectomy in disseminated prostatic cancer. In Castro, J. E. (ed.) *The Treatment of Prostatic Hypertrophy and Neoplasia.* pp. 171–192. (Lancaster: MTP Press)

Holland, J. M. and Grayhack, J. T. (1976). Basis of hormone treatment. In Williams,

D. I. and Chisholm, G. D. (eds.) *Scientific Foundations of Urology*. pp. 338–346. (London: Heinemann)

Horton, R., Hsieh, P., Barberia, J., Pages, L. and Cosgrave, M. (1975). Altered blood androgens in elderly men with prostatic hyperplasia. *J. Clin. Endocrinol. Metab.*, **41**, 793

Huggins, C. (1947). The etiology of benign prostatic hypertrophy. *Bull. NY, Acad. Med.*, **23**, 696

Huggins, C. and Clark, P. J. (1940). Quantitative studies of prostatic secretion. II. The effect of castration and of estrogen injection on the normal and on the hyperplastic prostatic glands of dogs. *J. Exp. Med.*, **72**, 747

Huggins, C. and Hodges, C. V. (1941). Studies on prostatic cancer. I. The effect of castration, of estrogen and of androgen injection on serum phosphatase in metastatic carcinoma of the prostate. *Cancer Res.*, **1**, 293

Huggins, C., Scott, W. W. and Hodges, C. V. (1941). Studies on prostatic cancer. III. The effects of fever of deoxycorticosterone and of estrogen on clinical patients with metastatic carcinoma of the prostate. *J. Urol.*, **46**, 997

Huggins, C. and Stevens, R. A. (1940). The effect of castration on benign hypertrophy of the prostate in man. *J. Urol.*, **43**, 705

Jacobi, G. H., Gupta, D., Rathgen, G. H. and Altwein, J. E. (1980a). Hormone dependance of prostatic carcinoma: serum androgens, plasma SHBG and prostatic androstanediol formation in untreated patients. In Wittliff, J. L. and Dapunt, O. (eds.) *Steroid Receptors and Hormone Dependent Neoplasia*. pp. 156–160. (New York: Masson Publishing Inc.)

Jacobi, G. H., Rathgen, G. H. and Altwein, J. E. (1980b). Serum prolactin and tumours of the prostate: unchanged basal levels of correlation to serum testosterone. *J. Endocrinol. Invest.*, **3**, 15

Jenkins, J. S. and McCaffery, V. M. (1974). Effect of oestradiol-17β and progesterone on the metabolism of testosterone by human prostatic tissue. *J. Endocrinol.*, **63**, 517

Johnson, D. E., Kaesler, K. E. and Ayala, A. G. (1975). Megestrol acetate for treatment of advanced carcinoma of the prostate. *J. Surg. Oncol.*, **7**, 9

Kipling, M. C. and Waterhouse, J. A. (1967). Cadmium and prostatic carcinoma. *Lancet*, **1**, 730

Krieg, M., Bartsch, W., Janssen, W. and Voigt, K. D. (1979). A comparative study of binding, metabolism and endogenous levels of androgens in normal, hyperplastic and carcinomatous human prostate. *J. Steroid Biochem.*, **11**, 615

Leinonen, P., Hammond, G. L., Lukkarinen, O. and Vihko, R. (1979). Serum sex hormone binding globulin and testosterone binding after estradiol administration, castration and their combination in men with prostatic carcinoma. *Invest. Urol.*, **17**, 24

Lewis, J. D., Ghanadian, R. and Chisholm, G. D. (1976). Serum 5α-dihydrotestosterone and testosterone changes with age in man. *Acta Endocrinol.*, **82**, 444

Lloyd, J. W., Thomas, J. A. and Mawhinney, M. G. (1975). Androgens and estrogens in the plasma and prostatic tissue of normal dogs and dogs with benign prostatic hypertrophy. *Invest. Urol.*, **13**, 220

Mahoudeau, J. A., Delassalle, A. and Bricaire, H. (1974). Secretion of dihydrotestosterone by human prostate in benign prostatic hypertrophy. *Acta Endocrinol.*, **77**, 401

Mawhinney, M. G. and Neubauer, B. L. (1979). Actions of estrogens in the male. *Invest. Urol.*, **16**, 409

Moore, R. A. (1935). The morphology of small prostatic carcinoma. *J. Urol.*, **33**, 224

Moore, R. A. (1947). *Endocrinology of Neoplastic Disease*. p. 194. (New York: Oxford University Press)

Moore, R. J., Gazak, J. M., Quebberman, J. F. and Wilson, J. D. (1974).

Concentration of dihydrotestosterone and 3α-androstanediol in naturally occurring and androgen-induced prostatic hyperplasia in the dog. *J. Clin. Invest.*, **64**, 1003

Moore, R. J., Gazak, J. M. and Wilson, J. D. (1979). Regulation of cytoplasmic dihydrotestosterone binding in dog prostate by 17β-estradiol. *J. Clin. Invest.*, **63**, 351

Mostofi, F. K. and Price, E. B. (1973). Tumours of the male genital system. In *Atlas on Tumour Pathology*. Series 2, p. 196. (Washington: Armed Forces Institute of Pathology)

Nesib, R. M. and Baum, W. C. (1950). Endocrine control of prostate carcinoma: clinical and statistical survey of 1818 cases. *J. Am. Med. Assoc.*, **143**, 1317

Noel, G. L., Suh, H. K., Stone, J. G. and Frantz, A. G. (1972). Human prolactin and growth hormone release during surgery and other conditions of stress. *J. Clin. Endocrinol. Metab.*, **35**, 840

Pirke, K. M. and Doerr, P. (1973). Age related changes and inter-relationship between plasma testosterone, oestradiol and testosterone-binding globulin in normal adult males. *Acta Endocrinol.*, **74**, 792

Puah, C. M. and Ghanadian, R. (1981). Correlative studies between endogenous steroids and stromal-epithelial composition in human benign hypertrophied prostate. *Br. J. Cancer*, **44**, 308

Renswick, M. I. and Grayhack, J. T. (1975). Treatment of stage IV carcinoma of the prostate. *Urol. Clin. N. Am.*, **2**, 141

Reynoso, G. and Murphy, G. P. (1972). Adrenalectomy and hypophysectomy in advanced prostatic carcinoma. *Cancer*, **29**, 941

Robinson, M. R. G. and Thomas, B. S. (1971). Effect of hormonal therapy on plasma testosterone levels in prostatic carcinoma. *Br. Med. J.*, **4**, 391

Scott, W. W. and Veumeulen, C. (1942). Studies on prostatic cancer. V. Excretion of 17-keto-steroids, estrogens and gonadotrophins before and after castration. *J. Clin. Endocrinol.*, **2**, 450

Seppelt, U. (1978). Correlation among prostate stroma, plasma estrogen levels and urinary estrogen secretion in patients with benign prostatic hypertrophy. *J. Clin. Endocrinol. Metab.*, **47**, 1230

Shain, S. A. and Boesel, R. W. (1978). Androgen receptor of the normal and hyperplastic canine prostate. *J. Clin. Invest.*, **61**, 654

Shearer, R. J., Hendry, W. F., Sommerville, I. F. and Fergusson, J. D. (1973). Plasma testosterone: an accurate monitor of hormone treatment in prostatic cancer. *Br. J. Urol.*, **45**, 668

Shimazaki, J., Kurihara, H., Ito, Y. and Shida, K. (1965). Testosterone metabolism in prostate; formation of androstan-17β-ol-3-one and androst-4-ene-3,17-dione and inhibitory effect of natural and synthetic estrogens. *Gunma, J. Med. Sci.*, **14**, 313

Siiteri, P. K. and Wilson, J. D. (1970). Dihydrotestosterone in prostatic hypertrophy. I. The formation and content of dihydrotestosterone in the hypertrophic prostate of man. *J. Clin. Invest.*, **49**, 1737

Smith, C. B., Ghanadian, R. and Chisholm, G. D. (1978). Inhibition of the nuclear dihydrotestosterone receptor complex from rat ventral prostate by anti-androgens and stilboestrol. *Mol. Cell. Endocrinol.*, **10**, 13

Swyer, G. I. M. (1944). Post-natal growth changes in the human prostate. *J. Anat.*, **78**, 130

Vermeulen, A. and De Sy, W. (1976). Androgens in patients with benign prostatic hyperplasia before and after prostatectomy. *J. Clin. Endocrinol. Metab.*, **43**, 1250

Walsh, P. C. and Wilson, J. D. (1976). The induction of prostatic hypertrophy in the dog with androstanediol. *J. Clin. Invest.*, **57**, 1093

Wendel, E. F., Brannen, G. E., Putong, P. B. and Grayhack, J. T. (1972). The effect of orchidectomy and estrogens on benign prostatic hyperplasia. *J. Urol.*, **108**, 116

White, J. W. (1895). The results of double castration in hypertrophy of the prostate. *Ann. Surg.*, **22**, 1

Yamihara, T. and Troen, P. (1972). Effect of estrogen on testosterone formation in human testis *in vitro*. *J. Clin. Endocrinol.*, **34**, 968

Zuckerman, S. and Groome, J. R. (1937). The aetiology of benign enlargement of the prostate in the dog. *J. Pathol. Bacteriol.*, **44**, 113

5

Biochemical and morphometric evaluations of prostatic epithelial and stromal cells

R. GHANADIAN AND C. M. PUAH

The current understanding of the zonal anatomy of the prostate and its possible relationship to the origin of the development of prostatic tumours has emphasized the need for a thorough investigation into the biochemical factors affecting these zones. Differences in these zones are further complicated by a diversity of cells which are present in this gland. The interaction between the two major prostatic cell types, namely the epithelium and stroma, has gained much attention and is thought to be a critical factor in the understanding of the normal and abnormal growth of this gland, but there is a paucity of information with regard to the hormonal response of each cell type. Preliminary studies from a number of laboratories do suggest differential hormonal responses associated with individual types of cell. A vivid example of these studies is the finding that the stromal growth is under oestrogenic influence. Such findings have great implications for the understanding of the aetiology of prostatic tumours and highlight the importance of the qualitative and quantitative analyses of a number of biochemical parameters associated with these cells. This field of prostate research has been seriously hampered by the lack of applicable separation techniques or methods which can be reliably utilized to assess the biochemical constituents of each cell type in intact tissues. In the past, techniques for the physical separation of these cells and morphometric analysis have been extensively utilized within other disciplines. However, their application to the study of prostatic tissues has been limited. More recently these techniques, and in particular morphometry and stereology, have attracted the attention of a number of research groups in the field of prostate research. However, these techniques have been complicated by the types of available prostatic specimens removed by different surgical procedures. This chapter is an attempt to highlight the importance of different cell types and the methodological problems associated with the study of these cells.

5.1   THE INTERACTION BETWEEN EPITHELIUM AND STROMA

As described in chapters 1 and 2, the cellular composition of prostatic tissue is not homogenous. Indeed, it is composed of at least two cell types, namely the epithelium and stroma. For many years the latter has been considered an inactive matrix and the functional activity of the gland has been attributed to the epithelium. However, this assumption has been seriously questioned by several research groups, who have clearly demonstrated the important interaction between those two matrices and have found the stromal elements playing a major role in the development of normal and abnormal growth of the prostate. Franks et al. (1970) have separated the epithelial and stromal components of human BPH tissues and found that the growth of the epithelium in culture is dependent upon the presence of stromal elements. The interaction between these two types of cells has been elegantly demonstrated by Cunha (1973) using embryonic mouse tissues, and has shown the dependence of embryonic mouse urogenital sinus epithelium upon urogenital mesenchyme (stroma) for its normal development. The importance of stroma in morphogenesis and the functional activity of the urogenital epithelium has recently been re-emphasized by the same group of investigators (Cunha and Lung, 1979). An important consideration is the role of biochemical elements and, in particular, the hormonal contents of each cell type which may influence this interaction. These factors have stimulated the development of techniques for separating and quantitating these two components of prostate tissues, in order to achieve a better understanding of these relationships. From the outset of these studies, two basic approaches have been adopted for the analysis of epithelium and stroma in the prostate, namely, the separation of the two types of cells by physical or chemical means and the morphometric analysis of the tissue.

5.1.1 Mechanical separation of epithelium and stroma

A simple method for the separation of prostatic cell types is to apply a constant pressure, but avoiding torsion, on prostatic tissues. Based on this principle several devices have been designed. Franks *et al.* (1970) were the first to introduce a screw-type press (Latapie press) for the separation of prostatic epithelial and stromal cells. Harper *et al.* (1974) separated prostatic cells based on the Latapie press. The material remaining in the press was considered to be the stromal elements, whilst the brei is a mixture of epithelial and stromal cells. This latter fraction was further subjected to filtration by using a nylon gauze in order to separate the epithelial elements. More recently a modified method was used by Romijn *et al.* (1980b). Other alternatives have been tried including the mincing of the tissue prior to mechanical separation through either cheese cloth (Katzenellenbogen and Leake, 1974) or nylon gauze (Cowan *et al.*, 1977; Sirett *et al.*, 1980; Krieg *et al.*, 1981), whilst other adaptations include the use of stainless steel wire screen with a teflon pestle (Bruchovsky *et al.*, 1980) or direct dissection of the prostatic specimen under a dissecting microscope (Bashirelahi *et al.*, 1980). With the exception of the last procedure which was reported to yield highly purified epithelial and stromal fractions, the other procedures have produced fractions with varying degrees of purity. In general, the purity of the separated stromal fraction has been higher than that of the epithelial cells irrespective of the type of mechanical devices employed. Bruchovsky *et al.* (1980) and Krieg *et al.*, (1981), have reported the purity of the epithelial fraction to vary between 50 and 100 %. In addition to the purity data, the percentage recovery of these separated fractions has also been evaluated. Cowan *et al.* (1977) have estimated the recovery of the epithelial fraction in BPH tissues to be approximately 30 %. Using these separation techniques a number of investigators have measured several biochemical parameters such as enzymes, nucleic acids, proteins, steroids and receptors in the two cell types of the prostate. A summary of this data is shown in Table 5.1. As already discussed by these authors the mechanically prepared epithelial and stromal cells may suffer from at least two major disadvantages, namely, cell damage during preparation (Franks *et al.*, 1970) and the cross-contamination of the two fractions. A close examination of Table 5.1 would reveal significant discrepancies between the reported values for some of the biochemical measurements, which could be attributed to the shortcomings of these techniques.

In these studies the activities of various enzymes have been estimated not only as biochemical constituents of the cell types but also as possible discriminant markers, to monitor the purity and recovery of the two cell types. However, a number of enzymes were found to be unsuitable for these purposes. Indeed, Cowan *et al.* (1977) have noted that both acid phosphatase

Table 5.1 Biochemical measurements in the epithelial and stromal cells of tissues obtained from benign hypertrophied, normal or malignant prostates. Separation of cell types has been achieved by mechanical means. Values are mean, mean ± SEM or expressed in range. Number of estimations are in parentheses

Measurement	Unit	Epithelia	Stroma	Reference
Benign hypertrophied prostate				
β-glucuronidase	μg phenolphthalein formed/hour	20–24(6)	0–12(9)	1
	% recovered*	14 ± 2.1(8)	18 ± 3.8(8)	2
Acid phosphatase	μmol p-nitrophenol formed/min per μg DNA	0.11(6)	0.02(6)	3
	Sigma unit; % recovered*	10 ± 1.7(11)	20 ± 4.4	2
	mU/mg protein	885(20)	162(22)	4
Hydroxyproline	cpm [³H]H₂O liberated/30 min per μg DNA	4.8(6)	10.9(6)	3
	Organon unit; % recovered*	1.0 ± 0.2(6)	95 ± 1.5	2
	pg/μg DNA	50(NA)	110(NA)	5
	μg/mg wet tissue	0.52(17)	3.0(17)	4
Arginase	Worthington Unit % recovered*	31 ± 9.0(6)	18 ± 4.2(6)	2
5α-reductase	pmol metabolites formed /mg DNA (min)⁻¹	2.4 ± 0.6(6)	27.3 ± 6.9	2
	pmol metabolites formed /mg protein ½ hourly	11.3 ± 1.9(21)	84.6 ± 13.1	6
	pmol metabolites formed /mg protein hourly	66 ± 4.6(20)	161 ± 28(20)	4
	nmol metabolites formed /mg protein hourly	0.6(NA)	2.5(NA)	7
3α (3β) hydroxysteroid dehydrogenase (reductive)	pmol metabolites formed /mg protein ½ hourly	11.7 ± 2.5(9)	20.9 ± 2.6(8)	6
(oxidative)	pmol metabolites formed /mg protein ½ hourly	4.9 ± 2.1(8)	12.7 ± 1.7(8)	6
Dehydroepiandrosterone sulphate sulphatase	pmol DHEA formed /mg protein hourly % recovered*	22 ± 5.5(9)	46 ± 7.3(9)	2
DNA	% recovered**	15 ± 2.1(12)	60 ± 3.7(12)	2

RNA	% recovered**	5.5±0.7(13)	57±3.7(13)	2
Sex hormone binding globulin	fmol/mg protein**	ND	26(NA)	3
Corticosteroid binding globulin	fmol/mg protein**	23(NA)	230(NA)	3
5α-dihydrotestosterone	pmol/mg DNA	7.1–20(4)	5.4–11.8(4)	6
	ng/mg DNA	6.2±2.6(6)	5.0±1.2(6)	8
	pg/mg protein	468±98(6)	93±15(6)	8
Androgen receptors (cytosol)	fmol/mg protein	0–115.4(23)	0–130.7(20)	9
	fmol/mg protein	19±2(NA)	25±3(NA)	4
	fmol/mg protein	30±6(5)	27±5(5)	8
Normal prostate				
5α-reductase	pmol metabolites formed /mg protein ½ hourly	9.2±3.0(3)	31.6±7.2(3)	6
	pmol metabolites formed /mg protein ½ hourly	53(2)	88(2)	4
3α(3β) hydroxysteroid dehydrogenase (reductive)	pmol metabolites formed /mg protein ½ hourly	19.7±5.5(3)	15±4.5(3)	6
(oxidative)	pmol metabolites formed /mg protein ½ hourly	7.2±2.5(3)	7.8±1.3(3)	6
5α-dihydrotestosterone	pmol/mg DNA	3–4.3(2)	4.9(2)	6
Androgen receptor (cytosol)	fmol/mg protein	7–18.6(3)	7–13(3)	9
Malignant prostate				
5α-reductase	pmol metabolites formed /mg protein ½ hourly	3.7(2)	12.4(2)	6
3α(3β) hydroxysteroid dehydrogenase (reductive)	pmol metabolites formed /mg protein ½ hourly	17.8(2)	13.2(2)	6
(oxidative)	pmol metabolites formed /mg protein ½ hourly	6.8(2)	8.4(2)	6
5α-dihydrotestosterone	pmol/mg DNA	5.1–15(2)	5.6–5.9(2)	6

* relative activity; ** relative concentration; NA not available; ND not determined

1. Nilsson et al. (1973), 2. Cowan et al. (1977), 3. Cowan et al. (1976), 4. Krieg et al. (1981), 5. Romijn et al. (1980a), 6. Bruchovsky et al. (1980), 7. Romijn et al. (1980b), 8. Sirett et al. (1980), 9. Bashirelahi et al. (1980)

and β-glucuronidase were poor markers for assessing the recovery of the intact epithelial cells. This was attributed to the dual localization of these enzymes which escaped into the washed fraction during purification. Similarly Romijn *et al.* (1980b) have found that hydroxyproline is a weak marker for stromal cells, possibly because of the extracellular presence of this enzyme. With regard to 5α-reductase, there is a general consensus that the activity of this enzyme is significantly higher in the stromal cells than that of epithelial. However, data on the product of this enzyme, i.e. 5α-dihydrotestosterone (DHT) is less clear. Bruchovsky *et al.* (1980) have measured the DHT concentration of epithelial and stromal fractions from four BPH tissues and found no significant differences in their DHT contents. A similar finding was also reported by Sirett *et al.* (1980). However, these workers found considerably higher levels of DHT in the epithelial fraction when the results were expressed in terms of protein content. The concentration of cytoplasmic androgen receptors has been estimated in the two cell types of BPH tissues (Sirett *et al.*, 1980) and an equal distribution of androgen receptor was found in both cell types.

Other biochemical data including nucleic acids, proteins and, in particular, steroid binding proteins, namely sex hormone binding globulin (SHBG) and corticosteroid binding globulin (CBG), were found to be significantly higher in the stromal fraction (Cowan *et al.*, 1976 Cowan *et al.*, 1977).

In the normal and malignant prostates, data obtained for the distribution of the biochemical constituents in the epithelial and stromal cells are less than those for BPH tissues. Whilst the activity of 5α-reductase follows the same pattern as that in BPH tissues, no apparent differences in the distribution of the activities of 3α (3β)-hydroxysteroid dehydrogenase in normal, benign and malignant prostates can be observed. However, data on normal and carcinomatous tissues are sparse and at present insufficient for a reliable comparison.

5.1.2 Non-mechanical separation of epithelium and stroma

These techniques are based on the utilization of either proteolytic enzymes or chelating agents such as Versene, to separate the desired components and have been used mainly in conjunction with tissue or organ cultures. However, they do not appear to be an attractive alternative to mechanical techniques, as these agents are known to cause damage to the cell membrane as well as producing secondary cellular changes in the cell organelles (Hilfer and Hilfer, 1966).

5.2 MORPHOMETRIC ANALYSIS

'Morphometry' which is a means of quantitatively describing structural features is becoming an acceptable approach in bridging the gap between morphological and biochemical data in biological research. A related term, but by no means synonymous is 'stereology' in which three-dimensional information on structures can be derived from two-dimensional sections of these structures. This is also becoming important in prostate research, as stereology can be applied to the study of structures independently of their size or their compositions, by providing relative values so that one can obtain more useful information about the structures of the organ under investigation. Data obtained by morphometry and stereology are interchangeable and have found wide applications in the analysis of a variety of human and experimental animal tissues. However, it is only recently that these techniques have emerged as viable alternatives in some aspects of prostate research, such as the epithelial-stromal interaction in relation to hormonal manipulation. Despite the advantages offered by morphometric techniques in the study of biological samples, these methods are not capable of measuring the absolute numbers of different cell types in the total organ (DeKlerk and Coffey, 1978). This is partly due to the differential effects of fixation, dehydration and embedding of the sections on the volume and shape of different tissue components (Bahr et al., 1957; Peutilla et al., 1975).

5.2.1 Principles of morphometric analysis

There are certain principles which govern the morphometric analysis of biological specimens. These principles have been discussed extensively by a number of investigators (Weibel, 1963; Weibel et al., 1966; Rohr et al., 1976) and can be summarized as follows:

(1) The structure which is to be quantitated must have a homogenous distribution within the tissue and must be present in sufficient numbers.

(2) Under a light or electron microscope a section of a structure with a dimension (N) appears to have the dimension (N−1).

(3) A strict random sampling of the specimen should be applied.

(4) Structures must be of similar size and shape from one part of the tissue to another.

(5) Sample preparation should be standardized. This should include fixation, buffering and embedding. A sufficiently thin section of constant thickness is most essential, in order to obtain a reliable assessment.

The above morphometric principles also apply to stereology. Indeed, stereology, which is an extension of morphometry and deals with three-dimensional analysis of structures based on two-dimensional measurements, requires similar considerations as for morphometry.

5.2.2 Application of morphometric analysis to human prostate

The simplest and most practical application of morphometric analysis is in the estimation of cell types, such as epithelium and stroma, in human prostatic tissues and in relating the distribution of these cells to biochemical data obtained on these specimens, such as the concentration of hormones or receptors. This quantitative approach avoids some of the disadvantages already discussed for mechanical separations. As described previously, a quantitative knowledge of the make-up of the tissue is most essential when the significance of the biochemical and, in particular, hormonal data is to be evaluated. This important consideration has prompted several research groups to quantify the percentages of the stroma and epithelium in prostatic tumours and to examine their relationships to the endogenous biochemical constituents. Based on the principles already outlined, we have estimated the percentages of epithelial and stromal cells of human benign hypertrophied prostate and have correlated this data with that of steroids including a number of testosterone metabolites and oestradiol-17β. The estimation of the percentages of the epithelium and the stroma was based on the volume occupied by the respective components when analysed by light microscopy. The principle behind this measurement was suggested by the French geologist, Delesse (1847) in which he stated that fractional volume v occupied by a component i was equalled to fractional area A in a random cross-section. This original method of calculation which involved planimetry of the combined area was subsequently replaced by point counting as suggested by Glagoleff (1933). The latter carried out his point counting by superimposing a regular point lattice on the section. This type of point counting was extended to biological specimens by Haug (1955) and Henning (1957). Since then this procedure has been widely used for the estimation of various components of different types of tissues. In general, the samples were processed according to the principles described for morphometric analysis and stereology and examined under a light or electron microscope in conjunction with an ocular grid (graticule). A number of different types of graticules are available commercially and the choice is dependent on the type of components within the specimen. Counting is based on the number of points which coincide with the component under investigation, and can either be carried out directly under the microscope or alternatively from micrographs of the specimen with the aid of a differential counter. The latter procedure is commonly employed with electron microscopic studies. The calculation of the percentages of various components is simply based on the number of points which coincide with the component when related to the total number of points projected by the graticule over the entire section.

Although the application of a morphometric technique to the study of human prostatic tumours follows the same principles as previously described, there are a number of considerations which have to be taken into account when analysing these tissues. The sampling procedure for these tumours is dependent upon the type of surgical techniques used for their removal. Whilst prostatic samples obtained by open prostatectomy, such as retropubic prostatectomy (RPP), are generally large and free from exposure to heat denaturation, the more commonly used transurethral resection (TUR) technique provides tissue in the form of small samples. Frequently the size of these samples is not uniform and only large ones are suitable for analysis. The burnt section of the outer region of TUR samples should be removed before applying any sampling procedure. Additionally a representative section of each sample is removed for morphometric analysis, whilst the rest of the samples are pooled for biochemical analyses. Samples removed for morphometric analysis can be kept in buffered formalin prior to histological preparation and subsequently be embedded in paraffin, cut into sections of 4 μm thickness and stained with haemotoxylin and eosin. This sampling procedure is generally suitable for those specimens in which the number of prostatic chips are limited to 10–15. In cases where a large prostate tumour has been removed by TUR procedure, a modified sampling technique should be applied. This would entail pooling all the cleaned operative material and systematically selecting representative samples from imaginary quadrants. This procedure is basically similar to the simple random sampling as described by Weibel (1969). This sampling technique for TUR samples could be improved if representative tissues from each area of the enlarged gland could be provided. However, such a differential sampling technique may not always be practical for the surgeon. Only samples obtained by open prostatectomy could be subjected to such a systematic random sampling (Weibel, 1969). If on the other hand, the operation specimen is relatively small and in the region of 1–5 g then a simple rather than systematic random sampling could only be applied.

In our studies using human BPH samples, the prepared sections were examined under a light microscopic field (× 63) with an aid of a superimposed graticule (100 sq). The entire section of each representative sample was counted and the results obtained were expressed as percentages of stromal, epithelial, acinar and glandular (sum of epithelial and acinar) elements. An example of a histologically prepared section of BPH tissue under light microscopy with a superimposed graticule is shown in Figure 5.1.

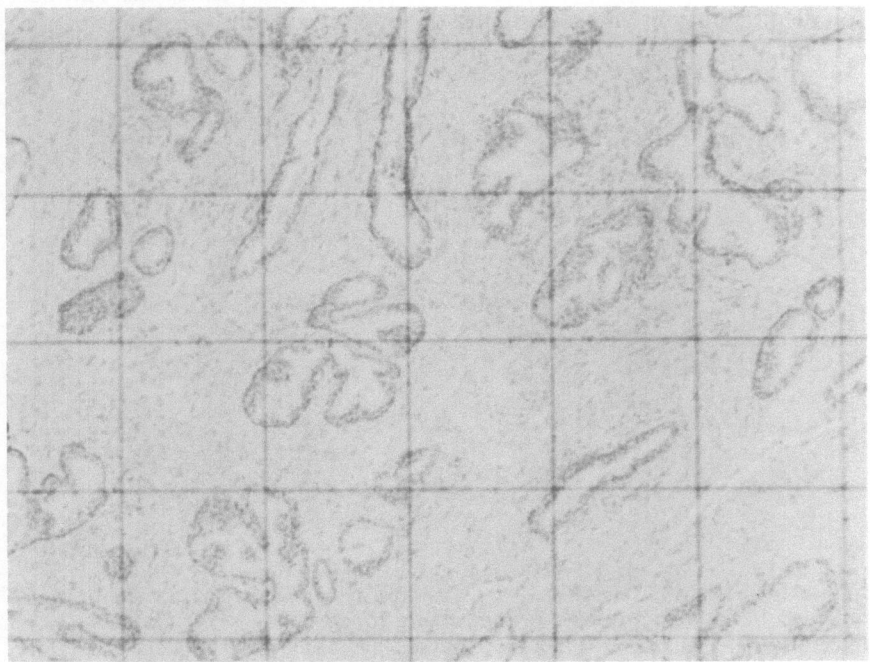

Figure 5.1 Light microscopy of a human benign hypertrophied prostate with a superimposed graticule (100 sq) for point counting of cell-types (H & E × 63)

5.3. THE COMPOSITION OF EPITHELIAL AND STROMAL CELLS IN HUMAN BPH

Despite the numerous reports on the biochemical data on normal and abnormal human prostates, data on the quantitative aspects of the cellular composition of human prostatic tissue is sparse. Data based on mechanical separation of the epithelial and stromal elements is only semi-quantitative, mainly due to poor recoveries and cross-contamination of the prepared fractions. Moreover, these techniques are unable to quantify the space occupied by these components (volume) as the latter may provide more precise information on the hypertrophy of the tumour. Using morphometry, we have investigated and compared the distributions of stromal, epithelial, acinar and glandular (epithelial and acinar) elements in BPH tissues obtained by either retropubic prostatectomy or transurethral resection (Figure 5.2). In both RPP and TUR samples the stromal cells constitute the bulk of tissue components whilst approximately equal amounts of epithelia and acinar lumina are found. In 14 RPP samples the mean percentage of stroma was 69.8 % and the corresponding value for 28 TUR samples was 81.5 %. The remaining 20–30 % represents the glandular elements. There was, however, a wide range of variation in the cellular composition of BPH tissues, but, in general, it was observed that BPH tissue consisted predominantly of stroma. A similar conclusion has been reached by Bartsch *et al.* (1979) using light microscopic stereological analysis on BPH tissue. Additionally these authors found a significant increase in the volumetric amount of stroma, and a

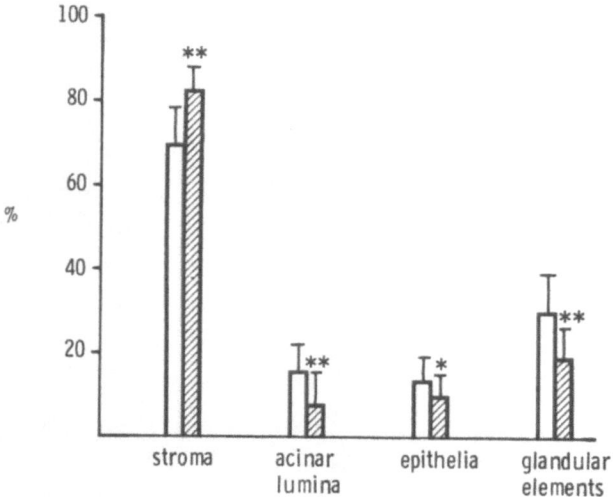

Figure 5.2 Distribution of cell types in human benign hypertrophied prostates obtained by either retropubic prostatectomy (open bars $n = 14$) or transurethral resection (hatched bars $n = 28$) and analysed by morphometry in our laboratory. Heights represent mean percentage of the cell types and vertical bars as standard deviations. Statistical differences (*t*-test) between the two types of specimens are *$p < 0.05$, **$p < 0.001$. Glandular elements are the sum of epithelia and acinar lumina

decrease in the glandular area in the BPH tissue when compared to the outer region of the normal prostate or the whole normal gland. At the present time morphometric studies of the malignant prostate are only in the preliminary stages.

5.4 SOURCE OF PROSTATIC TISSUE; TRANSURETHRAL RESECTION OR OPEN PROSTATECTOMY

An important consideration in the study of human prostatic tissues is the type of surgical specimen which is to be utilized for biochemical assessments. In general, apart from biopsy samples, there are at least two main categories of surgically removed human prostatic tissues. The first category consists of samples in which the tumour was removed by open procedures such as retropubic, suprapubic, radical and Millin's prostatectomy. These procedures usually provide large nodules which are suitable for strict random sampling. The second category of prostatectomy which is now commonly in use in most urological centres is that of transurethral resection, which involves the use of electroresection to remove sections of human prostatic tissue. This technique causes some damage to the periphery of the tissue samples, which raises the question as to the usefulness of such tissues for biochemical studies. There is little or no controversy regarding the use of material obtained by open prostatectomy. However, regarding TUR samples, no general consensus prevails. Whilst some investigators do not consider TUR samples suitable for biochemical analysis, others have utilized such tissues and reported satisfactory results. Despite the obvious influence that the source of tissue may have on the biochemical values, little information is available on this aspect of prostate research.

There are several important considerations which have to be taken into account, when using TUR material. At least two important factors are involved here, namely the effects of the surgical procedure and the location from which TUR samples were removed.

5.4.1 The effect of electroresection on TUR samples

Perhaps the most obvious concern with TUR samples is the damage incurred through the intense heat generated during electroresection of the prostate. Therefore, it is of paramount importance to know the extent to which the heat has penetrated these specimens. Using enzyme histochemistry de Voogt and Dingjan (1978) have reported that coagulation necrosis of TUR samples is less than $0.2 \, \mu m$ thick. In another histochemical study, Pertschuk et al. (1979) have shown that severely burnt TUR samples showed bright golden autofluorescence at the periphery of each sample; whilst beneath was a variable zone up to $200 \, \mu m$ wide, where non-specific uptake of ligand conjugate had occurred. They excluded from their studies badly burnt specimens that showed the described artifact which were also shown to be receptor negative. These studies clearly indicate that those tissues which are badly burnt are unreliable for biochemical assays. However, these studies also suggest that large TUR samples could easily withstand the heat generated by the electroresection and that, provided the outer burnt layer is removed, the sample can be used for biochemical analysis. Therefore, two critical factors should be considered when handling TUR materials: firstly, the size of the samples must be relatively large and, secondly, the burnt tissue must be removed. In general samples thicker than 5 mm are considered safe from heat denaturation provided the burnt tissue is removed prior to biochemical assays.

5.4.2   The location of the removed TUR samples

Another important consideration which could influence the outcome of biochemical measurements using TUR samples, is the incomplete removal of BPH tissue by transurethral resection. Whilst open prostatectomy removes most of the adenoma down to and beyond the verumontanum, transurethral resection of the gland confines itself to removing BPH intrusion down to but not usually below the veromontanum, due to the fear of injuring the sphincter (see Chapter 1). Indeed, Shah *et al.* (1979) have shown that up to 50 % of the total adenoma weight could be found below the verumontanum which could escape resection during TUR procedures and thus have concluded that prostatectomy by transurethral route is less complete due to residual subverumontanal prostatic tissues. These differences in surgical approaches would result in removing a varying proportion of the adenoma from areas that often are not quite comparable. This gives rise to two major problems which can eventually influence the biochemical results. Firstly, unlike samples obtained by open prostatectomy, a strict random sampling procedure cannot be applied to TUR samples and only simple random sampling can be employed. This can easily affect the accuracy of any biochemical studies. Secondly, anatomical differences in the location of the removed tissue could also influence the biochemical data. This is an important factor in relation to those biochemical parameters which display a differential regional distri-bution. A vivid example is that of distribution of 5α-dihydrotestosterone in the periurethral and outer regions of the gland. Indeed, Siiteri and Wilson (1970) have demonstrated that the content of this androgen in the periurethral region of the normal and benign prostates is two to threefold higher than that of the outer region. It is, therefore, quite clear that partial or total regional differences present in the resected samples could influence biochemical measurements. The problems relating to regional differences and the partial removal of tissue from the gland by TUR are extremely important when the biochemical results are to be compared to those obtained using RPP specimens. Indeed some of the differences in the biochemical data between TUR and RPP specimens could be attributed to the types of tissue removed from different regions of the gland rather than through their association with heat denaturation.

5.5   EVALUATION OF BIOCHEMICAL PARAMETERS IN TUR AND RPP SAMPLES

Despite the differences which exist between TUR and RPP samples, there are few or no comparative studies in terms of biochemical constituents of these specimens. In our laboratory such a study was initiated to detect possible changes in total proteins, nucleic acids and water content. This study was carried out in 26 RPP and 27 TUR specimens obtained from patients with BPH. The results are shown in Table 5.2. These results suggest that with the exception of RNA there is no significant difference in the biochemical constituents of TUR and RPP samples. An important aspect of this data is the similarity in water content of the two types of specimens, which suggests that, provided the TUR samples are cleaned and the burnt tissue removed, the water content is unaffected during transurethral resection. Furthermore, neither the protein nor the DNA content of the TUR specimens were affected. The comparable values of DNA between the two types of specimen also suggest that in general cellular damage in TUR samples is insignificant and tends to be confined to the outer layer of each burnt sample. Regarding the total RNA content the mean concentration of this nucleic acid in RPP samples (3.5 mg/g wet weight) was slightly higher than that of TUR specimens (3.2 mg/g wet weight). Although the difference is statistically significant, the interpretation of this difference is not understood.

Table 5.2 The concentrations of total protein, nucleic acids and water content in human benign hypertrophied prostate obtained by either retropubic prostatectomy (RPP) or transurethral resection (TUR). Values are either Mean $\pm$ SEM or in range. Number of estimations are shown in brackets

	RPP	TUR
Protein (mg/g wet weight)	95 ± 27 57–122 (27)	103 ± 5 19–137 (27)
DNA (mg/g wet weight)	3.2 ± 0.1 1.8–5.2 (26)	3.5 ± 0.2 1.8–6.1 (27)
RNA (mg/g wet weight)	3.5 ± 0.1 2.9–4.2 (26)	3.2 ± 0.1* 2.3–4.7 (25)
Water content (%)	83.5 ± 0.4 77.8–89.1 (26)	82.8 ± 0.6 75.4–91.1 (27)

* Significantly different from RPP, $p < 0.05$
Data from author's laboratory

In addition to biochemical parameters we have also compared the content of steroids in TUR and RPP samples. In 26 specimens of RPP and 27 TUR specimens, the concentrations of testosterone, 5α-dihydrotestosterone, 5α-androstane-3α, 17β-diol, androstenedione and oestradiol-17β, were estimated. These steroids were measured by radioimmunoassay procedures as described by Ghanadian and Puah (1981) and Puah and Ghanadian (unpublished). The results are shown in Table 5.3. Except for 5α-androstane-3α, 17β-diol the results revealed significant differences in the levels of steroids in these two types of specimens. Whilst the concentration of 5α-dihydrotestosterone is significantly higher ($p < 0.001$) in RPP samples, the levels of testosterone, androstenedione and oestradiol-17β are higher in TUR specimens. Values for significance were $p < 0.01$, $p < 0.02$ and $p < 0.001$ respectively. The significantly higher level of DHT in RPP samples is a reflection of the higher proportion of adenomatous tissues obtained by RPP. The TUR samples are a mixture of tissues obtained from more than one region of the prostate and may include surgical capsule. The higher concentration of oestradiol-17β, in the TUR specimen, may be due to the relatively higher percentage of stroma in these samples.

Table 5.3 The concentrations of endogenous steroids in human benign hypertrophied prostate obtained by either retropubic prostatectomy (RPP) or transurethral resection (TUR). Values are either Mean ± SEM or in range. Number of estimations are shown in brackets

	RPP	*TUR*
Testosterone (nmol/kg wet weight)	1.26 ± 0.07 0.53–1.98 (24)	1.60 ± 0.09* 0.72–2.54 (27)
5α-dihydrotestosterone (nmol/kg wet weight)	25.54 ± 1.07 17.27–39.73 (24)	19.39 ± 0.75*** 11.08–28.41 (27)
5α-androstane-3α,17β-diol (nmol/kg wet weight)	1.51 ± 0.09 0.82–2.26 (23)	1.58 ± 0.13 0.78–3.12 (25)
Androstenedione (nmol/kg wet weight)	1.85 ± 0.12 0.72–3.11 (26)	2.37 ± 0.16** 0.68–3.71 (27)
Oestradiol-17β (pmol/kg wet weight)	217.0 ± 7.8 156.7–305.0 (24)	258.4 ± 8.1*** 160.8–326.3 (27)

Significantly different from RPP;   * $p < 0.01$,   ** $p < 0.02$,   *** $p < 0.001$
Data from author's laboratory

It appears that differences in the concentration of some of the biochemical parameters, such as steroids, between TUR and RPP specimens are partially due to regional differences of these constituents and the concentrations of those biochemical constituents, which are equally distributed within the different regions of the gland, are less affected regardless of the type of specimens used. However, such a tentative conclusion requires further experimental support with a large number of RPP and TUR specimens including a more strict sampling procedure based on the regional difference within each prostate.

5.6 CORRELATION BETWEEN MORPHOMETRIC AND BIOCHEMICAL DATA

The majority of the available biochemical data on the prostate has been obtained by the use of whole tissue and with limited information as to the distribution of the biochemical substances within the different cell types. In this section the biochemical data obtained from TUR and RPP samples in relation to the morphometric composition of the same samples are discussed. There is no significant correlation between the concentrations of proteins, DNA, RNA or water content of either TUR or RPP specimen with any of the cell types. This would suggest that irrespective of the type of prostatic specimens used, these biochemical constituents do not exhibit any preferential distribution within different cell types. In contrast the steroid hormones in RPP samples revealed significant correlations with various cell types. The results are shown in Table 5.4. The significant correlation between oestradiol-17β and stroma may suggest a preferential localization of this steroid in the stroma. It is important to consider this finding in relation to the role of oestradiol-17β, in stimulating the stromal elements in the prostate as well as in other sex accessory organs of various experimental animals. Several studies have demonstrated that the growth of stroma from a variety of species is under oestrogenic influence (Mawhinney and Neubauer, 1979; Neubauer et al., 1981). Furthermore, the administration of a combination of pharmacological doses of oestradiol-17β, with either DHT or 5α-androstane-3α,17β-diol given to young castrated dogs, can induce glandular hyperplasia of the prostate which is indistinguishable from that of spontaneous tumour (DeKlerk et al., 1979). Similarly Tunn et al. (1980) have also been able to induce glandular hyperplasia in the prostate of dogs treated with 5α-androstane-3α,17β-diol. When these authors treated the animals with a combination of 5α-androstane-3α,17β-diol and oestradiol-17β, they developed stromal hyperplasia with squamous metaplasia of the epithelium and secondary cyst formation. These studies should be compared with the data on the correlation between the percentage of glandular elements and the amount of 5α-androstane-3α,17β-diol as well as the percentage of glandular cells and the ratio of 5α-androstane-3α,17β-diol to oestradiol-17β (Table 5.4). In these RPP specimens, there was no significant correlation between the content of DHT with any of the cell types. However, when the combined results of RPP and TUR samples were analysed there was a significant correlation between the percentage of glandular elements with the ratio of DHT to oestradiol-17β. There was also a strong relationship between the percentage of stromal cells and the content of oestradiol-17β. In contrast there was a lack of correlation between the percentage of cell types and the amount of steroids measured in the TUR samples. This may be partly due to the inclusion of non-adenomatous tissue in these TUR specimens. However, these findings require further experimental evidence to establish the significance of these relationships between the cell types and the contents of steroids in benign prostatic tumours.

Other investigators have also reported relationships between prostatic stroma and plasma oestradiol-17β, as well as total urinary oestrogens in patients with BPH (Seppelt, 1978). However, this relationship was not

Table 5.4 Correlations between the concentrations of testosterone (T), 5α-dihydrotestosterone (DHT), 5α-androstane-3α,17β-diol (diol) and oestradiol-17β(E_2) and percentages of stromal, glandular (acinar + epithelial) elements in 14 and 28 human benign hypertrophied prostates obtained by retropubic prostatectomy (RPP) and transurethral resection (TUR) respectively

| | Significance (value for p) | | |
	RPP	TUR	RPP+TUR
E_2/stroma	<0.02	NS	<0.001
E_2/epithelia	<0.005	NS	<0.02
E_2/acinar lumina	NS	NS	<0.001
E_2/glandular elements	<0.05	NS	<0.001
DHT/acinar lumina	NS	NS	<0.05
diol/stroma	NS	NS	<0.05
diol/glandular elements	<0.05	NS	<0.05
DHT/E_2/stroma	NS	NS	<0.005
DHT/E_2/acinar lumina	NS	NS	<0.005
DHT/E_2/glandular elements	NS	NS	<0.005
diol/E_2/stroma	<0.005	NS	<0.001
diol/E_2/epithelia	<0.05	NS	<0.005
diol/E_2/acinar lumina	NS	NS	<0.001
diol/E_2/glandular elements	<0.01	NS	<0.001
androgens*/E_2/stroma	NS	NS	<0.005
androgens/E_2/epithelia	NS	NS	<0.05
androgens/E_2/acinar lumina	NS	NS	<0.005
androgens/E_2/glandular elements	NS	NS·	<0.005

* androgens = T + DHT + diol
Data from author's laboratory

observed with plasma testosterone. Although this author employed both TUR and enucleated prostatic samples for the morphometric analysis of the tissues, the study lacked comparative data between the two types of surgical specimens. It appears that whilst androgens may be associated with non-stromal elements, oestradiol-17β is preferentially localized in the stroma, and that the activity of the important enzyme 5α-reductase appears to be relatively higher in the stromal than non-stromal cells.

Studies from our laboratory as well as findings by Bashirelahi et al. (1980) suggest that the receptor proteins for oestradiol-17β are also found to be higher in the stromal cells than in the epithelium. Indeed in our studies there was a significant correlation between the percentage of stromal cells and the concentration of oestrogen receptors in BPH tissues. Using specimens composed of mixed stromal and glandular hyperplasia, Shain et al. (1980) have found significant correlations between androgen receptors and epithelial cells. However, these authors excluded BPH specimens which were predominantly composed of stromal elements. Furthermore, these authors suggested that stromal cells may contain a considerable amount of androgen receptors.

5.7   STEREOLOGY

As described previously stereology is a scientific discipline based on the quantitative analysis of three-dimensional structures and textures extrapolated from two-dimensional measurements. The latter are based on morphometric analysis which can be obtained by a variety of quantitative procedures performed on any type of tissue. Although the two terms, morphometry and stereology, are closely related they are not synonymous (Weibel, 1969). Basically stereology follows the same principles as outlined for morphometry (see Principles of morphometric analysis, 5.2.1), but employs different procedures and definitions.

5.7.1   Symbols and definitions

In the studies of cellular structures by stereology there are at least three basic parameters which need to be defined. These are the volume, the surface and the number of profiles of the structures. The stereological data is usually expressed in terms of density in which the density of each parameter such as volume, surface or the number of structure profiles could be obtained by representative counting of test points and expressed in terms of a reference space. This reference space can be either the tissue or cytoplasm of different cell types. The basic symbols for stereological analysis applicable to most of the structural studies have been stated by a number of investigators (Weibel, 1969; Weibel, 1973; Rohr et al., 1976). Symbols related to the three main parameters are as follows: (1) volume density (V_{vi}) which is the volume fraction occupied by component i, (2) surface density (S_{vi}) which is collective surface area per volume, and (3) numerical density (N_{vi}) which is the number of component i per volume. As previously described for morphometric analysis these three stereological parameters could also be obtained by superimposing a systematic set of points over the histological sections or over the photomicrograph and counting the number of points lying over the different cellular components. Therefore, the above three parameters relating to the three-dimensional analysis are based on two-dimensional measurements and can be summarized as follows:

Two-dimensional measurements (2D)	*Three-dimensional measurements* (3D)
Counting of points (P)	→ Calculation of volume densities (V_{vi})
Counting of intersections (I)	→ Calculation of surface densities (S_{vi})
Counting of structure profiles (N)	→ Calculation of the numerical densities (N_{vi})

5.7.2   Counting of points (P)

As outlined for morphometric analysis the method for achieving volumetric measurement based on area estimation (A_{Ai}), namely planimetry, which was originally suggested by Delesse (1847), is still in use: ($V_{vi} = A_{Ai}$). However, planimetry is not convenient in stereological analysis. The introduction of point counting (P_{pi}) by superimposing over the sample section ($A_{Ai} = P_{pi}$) as suggested by Glagoleff (1933) has replaced the previous procedure. This method is generally used by biologists for volumetric quantitation of cellular components in a histological section.

5.7.3 Counting of intersections (I)

This measurement is based on the original equation suggested by Saltykov (1958) in which the total length of the boundaries of all structure profiles (B_{Ai}) per unit area of the object profile is proportional to the surface density of the structure, i.e. $S_{vi} = (4/\pi) B_{Ai}$. Since then, this equation has been modified by several investigators in which they have reduced the calculation of B_{Ai} to a count of the intersections of testlines with the surface (I_L) of the structure i which is $B_{Ai} = (\pi/2)I_{Li}$ (Weibel, 1969). An alternative equation for the quantitation of S_{vi} is that proposed by Chalkley et al. (1949) in which they project a line segment of known length (l) randomly and repeatedly on a microscopic field and count the number of times (h) a line endpoint falls on the component, as well as the number of times (c) the line intersects the boundary of the components. This equation is as follows: $V_{vi}/S_{vi} = lh/4c$. Since V_{vi} can be obtained by point counting S_{vi} can easily be computed.

5.7.4 Counting of structure profiles (N)

The number of structure profiles (N) can be determined directly by using the equation as suggested by DeHoff and Rhines (1961). This equation applies only when the shape and size distribution of the structures are approximately constant: $N_{vi} = N_{Ai}\overline{D}_i$ in which $\overline{D}_i$ is the mean particle diameter and N_{vi} is dependent on the shape and size distribution of the structure. Weibel and Gomez (1962) have introduced a modified equation for the estimation of N_{vi} which is:

$$N_{vi} = (K/\beta_i)(N_{Ai}^{3/2}/V_{vi}^{1/2})$$

where β is a dimensionless coefficient relating to the shape of the structure and K is another dimensionless coefficient relating to the distribution of the structure. For most biological systems K is between 1.01 and 1.10 and β can be obtained graphically. Other alternative procedures for the estimation of structure profiles (N) are those of Loud et al. (1965) and Aherne (1967). These two latter procedures do not require actual counting of the structure profiles and only require point counting of the section.

5.8 APPLICATION OF STEREOLOGY TO THE PROSTATE

The use of stereology in the studies of prostatic tissues was initially carried out on the rat ventral prostate (Bartsch et al., 1975; Rohr et al. 1976). The stereological analysis of the rat ventral prostate by light and electron microscopy revealed that this organ is basically 'hollow', consisting of more than 76% of glandular parenchyma and 24% of extracellular space (connective tissues, smooth muscles, nerve tissues and blood vessels). The glandular lumina accounted for 53% whilst the functional glandular parenchyma actually consisted of only 23%. The absolute mean cell volume of the prostatic acinar cells is 1950 μm^3,.which is similar to that of the absolute volume of the pancreatic cell. The volume of the rough endoplasmic reticulum consisted of 31% of the total cytoplasmic space, which reflects the function performed by prostatic cells. The main function of prostatic acinar cells involves the synthesis and the secretion of proteins. Both these two functions are androgen-dependent and have been shown by organ culture to be under the influence of testosterone metabolites (Baulieu et al., 1968; Lasnitzki, 1970).

The use of stereological analysis of the prostate has been extended to assess the effects of drugs on the prostate. Using rat prostate, the morphometrically defined space and membrane compartments of the gland and the glandular cells were examined following the administration of ethinyl-norgestrienone (Bartsch and Rohr, 1977). These authors showed a reduction of acinar parenchyma, glandular cells and their various compartments involved in the synthesis and secretion of proteins and enzymes. Furthermore, the volume density was shown to be reduced, whilst that of interacinar tissue remained unaltered. Electron microscopic studies also revealed that the columnar cells of the glandular elements became smaller, and the rough endoplasmic reticulum and mitochondria were significantly diminished. However, the volume of Golgi apparatus remained unaltered. DeKlerk and Coffey (1978) have studied the rat ventral prostate using a biomorphometric technique based on a combination of stereology and biochemical determination of RNA and DNA. These authors suggested that their technique could avoid some of the disadvantages encountered during histological preparations such as differential shrinkage of cellular components. In this technique, the determination of the ratio of various cell types, which were obtained by the standard morphometric analysis under light microscopy, were related to the total number of cells in the gland based on the total amount of DNA in the gland and the DNA content per cell nucleus. They have found that in 7 day castrated rats there was a general reduction of the total epithelial cell number (92%), epithelial cell size (85%), stromal cell number (39%) and stromal cell size (23%). The treatment of castrated rats with testosterone for 10 days had completely restored the epithelial cell size and the stromal cell number and size but not epithelial cell number.

Stereological analysis has also been extended to the study of the dog prostate as this species shares with man the phenomenon of developing benign hyperplasia with age. Tunn et al. (1980) have induced benign hyperplasia in the adult male dog by the administration of either 5α-androstane-3α,17β-diol alone or in combination with oestradiol-17β, and have studied the induced tumour stereologically. The intact untreated dog prostate consisted of 75% acinar parenchyma and 25% stromal tissue. The acinar parenchyma itself was comprised of two fractions, namely acinar cells and acinar lumina of which the former occupied more than 51% of the whole prostate. The 25% stromal tissue was found to be composed of smooth muscle and other residual stroma. It is interesting to note that the distribution of acinar parenchyma and stroma in this study followed the same pattern as reported for the rat ventral prostate by Bartsch *et al.* (1975). In the castrated dogs treated with 5α-androstane-3α,17β-diol there was an increase in volume density of acinar parenchyma reaching 84 % of the whole gland whilst the stromal compartment decreased to 16 %. The morphometric integrity of the interacinar stroma after castration and replacement with androgen remained unchanged when compared to the intact untreated dog. A combined treatment of the castrated dog with 5α-androstane-3α,17β-diol and oestradiol-17β, gave extensive stratified squamous metaplasia of the entire epithelium. This reduction of metaplastic epithelia was significant when compared to those castrated animals which were treated with 5α-androstane-3α,17β-diol alone. There was also a significant increase in acinar lumina in dogs receiving a combination of androgen and oestrogen. In this group of animals the volume density of stroma also increased significantly. This was possibly due to oestrogen stimulation of the stroma. Tunn *et al.* (1981) also studied the effect of the antiandrogen, cyproterone acetate, on the tumours induced experimentally in these animals. The effect of cyproterone acetate on adrogen induced tumours led to a significant reduction of the volume density of acinar parenchyma, which fell to 12 %, as well as a reduction of the smooth muscle cells with a substantial increase of stromal compartment of up to 88 %. This suggests that cyproterone acetate could reduce the epithelial proliferation induced by 5α-androstane-3α,17β-diol and the synergistic effects of this androgen with oestradiol-17β, on stromal proliferation. Tunn *et al.* (1981) have also shown that the antioestrogenic effect of tamoxifen can be monitored by this system. In addition, this compound reduced the stromal proliferation caused by oestradiol-17β. These findings should be considered in relation to the studies by DeKlerk *et al.* (1979) who were able to demonstrate the induction of benign hyperplasia in the intact dogs with either DHT or 5α-androstane-3α,17β-diol or a combination of any of these androgens with oestradiol-17β, in the castrated animals. This study together with that of Moore *et al.* (1979) suggest that the changes which have occurred in these animals following hormonal manipulation and leading to the induction of the tumour are a result of DHT accumulation within the gland.

Both normal and benign hypertrophied prostates have also been studied by stereology. These studies have indicated distinct differences between the prostates of rat and dog with that of man. The human prostate contains more interstitial fibromuscular tissue with a high amount of smooth muscle cells (Bartsch *et al.*, 1976) when compared to either rat or dog prostates. In the normal human prostate, the glandular elements of the inner part occupy 45 % of its volume and this increases to 55 % in the outer region of the gland. The volumetric amount of the interstitial fibromuscular tissue is higher in the inner part (55 %) than that of the outer region (45 %) of the gland (Bartsch *et al.*, 1979). In BPH tissues more than 60 % of the gland is composed of fibromuscular tissues with only 17 % related to acinar parenchymá. When BPH tissue was compared with normal gland, there was a significant fall in the volume density of the rough endoplasmic reticulum, Golgi apparatus, secretory droplets and lysosomes, indicating diminished secretory activity of these glandular cells in benign prostates. These stereological findings (Table 5.5) are in agreement with the descriptive morphology of BPH.

Table 5.5 Stereological data (% mean volumetric density) of human prostate under light and electron microscopy (data based on Bartsch *et al.* (1979), *J. Urol.*, **122**, 481)

	Normal	*BPH*
Light microscopy		
Whole gland		
Stroma	45	60*
Glandular cells	21	12*
Acinar lumina	28	28
Inner part		
Stroma	55	—
Glandular cells	45	—
Outer part		
Stroma	45	—
Glandular cells	55	—
Electron microscopy		
Rough endoplasmic reticulum	13.1	17.8
Golgi apparatus	4.1	2.6
Secretory droplets and lysosomes	35.1	25.3
Mitochondria	4.6	8.4
Fat droplets	0.9	0.3
Ground substance	42.0	45.6

* significantly different from normal gland, $p < 0.05$

The stereological analysis of the human prostate has also been employed for the evaluation of the efficacy of various drugs on BPH tissues and has been performed in similar manner to that described for experimental animals. Both cyproterone acetate and bromocriptine produced significant changes in human BPH tissues when analysed by stereological methods. The prominent effect of cyproterone acetate was the reduction of the volumetric amount of glandular tissue. This was in contrast to the effect of bromocriptine which actually produced an increase in the volumetric amount of glandular elements. The electron microscopic studies of the effects of bromocriptine on BPH tissues also revealed the activation of smooth muscles by this drug. In addition to the above mentioned synthetic compounds, the effect of tamoxifen was also assessed in this system. Tamoxifen when given to patients in a dosage of 20 mg twice a day appears to have no significant effect on the prostate (Bartsch *et al.*, 1981). It is quite apparent from these studies that stereology is a useful tool in combining the two disciplines of biochemistry and morphology in order to provide a better understanding of the changes associated with the cellular components of prostatic tissues.

5.9 CONCLUSIONS

The importance of the interaction between epithelial and stromal elements of prostatic cells has prompted attempts by many research groups to investigate the biochemical and morphological changes associated with these cellular elements. The suggestion that the functional activity of the urogenital epithelium is much dependent on that of stroma has stimulated interest in developing techniques capable of separating these two components. Many efforts have been made to develop mechanical or enzyme based techniques for separation of these cells. Despite the useful information provided by these techniques, several shortcomings, including cell damages, low degree of purity as well as poor recovery and initial requirement for large amounts of starting materials, have curbed the potential of these techniques. The use of morphometry and stereology has overcome a number of these disadvantages, and has introduced a new dimension to the quantitative aspects of prostate research. Whilst the former technique is essentially based on two-dimensional measurements, the latter deals with three-dimensional measurements of structures. The data obtained by these two techniques are interchangeable, and are based on random sampling of prostatic tissues. Principles behind these techniques have been discussed. Whilst morphometry has more potential in light microscopy studies of prostatic samples, stereology is applicable to both low and high power microscopy. Using these two techniques, biochemical findings related to normal and BPH tissues have been correlated with the various cellular components. In this chapter, the problems associated with tissue sampling and, in particular, the source of surgical samples have been discussed and much attention is given to differences in the biochemical parameters of the two main types of tissues, i.e. TUR and RPP samples. Biochemical and hormonal correlations with these two types of surgical specimen are discussed. Despite a number of shortcomings associated with the use of TUR samples, it appears from available evidence that they can provide satisfactory results provided certain precautions are taken in the handling of this material. In addition, this chapter has dealt with the application of both morphometry and stereology to both experimental animals as well as human prostatic tissues. The advantages and disadvantages of these techniques compared to other physical and chemical techniques are discussed. Using these techniques, the main feature of the rat ventral prostate and the dog prostate is shown to be the predominance of glandular elements compared to stroma, whereas the human prostate and in particular BPH tissues are shown to be more stromal than glandular. Additionally, stereological models developed for rat, dog and the human prostates have been found to be useful in evaluating the efficacy of various drugs.

5.10 REFERENCES

Aherne, W. (1967). Methods of counting discrete tissue components in microscopical sections. *J. R. Microscop. Soc.*, **87**, 493

Bahr, G. F., Bloom, G. and Friberg, U. (1957). Volume changes of tissues in physiological fluids during fixation in osmium tetroxide or formaldehyde and during subsequent treatment. *Exp. Cell Res.*, **12**, 342

Bartsch, G., Fisher, E. and Rohr, H. P. (1975). Ultrastructural morphometric analysis of the rat prostate (ventral lobe). *Urol. Res.*, **3**, 1

Bartsch, G., Frick, J. and Rohr, H. P. (1976). Stereology, a new morphological method of study of prostatic function and disease. In Marberger, H., Haschek, H., Schirmer, H. K. A., Colston, J. A. C. and Witkin, E. (eds.) *Progress in Clinical and Biological Research: Prostatic Disease.* vol. 6, pp. 123–141. (New York: Alan R. Liss)

Bartsch, G., Müller, H. R., Oberholzer, M. and Rohr, H. P. (1979). Light microscopic stereological analysis of the normal human prostate and of benign prostatic hyperplasia. *J. Urol.*, **122**, 487

Bartsch, G., Oberholzer, M. and Rohr, H. P. (1981). The effect of antiestrogen, antiandrogen and the prolactin inhibitor 2 bromo-α-ergocriptine on the stromal tissue of human benign prostatic hyperplasia. *Invest. Urol.*, **18**, 308

Bartsch, G. and Rohr, H. P. (1977). Ultrastructural stereology. A new approach to the study of prostatic function. *Invest. Urol.*, **14**, 301

Bashirelahi, N., Young, J. D., Sidh, S. M. and Sanefuji, H. (1980). Androgen, oestrogen and progestogen and the distribution in epithelial and stromal cells of human prostate. In Schroder, F. H. and de Voogt, H. J. (eds.) *Steroid Receptors, Metabolism and Prostatic Cancer.* pp. 240–256. (Amsterdam: Excerpta Medica)

Baulieu, E. E., Lasnitzki, I. and Robel, P. (1968). Metabolism of testosterone and action of metabolites on prostate glands grown in organ culture. *Nature (London)*, **219**, 1155

Bruchovsky, N., Rennie, P. S. and Wilkin, R. P. (1980). New aspects of androgen action in prostatic cells: stromal localization of 5α-reductase, nuclear abundance of androstanolone and binding of receptor to linker deoxyribonucleic acid. In Schroder, F. H. and de Voogt, H. J. (eds.) *Steroid Receptors, Metabolism and Prostatic Cancer.* pp. 57–76. (Amsterdam: Excerpta Medica)

Chalkley, H. W., Cornfield, J. and Park, H. (1949). A method for estimating volume–surface ratios. *Science*, **110**, 295

Cowan, R. A., Cowan, S. K., Giles, C. A. and Grant, J. K. (1976). Prostatic distribution of sex hormone-binding globulin and cortisol-binding globulin in benign hyperplasia. *J. Endocrinol.*, **71**, 121

Cowan, R. A., Cowan, S. K., Grant, J. K. and Elder, H. Y. (1977). Biochemical investigation of separated epithelium and stroma from benign hyperplastic prostatic tissue. *J. Endocrinol.*, **74**, 111

Cunha, G. R. (1973). The role of androgens in the epithelio-mesenchymal interactions involved in prostatic morphogenesis in embryonic mice. *Anat. Rec.*, **175**, 87

Cunha, G. R. and Lung, B. (1979). The importance of stroma in morphogenesis and functional activity of urogenital epithelium. *In Vitro*, **15**, 50

DeHoff, R. T. and Rhines, F. N. (1961). Determination of the number of particles per unit volume from measurements made on random plan sections: the general cylinder and the ellipsoid. *Trans. Am. Inst. Metal. Eng.*, **221**, 975

DeKlerk, D. P. and Coffey, D. S. (1978). Quantitative determination of prostatic epithelial and stromal hyperplasia by a new technique. Biomorphometrics. *Invest. Urol.*, **16**, 240

DeKlerk, D. P., Coffey, D. S., Ewing, L. L., McDermott, I. R., Reiner, W. G., Robinson, C. H., Scott, W. W., Strandberg, J. D., Talalay, P., Walsh, P. C., Wheaton, L. G. and Zirkin, B. R. (1979). Comparison of spontaneous and experimentally induced canine prostatic hyperplasia. *J. Clin. Invest.*, **64**, 842

Delesse, M. A. (1847). Procédé mécanique pour determiner la composition des roches. *C. R. Acad. Sci. (Paris)*, **25**, 544

de Voogt, H. J. and Dingjan, P. (1978). Steroid receptors in human prostatic cancer. A preliminary evaluation. *Urol. Res.*, **6**, 151

Franks, L. M., Riddle, P. N., Cartonell, A. W. and Grey, G. O. (1970). A comparative study of the ultrastructure and lack of growth capacity of adult human prostate epithelia mechanically separated from its stroma. *J. Pathol.*, **100**, 113

Ghanadian, R. and Puah, C. M. (1981). Relationships between oestradiol-17β, testosterone, dihydrotestosterone and 5α-androstane-3α,17β-diol in human benign hypertrophy and carcinoma of the prostate. *J. Endocrinol.*, **88**, 255

Glagoleff, A. A. (1933). On the geometrical methods of quantitative mineralogic analysis of rocks. *Trans. Inst. Econ. Mineral (USSR)*, **59**, 5

Harper, M. E., Pike, A., Peeling, W. B. and Griffiths, K. (1974). Steroids of adrenal origin metabolized by human prostatic tissue both *in vivo* and *in vitro*. *J. Endocrinol.*, **60**, 117

Haug, H. (1955). Die treffermethode, ein verfahren zur quantitativen analyse im histologischen schnitt. *Z. Anat. Entwickl-Gesch.*, **118**, 302

Henning, A. (1957). Fehler der oberflächenbestimmung von Kernen bei endlicher schnittdicke. *Mikroskopie*, **12**, 7

Hilfer, S. R. and Hilfer, E. K. (1966). Effects of dissociation agents on the fine structure of embryonic chick thyroid cells. *J. Morph.*, **119**, 217

Katzenellenbogen, B. S. and Leake, R. E. (1974). Distribution of the oestrogen-induced protein and of total protein between endometrial and myometrial fractions of the immature and mature rat uterus. *J. Endocrinol.*, **63**, 439

Krieg, M., Klotzl, G., Kaufmann, J. and Voigt, K. D. (1981). Stroma of human benign prostatic hyperplasia: preferential tissue for androgen metabolism and oestrogen binding. *Acta Endocrinol.*, **96**, 422

Lasnitzki, I. (1970). The rat prostate gland in organ culture. In Griffiths, K. and Pierrepoint, C. G. (eds.) *Some aspects of the aetiology and biochemistry of prostate cancer*. pp. 68–73. (Cardiff: Alpha Omega Alpha publishing)

Loud, A. V., Barany, W. C. and Pack, B. A. (1965). Quantitative evaluation of cytoplasmic structures in electron micrographs. *Lab. Invest.*, **14**, 996

Mawhinney, M. G. and Neubauer, B. L. (1979). Actions of estrogens in the male. *Invest. Urol.*, **16**, 409

Moore, R. J., Gazak, J. M., Quebbeman, J. F. and Wilson, J. D. (1979). Concentration of dihydrotestosterone and 3α-androstanediol in naturally occurring and androgen-induced prostatic hyperplasia in the dog. *J. Clin. Invest.*, **64**, 1003

Neubauer, B. L., Blume, C., Cricco, R., Greiner, J. and Mawhinney, M. (1981). Comparative effects and mechanism of castration, estrogen, anti-androgen and anti-estrogen-induced regression of accessory sex organ epithelium and muscle. *Invest. Urol.*, **18**, 229

Nilsson, T., Schueller, E. and Staubitz, W. (1973). β-glucuronidase activity of the epithelial cells and stroma cells in prostatic hyperplasia. *Invest. Urol.*, **11**, 145

Pertschuk, L. P., Zava, D. T., Tobin, E. H., Brigati, D. J., Gaetjens, E., Macchia, R. J., Wise, G. J., Wise, H. S., and Kim, D. S. (1979). Histochemical detection of steroid hormone receptors in the human prostate. In Murphy, G. P. and Sandberg, A. A. (eds.) *Progress in Clinical and Biological Research*. vol. *33*, pp. 113–132, (New York: Alan R. Liss)

Peutilla, A., McDowell, E. M. and Trump, B. F. (1975). Effects of fixation and post-fixations treatment on volume of injured cells. *J. Histochem. Cytochem.*, **23**, 251

Rohr, H., Oberholzer, M., Bartsch, G. and Keller, M. (1976). Morphometry in experimental pathology: methods, baseline data and applications. In Richter, G. W. and Epstein, M. A. (eds.) *International Review of Experimental Pathology*. pp. 233–325. (New York: Academic Press)

Romijn, J. C., Oishi, K., Bolt-de Vries, J., Schweikert, H. U., Mulder, E. and Schroder, F. H. (1980a). Androgen metabolism and androgen receptors in separated epithelium and stroma of the human prostate. In Schroder, F. H. and de Voogt, H. J. (eds.) *Steroid Receptors, Metabolism and Prostatic Cancer*. pp. 135–143. (Amsterdam: Excerpta Medica)

Romijn, J. C., Oishi, K. and Schroder, F. H. (1980b). Investigations on separated epithelium and stroma of human prostatic tissue. *The Prostate*, **1**, 118

Saltykov, S. A. (1958). *Stereometric Metallography*. 2nd Edn, p. 446. (Moscow: Metallurgizdat)

Seppelt, U. (1978). Correlation among prostate stroma, plasma estrogen levels and urinary estrogen excretion in patients with benign prostatic hypertrophy. *J. Clin. Endocrinol. Metab.*, **47**, 1230

Shah, P. J. R., Abrams, P. H., Feneley, R. C. L. and Green, N. A. (1979). The influence of prostatic anatomy on the differing results of prostatectomy according to the surgical approach. *Br. J. Urol.*, **51**, 549

Shain, S. A., Boesel, R. W., Lamm, D. L. and Radwin, H. M. (1980). Cytoplasmic and nuclear androgen receptor content of normal and neoplastic human prostates and lymph node metastases of human prostatic adenocarcinoma. *J. Clin. Endocrinol. Metab.*, **50**, 704

Siiteri, P. K. and Wilson, J. D. (1970). Dihydrotestosterone in prostatic hypertrophy. I. The formation and content of dihydrotestosterone in the hypertrophic prostate of man. *J. Clin. Invest.*, **49**, 1737

Sirett, D. A., Cowan, S. K., Janeczko, A. E., Grant, J. K. and Glen, E. S. (1980). Prostatic tissue distribution of 17 beta-hydroxy-5 alpha-androstan-3-one and of androgen receptors in benign hyperplasia. *J. Steroid Biochem.*, **13**, 723

Tunn, U. W., Funke, P. J., Senge, Th. and Neumann, F. (1981). Effects of cyproterone acetate and tamoxifen on experimentally induced epithelial and stromal proliferation of the canine prostate. Abs. 21 *Proceedings of the American Urological Association*, May 10–14, Boston

Tunn, U. W., Schuring, B., Senge, Th., Neumann, F., Schweikert, H. U. and Rohr, H. P. (1980). Morphometric analysis of prostates in castrated dogs after treatment with androstanediol, estradiol and cyproterone acetate. *Invest. Urol.*, **18**, 289

Weibel, E. R. (1963). Principle and methods for the morphometric study of the lung and other organs. *Lab. Invest.*, **12**, 131

Weibel, E. R. (1969). Stereological principles for the morphometry in electron microscopic cytology. In Bourne, G. H. and Danielli, J. F. (eds.), *International Review of Cytology*. vol. 26, pp. 235–302. (New York: Academic Press)

Weibel, E. R. (1973). Stereological techniques for electron microscopic morphometry. In Hayat, M. A. (ed.) *Principles and Techniques of Electron Microscopy: Biological Appplications*. vol. 3, pp. 237–296. (Princeton, New Jersey: Van Nostrand-Reinhold)

Weibel, E. R. and Gomez, D. M. (1962). A principle for counting tissue structures on random sections. *J. Appl. Physiol.*, **17**, 343

Weibel, E. R., Kistler, G. S. and Scherle, W. F. (1966). Practical stereological methods for morphometric cytology. *J. Cell. Biol.*, **30**, 23

6
Metabolism of steroids in the prostate

R. GHANADIAN AND C. B. SMITH

Although metabolism does not constitute an essential step in the mechanism of action of all steroids in the prostate, it is of paramount importance when considering the interaction of androgens and the mechanism by which this class of steroids exerts its biological action in the gland. This stage in the mechanism of action of androgens in the prostate is most vividly demonstrated in the metabolism of testosterone, which has attracted many experimental investigations with both animal and human prostatic tissues. The prerequisite for the metabolism of androgens in the prostate, as an essential part of their mechanism of action, is not typical of many target tissues for steroid hormones. Indeed apart from certain progestational steroids which can undergo metabolism as an essential part of their mode of action (Morgan and Wilson, 1970; Reel et al., 1971), the requirement for prior metabolism within the target cell, of the original secreted hormone in order to elicit its biological response, is confined to androgens. The target cell is usually able to take up naturally secreted steroid which binds to the specific receptor without being converted to a more active metabolite. An example of this may be seen in the case of the uterus which is an oestrogen dependent target tissue, and has been shown to retain tritiated oestradiol-17β basically unchanged (Jensen and Jacobson, 1962).

Despite the fact that androgen metabolism in the prostate has been investigated for many years, the first indication that the 5α-reductive enzymatic pathway, leading to the production of 5α-dihydrotestosterone from testosterone, was operative in this gland came from original work by Farnsworth and Brown (1963). In these classic experiments it was clearly demonstrated that in both the rat ventral prostate and human benign hypertrophied tissue, the predominant radiometabolite recovered was 5α-dihydrotestosterone. Later on in the same decade, the importance of this finding was succinctly revealed in the demonstration of a selective uptake and localization of this active androgen in the nuclei of rat ventral prostatic cells in two excellent reports by Anderson and Liao (1968) and Bruchovsky and Wilson (1968a). Subsequently these findings have been substantiated in numerous studies on the metabolism of testosterone by rat ventral prostate and human benign hypertrophied prostate. However, more recently with the extension of metabolic studies to carcinomatous tissues of the prostate the importance of the oxidative pathway has also been demonstrated (Morfin et al., 1977; Smith et al., 1980). The findings of these studies have contributed towards our present understanding of the mechanism of action of androgens in the prostate and continue to emphasize the extreme importance of these enzymatic activities in both the normal and tumour states found in this gland. Studies with both animal and human prostates have been performed by a variety of in vitro experimental techniques such as short term tissue or homogenate incubations, longer term organ culture or cell culture studies, perfusion and superfusion as well as in vivo experimentation. This wide spectrum of experimental designs can lead to differences which may arise from the natural interspecies variations and the choice of experimental technique employed. Therefore some degree of caution is necessary when interpreting the results. However, notwithstanding this cautionary note, research in this field has demonstrated comprehensively the metabolic fate of steroids and, in particular, androgens in the prostate.

6.1 ANDROGEN METABOLISM IN THE PROSTATE OF EXPERIMENTAL ANIMALS

A great deal of information about steroid metabolism in prostatic tissues has been derived from studies on experimental animals. Various species, but mostly rats and dogs, although occasionally mice, mastomys, guinea-pigs, cats, monkeys, lions and bulls, have been used. The choice of the rat ventral prostate as an experimental organ for metabolic studies lies in its availability and the ease with which this species may be subjected to hormonal manipulation, whilst studies on the dog prostate relate to the fact that this animal develops benign hyperplasia of the prostate.

Earlier attempts to demonstrate a specific uptake and the metabolism of androgen in the rat ventral prostate were inconclusive owing to the lack of radiolabelled steroid having appropriate specific activity. This apparent failure was due to the necessity of using hormone doses which were far in excess of physiological levels. Thus when Barry et al. (1952) and Holmes (1956) injected ^{14}C[testosterone] into male rats and mice, they found no specific localization in any organ other than that related to the excretion of hormone or its metabolites, whilst Pearlman and Pearlman (1961) identified a number of 5β-androstane derivatives in the prostate, following the infusion of tritiated androstenedione into adult male rats.

The first clear indication that the major metabolism of testosterone in the prostate was through its conversion to 5α-dihydrotestosterone came from the innovative studies of Farnsworth and Brown (1963). They perfused rat prostate with tritiated testosterone and were able to demonstrate the presence of 5α-reductase, 17β-dehydrogenase, 3α-dehydrogenase, and hydroxylase enzymes in this gland, with the major pathway being mediated through the first of these enzymes, resulting in the formation of 5α-dihydrotestosterone. Subsequent studies by Shimazaki et al. (1965a) using in vitro incubation of rat ventral prostate with ^{14}C[testosterone] substantiated these findings. Aliapoulios et al. (1965) infused ^{14}C[testosterone] in adult dogs and found that over 80% of the steroids recovered from the prostate were metabolic products with the major components being 5α-dihydrotestosterone and 5α-androstane-3α,17β-diol respectively. Despite the fact that at the time these investigations were in progress, the relative biological potency of 5α-dihydrotestosterone on the secondary sexual male organs was known to be greater than that of testosterone (Dorfman and Shipley, 1956), the significance of its presence in the rat ventral prostate was not fully realized until the publication of the original works by Anderson and Liao (1968) and Bruchovsky and Wilson (1968a). Their discovery that 5α-dihydrotestosterone was the active metabolite participating in the mechanism of action of androgens in the rat ventral prostate heralded a new era in the endocrinology of the prostate. They found that, following in vivo or in vitro administration of radiolabelled testosterone, over 80% of the radioactivity in the rat ventral prostate nuclei was accounted for by 5α-dihydrotestosterone. This stimulated an expansion of the investigations into the formation of this metabolite and its subsequent interactions with both cytoplasmic and nuclear components of prostatic tissues. Having ascertained that 5α-dihydrotestosterone was the principle androgen metabolite in the prostate, studies were concerned with the investigation of both its binding as well as its inter-relationship with other androgen metabolites in rat ventral prostate. Additionally the research was concerned with establishing whether or not such a metabolic pattern was common to the prostates of other species and equally to other androgen target organs. Most of these studies have supported the view that in the rat ventral prostate and those of several other species the general androgen pathway is similar to that detailed in Figure 6.1. Although this pathway demonstrates the most significant metabolites of testosterone commonly investigated in this gland, it does not attempt to cover the entire scope of the metabolic pathway which can occur in this gland. However it emphasizes those metabolites which are both quantitatively and qualitatively of greater importance in the prostate.

6.1.1   Steroid enzymes in the prostate of experimental animals

The enzymes involved in the metabolism of testosterone in the prostate can be divided into three main groups.

6.1.1.1   Δ⁴-3-Oxosteroid reductase

Two enzymes of this type have been demonstrated in the prostate. Firstly, a 5α-reductase which is responsible for the conversion of testosterone to 5α-dihydrotestosterone and can also convert androstenedione to 5α-androstanedione; this enzyme is extremely important as it is responsible for the formation of the majority of the 5α-dihydrotestosterone present in the tissue. It requires NADPH as an essential cofactor and its action is irreversible. It is predominantly located in the microsomal and nuclear fractions of the rat ventral prostate (Bruchovsky and Wilson, 1968b; Frederiksen and Wilson, 1971; Nozu and Tamaoki, 1973). The 5α-reductase enzyme is not only able to utilize testosterone as its substrate but also androstenedione, progesterone, 17β-hydroxy progesterone, corticosterone and 11-deoxy corticosterone. However, it is not effective on pregnenolone, dehydroepiandrosterone or 1.4 androstadiene-3,17-dione (Nozu and Tamaoki, 1974).

Secondly, the presence of a 5β-reductase has also been reported in this gland, although its activity is significantly less than that of its 5α-isomeric form. This enzyme also requires NADPH supplementation.

6.1.1.2   17β-hydroxysteroid oxidoreductase

This type of enzyme is frequently referred to as 17β-hydroxysteroid de-hydrogenase, but because of its readily reversible action is more aptly termed an oxidoreductase enzyme. 17β-hydroxysteroid oxidoreductases have been found in many tissues (Baulieu and Robel, 1970), have a reversible action, and require NAD, NADPH or their reduced forms as cofactors. Their ability, to interconvert an oxo group at the 17 position to an hydroxy group which possesses greater biological activity, gives these enzymes special importance in the prostate. These enzymes are notable for the conversion of testosterone to androstenedione as well as dihydrotestosterone to androstanedione, and can also convert androstane-3α,17β-diol to androsterone. These enzymes are located in both the soluble and microsomal fractions of the cell but in partieular are associated with the mitochondrial fraction (Shimazaki et al., 1965b; Hussein and Kochakian, 1968).

6.1.1.3 3α (3β)-hydroxysteroid oxidoreductase

This type of enzyme is also commonly referred to as an hydroxysteroid dehydrogenase, but due to its generally reversible action is termed an oxidoreductase enzyme. These enzymes require NAD, NADPH or their reduced counterparts as cofactors. The substrates for these enzymes in the rat prostate are the Δ^4 reduced 5α and 5β catabolites of testosterone and androstenedione. The 3α-oxido reductase is quantitatively by far the most important of these two enzymes and is located in the soluble fraction of the cell, with very little activity associated with the mitochondrial-microsomal fraction (Unhjem, 1970).

The combined action of these two enzymes can result in the production of several isomeric forms of androstanediol from dihydrotestosterone, of which the 5α-androstane-$3\alpha,17\beta$-diol is the most active. The 3α-oxido reductase is also responsible for the conversion of 5α-androstanedione to androsterone, and its isomeric form, epiandrosterone.

6.1.1.4 Other enzymes

In addition to the above three groups of enzymes, there are further conversions demonstrated in Figure 6.1, which relate to the metabolism of dehydroepiandrosterone and 5α-androstane-$3\beta,17\beta$-diol. Firstly, a Δ^5 ketosteroid reductase which appears to convert dehydroepiandrosterone to epiandrosterone and leads subsequently to the formation of 5α-androstane-$3\beta,17\beta$-diol when tritiated dehydroepiandrosterone is used as a substrate (Roy et al., 1972; Robel et al., 1975). Secondly, evidence has also been presented for the activities of 6α and 7α hydroxylase enzymes in the rat ventral prostate (Isaacs et al., 1979). The role of these enzymes and in particular 6α hydroxylase in the formation of 5α-androstane-$3\beta,6\alpha,17\beta$-triol and 5α-androstane-$3\beta,7\alpha,17\beta$-triol is important in forming a final pathway for terminating the androgenic effects of C_{19} androstane steroids in the prostate, via 5α-androstane $3\beta,17\beta$-diol.

6.1.2 Metabolism of testosterone and other androgens in the prostate of experimental animals

The presence of the above mentioned enzyme systems in the rat ventral prostate results in the formation of a diversity of metabolites following exposure of the tissue to radiolabelled testosterone (Figure 6.1). Metabolic studies have been performed using several experimental procedures including the in vitro techniques of direct short term incubation of tissue slices, minces or homogenates (Shimazaki et al., 1969; Gloyna and Wilson, 1969; Unhjem, 1970; Nozu and Tamaoki, 1974), explant culture (Baulieu et al., 1968; Lasnitzki and Franklin, 1972), and superfusion of tissue (Robel et al., 1975), and the in vivo studies by direct administration of labelled androgen (Tveter and Aakvaag, 1969; Bruchovsky, 1971; Buric et al., 1972; Ghanadian et al., 1977b; Smith et al., 1978b) or perfusion (Farnsworth and Brown, 1963). These studies have all contributed to the conclusion that the major metabolism of testosterone in this tissue is through the reductive pathway leading to the formation of 5α-

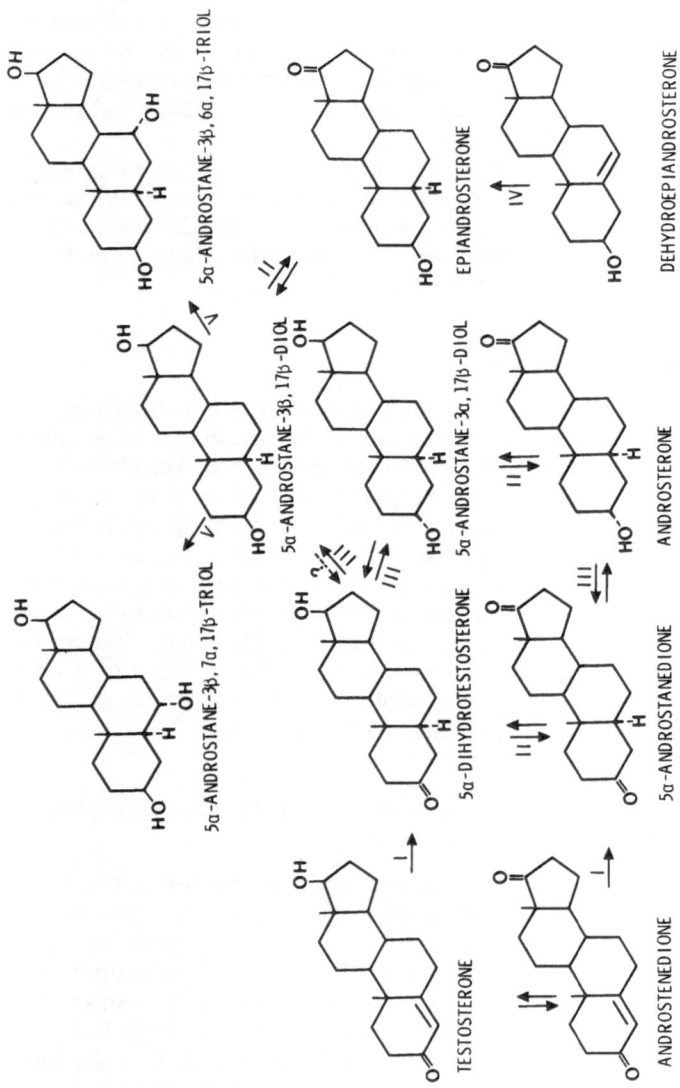

Figure 6.1 Major metabolic pathways of androgens in the rat ventral prostate. The enzymes are: I. Δ⁴-3-oxosteroid 5α-reductase, II. 17β-hydroxysteroid oxidoreductase, III. 3α(3β) hydroxysteroid oxidoreductase, IV. Δ⁵-ketosteroid reductase, V. 6α (7α) hydroxylase. Dotted arrow represents unconfirmed pathway

dihydrotestosterone as the major metabolite, and to a lesser extent the isomeric 5α-androstanediols. When these metabolites have been studied in organ culture, a differential action was observed between dihydrotestosterone and the androstanediols on the maintenance and growth of prostatic explants (Baulieu et al., 1968; Lasnitzki, 1970; Gittinger and Lasnitzki, 1971).

In these metabolic studies, apart from these aforementioned major reductive metabolites, additional reductive metabolites together with a number of oxidative metabolites have also been identified (Figure 6.1), but, depending on the technique employed, the contribution to the metabolite profile made by these compounds varies considerably. These differences in the levels of metabolites depend to a great extent on the activity of enzymic cofactors as well as on the temperature and nature of the tissue preparation employed.

In these types of metabolic studies, when radiolabelled dihydrotestosterone has been employed as the substrate the major recovered androgen has been found to be unaltered dihydrotestosterone (Bruchovsky, 1971; Buric et al., 1972; Robel et al., 1975). The principle metabolites of dihydrotestosterone in these studies have been found to be formed through the reductive pathway leading to androstanediols. Other notable metabolites were 5α-androstanedione and androsterone, although Buric et al. (1972) also recovered small amounts of radiolabelled testosterone and androstenedione. Robel et al. (1975) have clearly shown that the 5α-reduction is an irreversible pathway and hence the identity of these latter two metabolites reported by Buric et al. (1972) is questionable.

Several research groups have also studied the metabolism of 5α-androstane-3α,17β-diol (Bruchovsky, 1971; Robel et al., 1975). All these studies have demonstrated the formation of 5α-dihydrotestosterone as the major metabolic product indicating a readily interconvertible pathway between these two androgens. However, when 5α-androstane-3β,17β-diol has been utilized as the substrate, conflicting data has been obtained. Robel et al. (1975) found that most of the superfused 5α-androstane-3β,17β-diol was converted to several polar and less polar unidentified compounds. They did not find conversion of this androgen to 5α-dihydrotestosterone and the only uniquely identifiable metabolite was epiandrosterone, although small amounts of androstanedione were tentatively identified. However, Krieg et al. (1975) reported that thirty minutes after the injection of 5α-androstane-3β,17β-diol into male rats approximately 32% of the radiometabolite recovered in the prostate was 5α-dihydrotestosterone which is not in agreement with previous reports by Roy et al., (1972) and Robel et al. (1975). However, as this experiment was performed in vivo, this may suggest prior metabolism of the injected substrate at an alternative site in the rat.

Androstenedione has also been utilized as substrate for metabolic studies in the rat ventral prostate (Tveter and Aakvaag, 1969; Bruchovsky, 1971; Roy et al., 1972). These studies have shown the formation of 5α-dihydrotestosterone from androstenedione. They also demonstrated the formation of significant quantities of 5α-androstanedione and androsterone. However, depending upon the experimental procedures the concentration of these radiometabolites has varied considerably. The formation of 5α-dihydrotestosterone in this instance appears to be through the 5α-reduction of androstenedione to the intermediate androgen, namely 5α-androstanedione. The formation of 5α-dihydrotestosterone through testosterone seems to be less significant and, indeed, the formation of testosterone in these studies has been negligible.

The metabolism of 5α-androstanedione, androsterone, epiandrosterone and dehydroepiandrosterone has also been investigated in the rat ventral prostate (Bruchovsky, 1971; Roy et al., 1972). The two interconvertible androgens, 5α-androstanedione and androsterone, can both give rise to the formation of 5α-dihydrotestosterone. Small quantities of 5α-androstanediols are also formed indirectly with 5α-dihydrotestosterone as the intermediary product. When epiandrosterone and dehydroepiandrosterone have been used as substrate in this type of metabolic study, only minimal metabolism has been observed. Dehydroepiandrosterone is found to be partially converted to epiandrosterone and androst-5-ene-3β,17β-diol, whilst epiandrosterone is partially converted to 5α-androstane-3β,17β-diol (Roy et al., 1972). The limited degree of metabolism in this study appears to be due to the inability of the 3β-hydroxyl grouping in these two substrates to be oxidized to a 3-ketone group.

It would appear that the major conclusion which can be drawn from studies into the metabolism of androgens by the rat ventral prostate is that, irrespective of the androgenic precursor utilized as substrate, there is in most cases a tendency towards the formation of the 5α-reduced metabolites of testosterone, but notably 5α-dihydrotestosterone, in this gland. This important aspect of the metabolism of androgens whereby precursor androgens are transformed to their most active derivatives, which are functional in the mechanism of action of these steroids and thereby in controlling growth, has stimulated comparative studies to determine whether this metabolic pattern is a common feature in the prostates of other species. A comprehensive study on 11 different species was conducted by Gloyna and Wilson (1969) in which notable differences in the formation of 5α-dihydrotestosterone were found when using an *in vitro* experimental technique to assay testosterone metabolism. A surprisingly wide range of Δ^4-3-oxosteroid 5α-reductase activities was obtained in the prostates of different species. The highest level of 5α-dihydrotestosterone formation was found to be in the rat ventral prostate followed by the prostatic tissues of man, lion, dog, mouse, guinea-pig, cat, bobcat and finally the bull, in which the level of enzymic activity was virtually undetectable. The values ranged from 569 ± 69 in the rat down to 4 ± 3 pmol per 100 mg tissue hourly in the bull. However, the rate of 5α-dihydrotestosterone formation was distinctly higher in the calf than that of the mature animal. A similar situation has also been reported for the rabbit prostate. Whilst the adult rabbit prostate was found to have only a limited capacity for testosterone 5α-reduction, at birth 5α-reductase activity was detectable but declined with maturity (Wilson and Gloyna, 1970; Wilson and Lasnitzki, 1971; Booth and Jones, 1979).

The conversion of testosterone to its major 5α-reduced metabolites has also been demonstrated in the prostate of both the male and female of the African rodent *Praomys* (*Mastomys*) *natalensis*. The female of this species possesses a well developed prostate and thus this species has provided a useful model for prostatic research. (Ghanadian et al., 1975; Ghanadian et al., 1976). In a series of *in vivo* and *in vitro* studies utilizing tritiated testosterone, it was found that the major radiometabolite bound in the cytoplasmic and nuclear fractions of the prostate in both the male and female animals was 5α-dihydrotestosterone (Ghanadian *et al.*, 1977a, 1978; Smith *et al.*, 1978a, 1979). The levels of other metabolites in these studies were comparatively low as only the bound steroid fraction of the cytoplasmic and nuclear preparations were analysed. Nevertheless, the presence of the 5α-reductase in the prostate of the female in this species is particularly noteworthy.

More attention has been paid to the metabolism of androgens in the prostate of the dog. One of the main reasons for this is the fact that this animal shares with man an age-dependent tendency towards the development of benign prostatic hyperplasia and adenocarcinoma of the prostate (Moore, 1944; Huggins, 1945). Early studies on the metabolism of testosterone by the canine prostate using infusion techniques indicated the presence of the three major enzymes already described for the rat ventral prostate (Aliapoulios *et al.*, 1965). They found the major metabolites to be dihydrotestosterone and 5α-androstane-3α,17β-diol and confirmed the presence of 17β-hydroxysteroid and 3α-hydroxysteroid oxidoreductase as well as Δ⁴-3-oxosteroid 5α- reductase. Subsequent studies by this group (Morfin *et al.*, 1970; Ofner *et al.*, 1975) reported that whilst in the *in vivo* studies 5α-dihydrotestosterone remained the major radiometabolite of testosterone, the 3β-reduced metabolites isoandrosterone and 5α-androstane-3β,17β-diol predominated over the 3α epimers, androsterone and 5α-androstane-3α,17β-diol. Additionally using an *in vitro* technique a substantial interconversion between 5α-androstane-3α,17β-diol to 5α-dihydrotestosterone (40%) was found to occur, whilst in contrast only a low conversion of the 3β epimer was found (6%). This is in agreement with reports that the activity of the 3α-hydroxysteroid dehydrogenase in this tissue is exceedingly high, under conditions when prostate growth is stimulated (Jacobi *et al.*, 1978a). Using an *in vitro* incubation technique Griffiths *et al.*, 1970 and Harper *et al.*, 1971 also showed 5α-dihydrotestosterone to be the main metabolite of testosterone in canine prostatic tissues and suggested the presence of 17α-hydroxysteroid dehydrogenase and its possible localization in the nucleus. They found epitestosterone, 5α-androstane-3α,17α-diol and 5α-androstane-3β,17α-diol as well as the 17β-diol isomers reported by other groups. A functional role for 5α-androstane-3α,17α-diol in the mechanism of action of androgens in the dog prostate was later indicated by Evans and Pierrepoint (1975, 1976). However, this finding has not been confirmed by another group (Ofner *et al.*, 1979). Perfusion (Haltmeyer and Eik-Nes, 1972; Eik-Nes, 1975) and superfusion (Giorgi *et al.*, 1972) techniques have also provided further support for the conversion of testosterone to 5α-dihydrotestosterone in the canine prostate. In addition, the interconversion of androstenedione and testosterone and the ability of the dog prostate to secrete 5α-dihydrotestosterone into the superfusate with either of these precursors have also been reported by Giorgi *et al.*, 1972. Most of these studies have indicated a similarity between the metabolic pattern obtained with canine prostatic preparation and those with human prostatic tissues.

Apart from the studies which have been performed on the dog prostate which relate to the development of benign hypertrophy in this animal, recent work has also been reported on the metabolism of androgens by prostatic tissues of primates. The prostate of primates consists of two discrete lobes, namely a caudal and a cranial, which have been compared to the peripheral and central zones of the human prostate (Blacklock and Bouskill, 1977). *In vitro* studies on the entire gland by Arora-Dinakar *et al.*, 1977 indicated that 5α-dihydrotestosterone was the major radiometabolite of testosterone in this gland. Subsequent studies on the separate lobes of this prostate confirmed that 5α-dihydrotestosterone was the main metabolite in both the caudal and cranial lobes and that significant amounts of the 5α-androstanediols were also formed. Other metabolites identified were androsterone, 5α-androstanedione and androstenedione (Ghanadian and Smith, 1981; Ghanadian, 1981). No significant differences were noted between the metabolic pathways in the two lobes. It would appear that the main enzymes reported for the rat and dog prostates are also active in this tissue.

6.2 ANDROGEN METABOLISM IN THE HUMAN PROSTATE

Studies on androgen metabolism in the human prostate with regard to both the normal gland and its tumours, have been of particular importance in view of the complexity of this tissue. Since studies on the mechanism of action of androgens in the prostate have clearly demonstrated the important role of the initial conversion of testosterone to 5α-dihydrotestosterone, it has proved essential to investigate the scope of enzymic activity and the metabolic products of testosterone within the normal, benign hypertrophied and malignant tissues. Most studies have concentrated on the benign hyper-trophied gland since it has been readily available in both large numbers and quantities. In general, studies on this tissue have benefited from the more frequent use of surgical material obtained by retropubic prostatectomy. However, with the decline in the last decade in the use of this surgical technique, more data has been reported using tissue provided by transurethral resection. Whilst the tissue obtained from the former technique is preferable, in that it is both large and has not been exposed to unfavourable conditions, the latter is only obtained as relatively small chips with a burned periphery which must be effectively removed in order to obtain comparatively reliable material. Surgical specimens of malignant tumours are virtually always obtained by the latter technique and hence data obtained from this material require cautious interpretation. Another consideration which must be taken into account when analysing data of prostatic tumours and which is especially relevant to the malignant disease is any conservative treatment which patients have received prior to surgery such as endocrine or X-ray therapy. In contrast to the tumour tissues, most normal prostatic specimens are obtained either by total cystectomy on patients with bladder tumours or from cadavers. In relation to the former, consideration must again be given to conservative management of the bladder tumour which may have had an effect on the prostate, whilst in the latter the time interval between death and removal of the organ is an important aspect. Additionally, the presence of any form of prostatic disease and, in particular, the existence of benign hypertrophy in the elderly cases must be ruled out.

6.2.1   Normal prostate

Relatively fewer studies have been carried out on the normal human prostate due to the problems in having a readily available supply. Nevertheless, by employing a number of different techniques using tritiated testosterone as substrate, the formation of 5α-dihydrotestosterone as the principle metabolite has been established (Giorgi et al., 1971; Mainwaring and Milroy, 1973). Furthermore, as in the animal studies previously described, an important role has also been found for the 3α and 3β hydroxysteroid oxidoreductase in that the 5α-androstanediols contribute significantly to the metabolites in this tissue. The presence of other oxidative and reductive metabolites, namely androstenedione, androstanedione, androsterone and isoandrosterone, has also been reported (Djoseland et al., 1977; Morfin et al., 1978). The latter group have also indicated a role for 6β and 7α-hydroxylations of 5α-androstane-3α,17β-diol in the normal human prostate, resulting in the formation of significant quantities of 5α-androstane-3α,7α,17β-triol and 5α-androstane-3β,6β,17β-triol (Morfin et al., 1977). The possible formation of the latter compounds in relation to the predominant pathway of androgens in the normal human prostate is depicted in Figure 6.2. The in vitro criteria which may influence the metabolic pattern of androgens include the substrate concentration, enzymic cofactor requirement, the time and temperature of incubation and the buffering system used, all of which require careful examination (Bruchovsky and Lieskovsky, 1979). Another important factor which has considerable bearing on the metabolic profile is the nature of the cellular preparation. The use of minces, homogenates, microsomal, nuclear and cytoplasmic fractions has been reported by Morfin et al. (1978), and an indication that the possible discrete localization of some of the enzymes involved in androgen metabolism may lead to a distortion of the metabolic pattern. The wide range of experimental methodology employed by different research groups, varying from tissue or cell fraction incubation studies, referred to above, to the use of superfusion and long term organ culture methods, has given rise to a wide spectrum in the ratio of both reductive and oxidative metabolites in these studies. However, the general consensus with regard to androgen metabolism in the normal human prostate confirms a strong trend towards the reductive pathway and in particular the formation of 5α-dihydrotestosterone.

6.2.2   Benign hypertrophied prostate

Studies on androgen metabolism in this tissue have far exceeded those on either the normal or malignant prostate. As long ago as 1954, Wotiz and Lemon attempted to study testosterone metabolism in this tissue. However, the lack of high specific radiolabelled steroid prevented an adequate conclusion. The first breakthrough came from studies by Farnsworth et al., 1962 and Farnsworth and Brown (1963) who clearly demonstrated the presence of both reductive and oxidative pathways in both minces and slices of this tissue, and showed that the major metabolite is 5α-dihydrotestosterone, followed by 5α-androstane-3α,17β-diol and androstenedione. Other notable metabolites in these studies were androsterone and 5α-androstanedione. In common with studies of the metabolism of androgens by normal human prostate, a critical evaluation of the methodological approach is essential when studies are performed with the hypertrophied tissues. In general, *in vitro* studies may be classified into three types depending upon the nature of the tissue preparations and experimental conditions, namely, short term incubation of tissue slices (Farnsworth and Brown, 1963; Attramadal *et al.*, 1975) or minces (Acevado and Goldzieher, 1965; Shimazaki, *et al.*, 1965a; Jenkins and McCaffery, 1974; Harper *et al.*, 1974; Orestano *et al.*, 1974; Morfin *et al.*, 1975), short term incubation of homogenate (Chamberlain *et al.*, 1966; Ofner *et al.*, 1970; Becker *et al.*, 1975; Cowan *et al.*, 1977; Morfin *et al.*, 1978; Bruchovsky and Lieskovsky, 1979), subcellular fractions (Chamberlain *et al.*, 1966; Habib *et al.*, 1979) and finally longer term tissue culture procedures (Mabin *et al.*, 1970; Bard and Lasnitzki, 1977; Lasnitzki, 1979; Smith *et al.*, 1980). In addition, the use of superfusion techniques have also been reported (Giorgi *et al.*, 1971; Malathi and Gurpide, 1977). These reports have complemented each other, and resulted in the identification in this tissue of three major classes of enzymes namely:

  (i) Δ^4-3-oxosteroid 5α-reductase
  (ii) 17β-hydroxysteroid oxidoreductase
  (iii) 3α-and 3β-hydroxysteroid oxidoreductase

Additionally, evidence supporting the presence of 2β-,6β-and 7α-hydroxylases (Acevado and Goldzieher, 1965; Morfin *et al.*, 1980) has been presented. Farnsworth (1966) has reported the metabolism of testosterone to 19-nor androstane analogs, which suggests the presence of enzymes responsible for 10-demethylation and subsequent conversion to 2-methoxy oestrone, which is indicative of the aromatization of androgens to oestrogens in this tissue. The presence of dehydroepiandrosterone sulphate sulphatase was also first reported by Farnsworth (1975) and subsequently confirmed by Cowan *et al.* (1977) and was shown to be responsible for the conversion of dehydroepiandrosterone sulphate to dehydroepiandrosterone (DHEA). Some evidence that the latter may be further converted to 5α-reduced metabolites of testosterone has been provided by Collins *et al.*, 1970, and Harper *et al.*, 1974. This indicates the possible presence of a Δ^5-ketosteroid isomerase/3β-hydroxysteroid dehydrogenase complex and also a Δ^5-ketosteroid reductase which would be in keeping with the metabolic pattern exhibited by the rat ventral prostate. The presence of a 5β-reductase enzyme has also been reported by Chamberlain *et al.* (1966), but subsequent studies by Ofner *et al.* (1970) did not confirm their original suggestions.

The metabolic pathway of androgens and its related enzymes in the human tissue is demonstrated in Figure 6.2. The important feature of the metabolic pathway of androgens shown in this figure is the predominant role of the reductive pathway. Most studies using benign hypertrophied tissues have demonstrated substantial 5α-reductase and 3α(3β)hydroxysteroid oxidored-

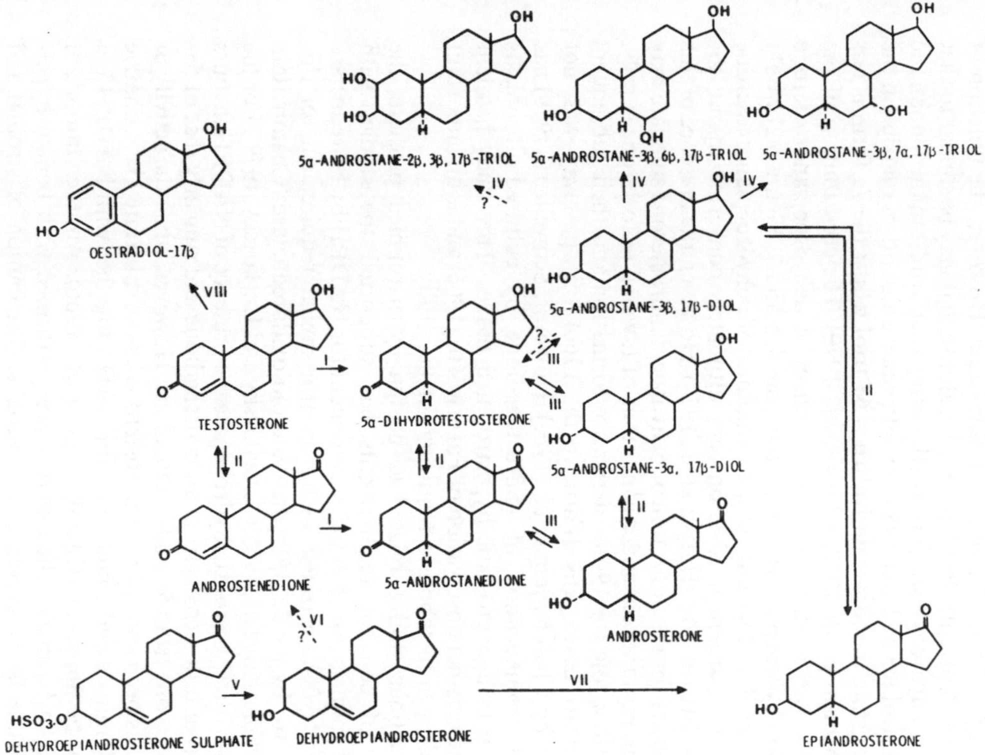

Figure 6.2 Major metabolic pathways in human prostatic tissues. Unconfirmed pathways are shown by dotted arrows

The enzymes are: I. Δ⁴-3-oxosteroid 5α-reductase, II. 17β-hydroxysteroid oxidoreductase, III. 3α(3β) hydroxysteroid oxidoreductase, IV. 2β(6β) or 7α-hydroxylase, V. Dehydroepiandrosterone sulphate-sulphatase, VI. Δ⁵-ketosteroid isomerase/3β-hydroxysteroid dehydrogenase, VII. Δ⁵-ketosteroid-reductase, VIII. 10 Demethylase/aromatization uctase activities, which result in the recovery of 5α-dihydrotestosterone and the isomeric 5α-androstanediols as the major metabolites. The oxidative metabolism in this tissue tends to be much less active, when compared to the reductive route, but does result in limited formation of androstenedione and 5α-androstanedione. The function of the hydroxylase enzymes acting at the 6β and 7α positions has been reported by Morfin et al. (1978) to be associated with the disposal of androgens through the conversion of 5α-androstane-3β,17β-diol to hydroxylated triol derivatives in this gland. However, the function of 2β-hydroxylase is currently less understood, although it may be similar to that of the other two hydroxylases. It is worth noting that, whilst in the human the predominant triol formed is the 7α triol with small amounts of 6β triol, in the rat ventral prostate the major derivative is 6α triol whilst the 7α form is less significant (Morfin et al., 1978; Isaacs et al., 1979). The contribution of the three enzymes associated with the metabolism of dehydroepiandrosterone sulphate and dehydroepiandrosterone (enzyme 4, 5 and 7, Figure 6.2) would appear to be small, in that only limited amounts of dehydroepiandrosterone sulphate and dehydroepiandrosterone are ultimately converted to the 5α-reduced derivatives in vitro (Harper et al., 1974). However, the presence of this potential capacity for the utilization of dehydroepiandrosterone sulphate may play a more important role under conditions of lowered testosterone supply. With regard to a role for 19-nor derivative formation and their subsequent aromatization to oestrogens (Farnsworth, 1966) this pathway was not demonstrable by Chamberlain et al. (1966). However, Schweikert (1979) has reported the aromatization of androstenedione by cultured fibroblasts obtained from benign prostatic hypertrophied tissues. This study has lent support to the original observation of Farnsworth (1966) and is an important aspect of androgen metabolism requiring further study.

In the metabolic studies related to benign hypertrophied prostate, the investigation of cofactor requirements has supported the studies with experimental animals. An essential requirement for NADPH by 5α-reductase has been clearly demonstrated, as has been a similar requirement for this reduced cofactor by the 3α(3β)hydroxysteroid oxidoreductase (Chamberlain et al., 1966; Shimazaki et al., 1965b; Bruchovsky and Lieskovsky, 1979). For the action of 17β-hydroxysteroid dehydrogenase the presence of NADPH favours the formation of testosterone from androstenedione and similarly that of 5α-dihydrotestosterone from 5α-androstanedione. However, when the activity of this enzyme has been studied with testosterone as the substrate, the oxidative role can predominate and a preference for NAD^+ together with $NADPH^+$ as cofactor may be apparent (Chamberlain et al., 1966). Another important consideration to be made when studies are performed with benign hyper-trophied prostate is the presence of a variable distribution of stromal and epithelial elements which contribute unevenly to the enzymic activities of this gland. Cowan et al., 1977, Romijn et al., 1980 and Bruchovsky et al., 1980 have separated prostatic tissues into stromal and epithelial fractions and found that the activity of 5α-reductase was considerably higher in the stromal than in the epithelial fraction. Romijn et al. (1980) also found that metabolism observed in a single cell suspension prepared by enzymic treatment of stromal tissue was different in both quantitative and qualitative aspects from that in untreated stromal tissue. The single cell suspension was not only more active with regard to 5α-reductase but also had a very high 17β-hydroxysteroid oxidoreductase activity and appeared to resemble the metabolism observed in fibroblasts derived from benign hyperplastic prostatic tissues as reported by Schweikert *et al.* (1980). The study by Bruchovsky *et al.* (1980) also found that the distribution of 3α(3β) hydroxysteroid oxidoreductase was more evenly divided between the two cell types. Cowan *et al.* (1977) studied the activity of dehydroepiandrosterone sulphate sulphatase in this tissue and found it to be predominantly a constituent of the epithelial cells.

Studies on the intracellular distribution of the three major enzymes present in benign hypertrophied human prostate, namely 5α-reductase, 17β-hydroxysteroid oxidoreductase and the 3α(3β)hydroxysteroid oxidoreductase, have indicated that the first enzyme is predominantly localized in the soluble fraction, although it is associated somewhat with the light microsomal particulate material. The 17β-hydroxysteroid oxidoreductase is mainly localized in the particulate material and appears to have an association with the mitochondrial fraction, whilst finally the 3α(3β)oxidoreductases are wholly found within the soluble cellular fraction (Chamberlain *et al.*, 1966).

6.2.3 Malignant prostate

The metabolism of androgens in malignant prostatic tissues warrants equivalent consideration to that of the benign tumours as its role in the mechanism of action of androgens in this tissue is equally important. Data obtained in early studies has provided a rather diverse picture of the metabolic pattern of androgens in this tumour (Lemon *et al.*, 1953; Wotiz and Lemon, 1954; Breuer *et al.*, 1959; Acevado and Goldzieher, 1965; Shimazaki *et al.*, 1965a). Despite the fact that these studies resulted in the demonstration of a number of the enzymes associated with androgen metabolism, no clear consensus as to the major metabolic pathway in the malignant tissue was obtained. Several factors, including the type, the extent and distribution of the malignant cells within the gland, as well as the existence of the benign tumours within the same specimen, may all have had a bearing on the diversity of these results. These considerations are additional to those relating to the methodology employed and previously discussed in relation to experimentation with the benign tumour. Undoubtedly the most critical consideration in this tissue must be given to the confirmation of malignancy within the tissue utilized for enzymic studies, in order to ensure that if the tumour is only confined to discrete focal regions a portion of these areas, and not regions of non-malignant tissue, are analysed. Secondly, within the broad spectrum of malignancy, the degree of cellular differentiation which ranges from well through to poorly differentiated carcinomas must be taken into account when considering the results.

More recent studies have established that, although most of the enzymes present in the normal and benign tumours are also functional in carcinomatous tissue, the overall metabolic activity is diminished in the less differentiated specimens (Jenkins and McCaffery, 1974; Djoseland *et al.*, 1977; Morfin *et al.*, 1977). Other groups have reported that this reduction in metabolic activity is a general feature of the malignant tumour (Bard and Lasnitzki, 1977; Bruchovsky and Lieskovsky, 1979; Ghanadian *et al.*, 1979; Krieg *et al.*, 1978; Habib, 1980; Smith *et al.*, 1980). This point has been clearly demonstrated by studies carried out on BPH and carcinomatous tissues with varying degrees of differentiation by Morfin *et al.* (1977). Whilst the overall metabolism was lower in general for the carcinomatous tissues, in those instances where significant metabolism was present, the metabolism was of an oxidative nature in contrast to the reductive metabolism seen in the benign tissue. Using organ culture for 20 hours, Bard and Lasnitzki (1977) also reported that most carcinomas produced less dihydrotestosterone from testosterone than found in benign hyperplastic tissues. However, no relationship was observed between metabolism and the degree of differentiation despite the fact that a proportion of the carcinoma samples formed higher levels of 17-oxo derivatives. Smith *et al.* (1980) using a similar organ culture technique for 48 hours have found a consistent formation of 17-oxo derivatives as the major metabolites of testosterone in carcinoma samples irrespective of the degree of differentiation. Androstenedione contributed more than 59 % of the overall recovered metabolites followed by 5α-androstanediols (16.8 %), dihydrotestosterone (14.3 %), 5α-androstanedione (4.5 %) and androsterone (1.8 %). In our studies, when 5α-dihydrotestosterone is used as substrate in this system, the ability of the carcinomatous tissue to form the 5α-androstanediols does not appear to be impaired. This would suggest that, whilst the 5α-reductase activity is reduced in cancer tumours, no apparent change in the activity of the 3α (3β)hydroxysteroid oxidoreductase could be observed. When androstenedione was used as substrate by Bard and Lasnitzki, 1977, small amounts of testosterone and 5α-androstanedione were formed together with their further reduced products. Kliman *et al.* (1978) have studied metabolism of testosterone by both primary and secondary metastatic carcinomatous prostatic tissues and found that, whilst metabolism by the primary tumour was lower than that observed under similar conditions in benign tumours, the metabolism from metastatic deposits of regional lymph nodes was significantly lower than that of the tissue from the primary sites. Thus it may be concluded that, whilst the metabolism of androgen is greatly decreased in malignant tumours, there is a shift in direction towards a more oxidative pathway with diminished reductive products, despite the clear presence of all the major enzyme systems shown in Figure 6.2.

6.2.4 Comparison between androgen metabolism in normal, benign and malignant prostates

Comparative studies between the three types of tissue have concentrated mostly on the benign hypertrophied and carcinomatous tissues, whilst studies involving the normal gland are fewer, this being generally due to the lack of supply of suitable normal tissue. As previously mentioned, normal tissue can be obtained either from operative procedures, in particular following total cystectomy for cancer of the bladder, or from cadaver sources which may suffer through the time interval elapsing between death and dissection of the gland. In the metabolic studies several factors, including the nature of the tissue preparation, the relationship between the levels of steroid substrate, cofactor and the enzyme, as well as differences in methods of presenting data, have contributed to the diversity of the results which have appeared in the literature. In order to overcome some of these differences and to present the results in a reasonably uniform fashion the percentage of the substrate metabolized can be taken as an indication of the overall metabolic activity present, whilst the relationship between the metabolites of the substrate in terms of percentage formed, leads to a clearer indication of any differences present in the metabolites produced by these three types of tissue. Despite the presence of a common enzymic pathway in the three types of tissue, it would appear that there are differences in the enzymic activity between the normal, benign hypertrophied and malignant prostates. From a close examination of the available data it may be seen that the metabolic activity in the benign hypertrophied tissue is greater than that in the normal gland which in turn has itself greater activity than the malignant tumours.

With regard to the enzymic activities present in the normal and benign hypertrophied prostate the general consensus is of the opinion that enzymes 1 and 2, i.e. 5α-reductase and $3\alpha(3\beta)$oxidoreductase, are the two most important enzymes, when one considers their relative contributions to the metabolites of testosterone in the gland. The role of these enzymes in the formation of dihydrotestosterone from either testosterone or by interconversion of 5α-androstane-$3\alpha,17\beta$-diol appears to be a central aspect in controlling the level of 5α-dihydrotestosterone, whilst the role of 3β-oxidoreductase in the formation of 5α-androstane-$3\beta,17\beta$-diol, which is an essentially irreversible reaction, is more involved in the formation of hydroxylated triol derivatives, which have been suggested to be a means by which androgens may be disposed of by the human prostate (Morfin et al., 1978; Morfin et al., 1980). The requirement of NADPH by both the 5α-reductase and the $3\alpha(3\beta)$ oxidoreductase enzymes has been established (Chamberlain et al., 1966) and appears to play a significant role in determining the amount of 5α-dihydrotestosterone in the gland. By giving consideration to some of the more detailed factors obtained from studies in the role of these enzymes and their cofactors in the rat ventral prostate and, in particular, those relating to the independence of the 3α- and 3β-reduction of 5α-dihydrotestosterone from hormonal control and additionally the maintenance of 5α-androstane-$3\beta,17\beta$-diol secretion by the prostate (Robel et al., 1971; Shimazaki et al., 1972; Moore and Wilson, 1976), it has been suggested that the endogenous reduced cofactors are utilized at first for the formation of constant levels of 5α-androstane-$3\beta,17\beta$-diol and its triol derivatives and thereby limiting the formation of 5α-androstane-$3\alpha,17\beta$-diol from 5α-dihydrotestosterone in the prostate (Morfin et al., 1978). Based on such a model it could be envisaged that an increase in 5α-reductase activity would be accompanied by a decline in the 3α-reduction of the 5α-dihydrotestosterone and since 3β-reduction of the latter would remain constant, this could lead to an increase of the level of 5α-dihydrotestosterone. Bruchovsky and Lieskovsky (1979) have reported such an increase in 5α-reductase activity in hypertrophied tissue which is associated with a decline in the combined activities of $3\alpha(3\beta)$ oxidoreductase when compared with the normal gland. This could possibly support the view discussed by Morfin et al. (1978) that dihydrotestosterone is able to accumulate in benign hyperplastic tissue mainly from back transformation of 5α-androstane 3α,17β-diol and 5α-androstane-dione involving available endogenous cofactors, whilst 5α-androstane-3β,17β-diol formation from 5α-dihydrotestosterone remains constant in both the normal and benign tissues and plays a role in prostatic secretion. However, the question as to whether or not the accumulation of androgen in benign hypertrophied tissue is, in itself, responsible for the raised 5α-reductase activity is also pertinent. Indeed the enhanced capacity of the benign tumour to take up androgen may be due to increased non-specific binding sites (Giorgi et al., 1974) which would allow an increase in the activity of 5α-reductase, as it has been indicated that pharmacological amounts of androgens can increase the activity of this enzyme in the rat (Shimazaki et al., 1972; Moore and Wilson, 1973). Although a heightened 5α-reductase activity is plainly apparent in benign hypertrophied tissue, whether this results directly from an enzymic disorder or indirectly through secondary stimulation of enzymic activity following the accumulation of androgen, or a combination of both, is not clear. However, if the second of these possibilities is operative in benign hypertrophied tissue, then the observation, that in malignant tumours there is slightly raised androgen concentration (Habib et al., 1976; Farnsworth and Brown, 1976; Geller et al., 1978) together with lowered 5α-reductase activity when compared to the normal, would necessitate the prediction of a fault in the relationship between androgen and its stimulation of enzymic activity in the malignant tumour.

As well as the importance of the comparative aspects of the 5α-reductase enzyme the activity of 3α(3β)hydroxysteroid oxidoreductase is equally important, when considering the fate of 5α-dihydrotestosterone. A comparison of the activity of this enzyme between the normal and benign hypertrophied tissues has been made by Jacobi and Wilson (1977) and Bruchovsky and Lieskovsky (1979). The former found the formation of 3α(3β) androstanediol to be significantly higher in microsomes and cytosol of the benign hypertrophied prostate than in the normal gland. Conversely the latter authors found the activity of this enzyme in tissue homogenate to be slightly but significantly ($p < 0.025$) lower in the benign tissue when compared to the normal gland. The discrepancy between these two well documented studies may lie in the nature of tissue preparations utilized. Morfin et al. (1978) have studied all three types of preparation in the same tissue samples and found that, whilst no significant difference was found in the enzyme activity of homogenate between the normal and hyperplastic tissues, microsomes of the former had significantly more enzymic activity than the latter, whilst the complete reverse was apparent in cytoplasmic preparation. However, the data reported by Shida et al. (1975) Djoseland et al. (1977) and Krieg et al. (1979) would suggest a trend towards a lower level of this enzyme in benign tissue relative to the normal gland. The comparison of activity of this enzyme between benign and carcinomatous prostate appears to show a tendency towards the level in carcinoma being marginally lower (Bruchovsky and Liekovsky, 1979; Krieg et al., 1979). Further studies on the comparative aspects of the 3α(3β) oxidoreductase would be advantageous in clarifying the role of this enzyme, particularly in view of the higher level of 5α-androstane-

$3\alpha,17\beta$-diol in carcinoma of the prostate compared with the benign tumour (Ghanadian and Puah, 1981) and the lower levels of the 5α-androstanediols reported in benign tumours when compared to the normal (Geller *et al.*, 1976).

When making a comparison between the malignant tumour and normal or benign hyperplastic tissues it is plainly evident that not only the 5α-reductase activity is markedly diminished but also a major contribution to the metabolites is made through the oxidative pathways in the malignant tissues, as compared to the predominantly reductive route in the benign hypertrophied tissue (Figure 6.3).

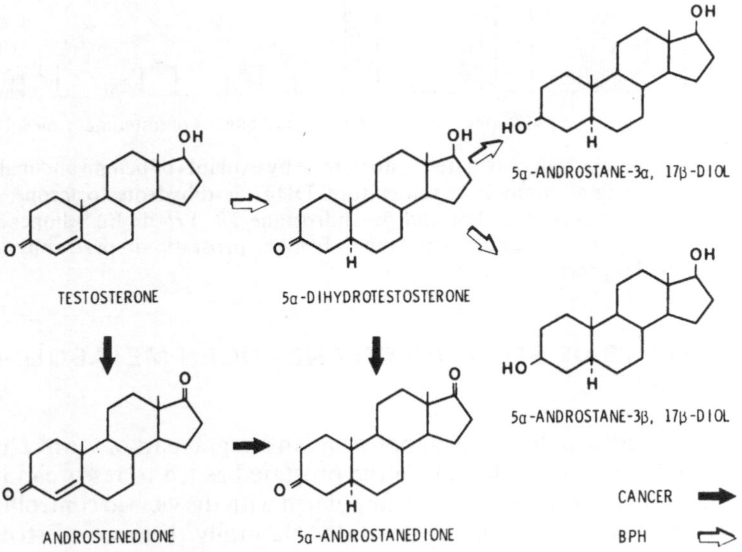

Figure 6.3 Predominant pathways of testosterone metabolism in benign and malignant human prostates

The oxidation of testosterone by 17β-hydroxysteroid oxidoreductase to androstenedione is a prominent feature in cancer tissue (Morfin *et al.*, 1977; Ghanadian *et al.*, 1979; Habib, 1980). It would appear that there is greater tendency towards this conversion in the less well differentiated carcinoma. However, some reports have not substantiated this trend (Bard and Lasnitzki, 1977). It must be emphasized that, whilst the reduced metabolic activity of androgens is the main feature of prostatic carcinoma, the ability of the tissue to utilize the oxidative enzymic pathway *in vitro* may be of great value as a discriminator in assessing prostatic carcinomas (Ghanadian *et al.*, 1981). This factor is graphically illustrated in the comparative study of testosterone metabolism between benign and malignant prostatic tissues carried out in our laboratory (Figure 6.4).

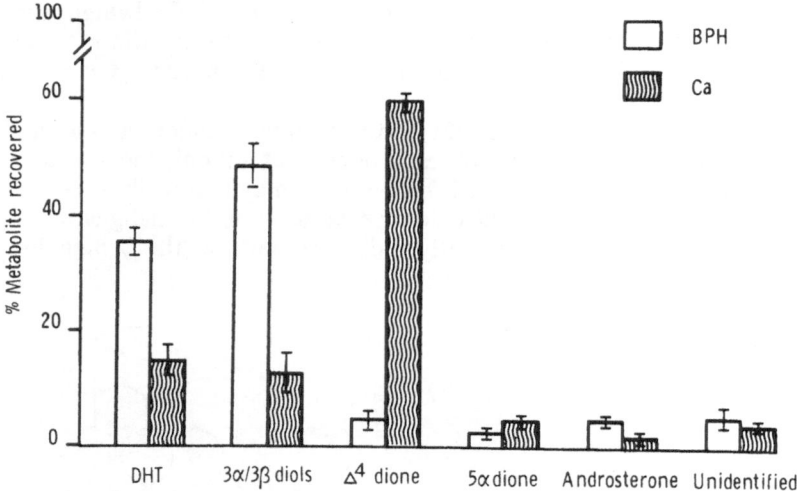

Figure 6.4 Metabolism of tritiated testosterone by explants of benign and malignant prostates following 48 hours in organ culture. DHT: 5α-dihydrotestosterone; 3α/3β-diols: 5α-androstane-3α, 17β-diol and 5α-androstane-3β, 17β-diol;Δ⁴-dione: androstenedione; 5α-dione: 5α-androstanedione; benign prostatic hypertrophy: BPH; carcinoma of the prostate: Ca

6.3 EFFECTS OF STEROIDS ON ANDROGEN METABOLISM IN THE PROSTATE

The importance of androgen metabolism as an integral part of the mechanism of action of this class of steroids in the prostate has led to research into the means by which this stage may be manipulated with the view to controlling the interaction of androgens in the prostate. Naturally, because of structural considerations, the main candidates for these types of inhibitory studies have been the natural and synthetic steroid hormones, although a number of non-steroidal compounds have also been employed. In both animal and human studies, the most commonly used hormones have been either oestrogens, androgens or progestational compounds of which the oestrogens have been most widely employed compounds. Lee *et al.* (1973) have examined the effect of more than 25 oestrogenic derivatives on the 5α-reduction of testosterone in the rat ventral prostate and have found that the majority were able to inhibit this enzyme to a marked extent. Oestradiol-17β was found to be the most effective with its ester derivatives being the next most potent group, the 17-glucoronide and 3-sulphate conjugates together with oestradiol isomers were all less effective inhibitors, whilst the 3-methoxy derivatives of oestradiol and oestriol were poor inhibitors. Additionally Nozu and Tamaoki (1974) found that diethylstilboestrol and etienic acid, as well as a number of other natural and synthetic compounds including progesterone, 17β-hydroxy progesterone and 11-deoxycorticosterone, were also effective in reducing the activity of 5α-reductase of the rat ventral prostate. However, the inhibitory effect of diethylstilboestrol on 5α-reductase has been a matter of some controversy. Whilst Lee *et al.* (1973) and Belham and Neal (1971) found negligible effect of stilboestrol on this enzyme, both Shimazaki *et al.* (1965a) and Groom *et al.* (1971) found some effect in this tissue. The *in vivo* studies have tended to indicate negligible effects by oestrogens on the activity of 5α-reductase (Fencl and Villee, 1973 and Lee *et al.*, 1975), although in *in vivo* studies oestrogens have several diverse effects which could account for the apparent discrepancy with the *in vitro* results. The effect of prolactin on the metabolism of testosterone has also been investigated by Thomas and Manandhar (1975). Although this hormone has been shown to act on the prostate, whether or not it exerts a direct effect on the activity of steroid enzymes requires further clarification.

More studies have been carried out with regard to the inhibition of 5α-reductase in human prostatic tumours. In general, most studies indicate that in both the benign and malignant human prostates oestrogens exert an inhibitory effect on the 5α-reductase activity of these tumours (Shimazaki *et al.*, 1965a; Farnsworth, 1969; Jenkins and McCaffery, 1974; Bard and Lasnitzki, 1977; Habib *et al.*, 1979). Similarly diethylstilboestrol has also been shown to be effective in reducing the activity of this enzyme. However, these studies should be considered in relation to the effective dose required in order to achieve enzymic inhibition. The high levels utilized to obtain *in vitro* inhibition may have little or no relevance to the clinical situation and are far in excess of the levels which are known to achieve hormonal suppression in clinical practice. This would suggest that, although oestrogens are plainly capable of inhibiting the 5α-reduction of testosterone, the major clinical manifestation of oestrogen treatment is via an alternative mechanism. The effect of progestational compounds on androgen metabolism has also been examined. Studies by Jenkins and McCaffery (1974), Orestano *et al.* (1974) and Morfin *et al.* (1975) have indicated a direct inhibitory effect of either progesterone or 19-nor-17α-hydroxy progesterone caproate on the conversion of testosterone to 5α-dihydrotestosterone in human prostatic tumours. Some of this effect is related to the direct competition by progesterone for the enzyme (Morfin *et al.*, 1975). In these studies a notably smaller quantity of progestational compound was required to achieve an equivalent inhibition to that observed with tested oestrogens. This would suggest that these compounds may prove more valuable in a clinical approach involving enzymic control of the tumour. It is noteworthy, however, that cyproterone acetate which is an antiandrogen with a 17α-hydroxy progesterone structure does not have any significant effect in reducing the 5α-reductase activity (Rennie and Bruchovsky, 1973; Giorgi *et al.*, 1974; Nozu and Tamaoki, 1974; Neumann *et al.*, 1975).

6.4 METABOLISM OF STEROIDS OTHER THAN ANDROGENS

The metabolism of oestrogens and progesterone has been studied using both benign and malignant tumours of the human prostate. Acevado and Goldzieher (1964) found evidence for the conversion of oestrone to oestradiol-17β, to oestriol, to 3-hydroxy oestrone and also to 2-methoxy oestrone. This would indicate the presence of 17β-hydroxy dehydrogenase, 16-hydroxylase, 2-hydroxylase and O-methyltransferase in both types of prostatic tumours. The reversibility of the oestrone and oestradiol-17β pathway has also been reported by Mabin *et al.* (1970) in benign hypertrophied prostate using an organ culture technique for their metabolic studies. The importance of this interconversion and, in general, the ability of prostatic tumours to metabolize oestrogens is related to the possible role of these steroid hormones in the aetiology of prostatic tumours, as has been demonstrated experimentally in the dog prostate (DeKlerk *et al.*, 1979).

The metabolism of progesterone has also been studied in benign hypertrophied prostate (Acevado and Goldzieher, 1965; Morfin *et al.*, 1975). The former group indicated the presence of enzymes for the 5α-reduction, 20α-oxido reduction and the 6β-hydroxylation of progesterone. Morfin *et al.* (1975) confirmed the presence of 5α-reductase and 6β-hydroxylase activities and additionally found evidence for a very active 3β-hydroxy C_{21} steroid dehydrogenase. They noted that 5α-reduction of progesterone was carried out by the same enzyme which converts testosterone to 5α-dihydrotestosterone. However, subsequent catabolism of the 5α-reduced products at the 3 position was not competitive and therefore did not involve the same enzymic pathways, thus explaining the lack of 3α-reduced pregnone derivatives. Since progesterone actively competes for 5α-reductase but does not require the same catabolic pathway for its 5α-reduced derivatives as 5α-dihydrotestosterone, the resultant effect of progesterone administration would be to diminish the overall level of 5α-dihydrotestosterone by inhibiting its production but not reducing its catabolism. The significance of this mechanism would lie in the requirement for relatively low levels of progesterone to reduce the 5α-dihydrotestosterone in the tissue, although the involvement of progesterone in areas other than its competition for 5α-reductase might complicate this rather simplified approach.

6.5 CONCLUSIONS

Our current knowledge regarding the role of steroid hormones in the prostate has highlighted the paramount importance of the metabolism of androgens as an integral part of their mechanism of action in this gland. The original observation that the metabolism of testosterone to 5α-dihydrotestosterone was an essential step in order that subsequent events leading to protein synthesis and cell division might occur, arose from studies on the rat ventral prostate, and emphasized the obligatory role of androgen metabolism. With a few minor exceptions this mandatory requirement for prior metabolism is confined to the mechanism of action of androgens and in particular to their role in the prostate. This phenomenon appears to be a general characteristic, since it has been demonstrated in prostates of several animal species, as well as the human prostate and its tumours.

In this chapter an attempt has been made to review our current understanding of steroid metabolism in the prostate with most emphasis directed towards that of androgens. The interrelation between the various enzymes and their products together with their subcellular localization and cofactor requirements in both experimental animals and human tissue has been discussed. The predominant feature of these studies is the demonstration of an active reductive metabolite pathway which involves Δ^4-3-oxosteroid reductase (5α-reductase) and $3\alpha(3\beta)$ hydroxysteroid oxidoreductase and leads to the formation of 5α-dihydrotestosterone and the isomeric forms of 5α-androstanediol, with a great tendency towards the formation of the former product which has a much higher level of androgenicity when compared to its precursor. Although this pattern of metabolic activity is a general feature in most experimental animal prostates and also present in all three types of human tissues, namely normal, benign and malignant prostates, there are certain differences in the relative activity of the reductive route in the human tumours. Whilst in the benign gland the reductive pathway appears to be more active than in the normal gland, in the malignant tumours the activity of this pathway is significantly reduced. On the other hand, the oxidative pathway would appear to be more predominant in the malignant glands and it has been suggested that this differential aspect of androgen metabolism between the benign and malignant tumour may be used as a discriminating factor. Based on the present findings, it is apparent that, despite reasonable consistency with regard to the functional activity of the major enzymic pathways in experimental animals and the normal human prostate, there are still some anomalies and disagreement as to the comparative aspects of the benign and malignant tumours, and more so with the degree of malignancy in the carcinomatous tissues. An important feature of the studies related to the androgen metabolism in benign and malignant tumours is the consistency between some of the findings on the hormone levels in prostatic tissues and serum from patients with these two diseases. The higher level of testosterone and dihydrotestosterone in malignant and benign tumours respectively is in good agreement with the metabolic studies using radiolabelled testosterone. Whilst in the benign tumour radiolabelled 5α-dihydrotestosterone appears to be the major metabolite, in the malignant tissue less testosterone is metabolized and relatively more androstenedione and lower 5α-dihydrotestosterone are produced. These findings in particular emphasize the significance of the metabolic studies and highlight their importance in future studies of prostatic tumours.

6.6 REFERENCES

Acevado, H. F. and Goldzieher, J. W. (1964). The metabolism of [^{14}C]estrone by hypertrophic and carcinomatous human prostate tissue. *Biochim. Biophys. Acta*, **82**, 118

Acevado, H. F. and Goldzieher, J. W. (1965). The metabolism of [^{14}C]testosterone by hypertrophic and carcinomatous human prostatic tissue. *Biochim. Biophys. Acta*, **97**, 571

Aliapoulios, M. A., Chamberlain, J., Jagarinec, N. and Ofner, P. (1965). Metabolism of [4^{14}C]testosterone by human and canine prostate. *Biochem. J.*, **98**, 15

Anderson, K. M. and Liao, S. (1968). Selective retention of dihydrotestosterone by prostatic nuclei. *Nature (London)*, **219**, 277

Arora-Dinakar, R., Dinakar, N. and Prasad, M. R. N. (1977). Metabolism in vitro of
³H-testosterone in testis, epididymis and sex accessories of the Rhesus monkey,
Macaca mulatta: effects of cyproterone acetate on androgen metabolism. *Indian J.
Exp. Biol.*, **15**, 953

Attramadal, A., Tveter, K. J., Weddington, S. C., Djoseland, O., Naess, O., Hansson,
V. and Torgersen, O. (1975). Androgen binding and metabolism in the human
prostate. *Vitam. Horm.*, **33**, 247

Bard, D. R. and Lasnitzki, I. (1977). The influence of oestradiol on the metabolism of
androgens by human prostatic tissue. *J. Endocrinol.*, **74**, 1

Barry, M. C., Eindinoff, M. L., Dobsiner, K. and Gallagher, T. F. (1952). The fate of
C¹⁴-testosterone and C¹⁴-progesterone in mice and rats. *Endocrinology.*, **50**, 587

Baulieu, E. E., Lasnitzki, I. and Robel, P. (1968). Metabolism of testosterone and
action of metabolites on prostate glands grown in organ culture. *Nature (London)*,
219, 1155

Baulieu, E. E. and Robel, P. (1970). Catabolism of testosterone and androstenedione.
In Eik-Nes, K. B. (ed.) *The Androgens of the Testis*, pp. 49–71. (New York: Marcel
Dekker)

Becker, H., Horst, H. J., Krieg, M., Steins, P. and Voigt, K. D. (1975). Uptake,
metabolism and binding of various androgens in human prostatic tissue: *in vivo* and
in vitro studies. *J. Steroid Biochem.*, **6**, 447

Belham, J. E. and Neal, G. E. (1971). Testosterone action in the rat ventral prostate.
Biochem. J., **125**, 81

Blacklock, N. J. and Bouskill, K. (1977). The zonal anatomy of the prostate in man and
in the Rhesus monkey (*Macaca mulatta*). *Urol. Res.*, **5**, 163

Booth, W. D. and Jones, R. (1979). Metabolism of testosterone and 5α-reduced
androgens by the rabbit prostate and epididymis: studies *in vitro* and *in vivo*. *J.
Endocrinol.*, **82**, 207

Breuer, H., Nocke, L. and Pechthold, I. (1959). Metabolism of testosterone in normal
and neoplastic human tissue. *Z. Vitamin, Hormon-ferment forsch*, **10**, 106

Bruchovsky, N. (1971). Comparison of the metabolites formed in rat prostate
following the *in vivo* administration of seven natural androgens. *Endocrinology*, **89**,
1212

Bruchovsky, N. and Lieskovsky, G. (1979). Increased ratio of 5α-reductase: (3α)β-
hydroxy steroid dehydrogenase activities in the hyperplastic human prostate. *J.
Endocrinol.*, **80**, 289

Bruchovsky, N., Rennie, P. S. and Wilkin, R. P. (1980). New aspects of androgen
action in prostatic cells: stromal localization of 5α-reductase, nuclear abundance of
androstanolone and binding of receptor to linker deoxyribonucleic acid. In
Schroder, F. H. and deVoogt, H. J. (eds) *Steroid Receptors, Metabolism and
Prostatic Cancer*. pp. 57–76. (Amsterdam: Excerpta Medica)

Bruchovsky, N. and Wilson, J. D. (1968a). The intranuclear binding of testosterone
and 5α-androstan-17-ol-3-one by rat prostate. *J. Biol. Chem.*, **243**, 5953

Bruchovsky, N. and Wilson, J. D. (1968b). The conversion of testosterone to 5α-
androstan-17β-ol-3-one by rat prostate *in vivo* and *in vitro*. *J. Biol. Chem.*, **243**, 2012

Buric, L., Becker, H., Petersen, C. and Voigt, K. D. (1972). Metabolism and mode of
action of androgens in target tissues of male rats. *Acta Endocrinol.*, **69**, 153

Chamberlain, J., Jagarinec, N. and Ofner, P. (1966). Catabolism of 4-¹⁴C testosterone
by sub-cellular fraction of human prostate. *Biochem. J.*, **99**, 610

Collins, W. P., Koullapis, E. N., Bridges, C. E. and Sommerville, I. F. (1970). Studies
on steroid metabolism in human prostatic tissue. *J. Steroid Biochem.*, **1**, 195

Cowan, R. A., Cowan, S. K., Grant, J. K. and Elder, H. Y. (1977). Biochemical
investigations of separated epithelium and stroma from benign hyperplastic
prostatic tissue. *J. Endocrinol.*, **74**, 111

DeKlerk, D. P., Coffey, D. S., Ewing, L. L., McDermott, I. R., Reiner, W. G., Robinson, C. H., Scott, W. W., Strandberg, J. D., Talalay, P., Walsh, P. C., Wheaton, L. G. and Zirkin, B. R. (1979). Comparison of spontaneous and experimentally induced canine prostatic hyperplasia. *J. Clin. Invest.*, **64**, 842

Djoseland, O., Tveter, K. J., Attramadal, A. and Hansson, V. (1977). Metabolism of testosterone in the human prostate and seminal vesicles. *Scand. J. Urol. Nephrol.*, **11**, 1

Dorfman, R. I. and Shipley, R. A. (1956). *Androgens; Biochemistry, Physiology and Clinical Significance.* (New York: John Wiley)

Eik-Nes, K. B. (1975). Infusion of the dog prostate. In Goland, M. (ed.) *Normal and Abnormal Growth of the Prostate.* pp. 156–159. (Springfield: Charles C. Thomas)

Evans, C. R. and Pierrepoint, C. G. (1975). Demonstration of a specific cytosol receptor in the normal and hyperplastic canine prostate for 5α-androstane-3α,17α-diol. *J. Endocrinol.*, **64**, 539

Evans, C. R. and Pierrepoint, C. G. (1976). Studies on the uptake and binding of 5α-androstane-3α,17α-diol by canine prostatic nuclei. *J. Endocrinol.*, **70**, 31

Farnsworth, W. E. (1966). Metabolism of 19-nortestosterone by human prostate. *Steroids*, **8**, 825

Farnsworth, W. E. (1969). A direct effect of estrogens on prostatic metabolism of testosterone. *Invest. Urol.*, **6**, 423

Farnsworth, W. E. (1975). Human prostatic dehydroepiandrosterone sulphatase. In Goland, M. (ed.) *Normal and Abnormal Growth of the Prostate.* pp. 160–170. (Springfield: Charles C. Thomas)

Farnsworth, W. E. and Brown, J. R. (1963). Testosterone metabolism in the prostate. In Vollmer, E. P. (ed.) *Biology of the Prostate and Related Tissues.* Vol. 12, pp. 323–329. Natl. Cancer. Inst. Monogr.

Farnsworth, W. E. and Brown, J. R. (1976). Androgen of the human prostate. *Endocr. Res. Commun.*, **3**, 105

Farnsworth, W. E., Brown, J. R., Lano, C. and Cross, A. (1962). Prostatic metabolism of testosterone. *Fed. Proc.*, **21**, 211

Fencl, M. de M. and Villee, C. A. (1973). Effect of estradiol in the metabolism of testosterone by rat prostate. *Steroids*, **21**, 537

Frederiksen, D. W. and Wilson, J. D. (1971). Partial characterization of the nuclear reduced nicotinamide adenine dinucleotide phosphate: delta 4-3 ketosteroid 5α-oxidoreductase of rat prostate. *J. Biol. Chem.*, **246**, 2584

Geller, J., Albert, J., Lopez, D., Geller, S. and Niwayama, G. (1976). Comparison of androgen metabolites in benign prostatic hypertrophy (BPH) and normal prostate. *J. Clin. Endocrinol. Metab.*, **43**, 686

Geller, J., Albert, J. de la Vega, D., Loza, D. and Stoeltzing, W. (1978). Dihydrotestosterone concentration in prostate cancer tissue as a predictor of tumour differentiation and hormonal dependency. *Cancer Res.*, **38**, 4349

Ghanadian, R. (1981). Androgen regulation in the prostate of Rhesus monkey (*Macaca mulatta*) In Hafez, E. S. E. and Spring-Mills, E. (eds.) *Clinics in Andrology*, Vol. 6: *Prostatic Carcinoma, Biology and Diagnosis.* pp. 160–164. (The Hague: Martinus)

Ghanadian, R., Holland, J. M. and Chisholm, G. D. (1975). Identification of a female prostate in *Praomys (Mastomys) natalensis* using ³H steroids. *Br. J. Urol.*, **47**, 77

Ghanadian, R., Holland, J. M. and Chisholm, G. D. (1976). Uptake and distribution of ³H testosterone in tissues of male *Praomys (Mastomys) natalensis*: an *in vivo* and *in vitro* study on the prostate. *Urol. Res.*, **4**, 77

Ghanadian, R., Masters, J. M. and Smith, C. B. (1979). Androgen metabolism in benign hypertrophy and carcinoma of the prostate. *Cancer Treat. Rep.*, **63**, 1153

Ghanadian, R., Masters, J. R. W. and Smith, C. B. (1981). Altered androgen metabolism in carcinoma of the prostate. *Eur. Urol.*, **7**, 169

Ghanadian, R. and Puah, C. (1981). Relationships between oestradiol-17β, testosterone, dihydrotestosterone and 5α-androstane-3α,17β-diol in human benign hypertrophy and carcinoma of the prostate. *J. Endocrinol.*, **88**, 255

Ghanadian, R. and Smith, C. B. (1981). Androgen metabolism within the lobes of Rhesus monkey prostate. *Eur. Urol.*, **7**, 89

Ghanadian, R., Smith, C. B. and Chisholm, G. D. (1977a). Identification of an androgen receptor in the cytosol of the female *Mastomys* prostate. *Mol. Cell. Endocrinol.*, **8**, 147

Ghanadian, R., Smith, C. B. and Chisholm, G. D. (1978). Receptor protein for dihydrotestosterone in nuclei of the female prostate of *Praomys (Mastomys) natalensis*. *Invest. Urol.*, **16**, 119

Ghanadian, R., Smith, C. B., Williams, G. and Chisholm, G. D. (1977b). The effect of antiandrogens and stilboestrol on the cytosol receptor in rat prostate. *Br. J. Urol.*, **49**, 695

Giorgi, E. P., Grant, J. K., Stewart, J. C. and Reid, J. (1972). Androgen dynamics *in vitro* in the canine prostate gland. *J. Endocrinol.*, **55**, 421

Giorgi, E. P., Moses, T. F., Grant, J. K., Scott, R. and Sinclair, J. (1974). *In vitro* studies of the regulation of androgen-tissue relationship in normal canine and hyperplastic human prostate. *Mol. Cell. Endocrinol.*, **1**, 271

Giorgi, E. P., Stewart, J. C., Grant, J. K. and Scott, R. (1971). Androgen dynamics *in vitro* in the normal and hyperplastic human prostate gland. *Biochem. J.*, **123**, 41

Gittinger, J. W. and Lasnitzki, I. (1971). The effect of testosterone and testosterone metabolites on the fine structure of the rat prostate gland in organ culture. *J. Endocrinol.*, **52**, 459

Gloyna, R. E. and Wilson, J. D. (1969). A comparative study of the conversion of testosterone to 17β-hydroxy-5α-androstan-3-one (dihydrotestosterone) by prostate and epididymis. *J. Clin. Endocrinol.*, **29**, 970

Griffiths, K., Harper, M. E., Groom, M. A., Pike, A. M., Fahmy, A. R. and Pierrepoint, C. G. (1970). Testosterone metabolism in the dog prostate with regard to its growth and function. In Griffiths, K. and Pierrepoint, C. G. (eds.) *Some Aspects of the Aetiology and Biochemistry of Prostatic Cancer*. pp. 88–94. (Cardiff: Alpha Omega Alpha)

Groom, M., Harper, M. E., Fahmy, A. R. and Griffiths, K. (1971). The effect of oestrogen on the prostatic metabolism of testosterone in tissue culture. *Biochem. J.*, **122**, 125

Habib, F. K. (1980). Studies on the *in vitro* binding and metabolism of testosterone in benign prostatic hypertrophy and carcinoma of the prostate: a correlation with endogenous androgen levels. In Schroder, F. H. and de Voogt, H. J. (eds.) *Steroid Receptors, Metabolism and Prostatic Cancer*. pp. 157–164. (Amsterdam: Excerpta Medica)

Habib, F. K., Lee, I. R., Stitch, S. R. and Smith, P. H. (1976). Androgen levels in the plasma and prostatic tissues of patients with benign hypertrophy and carcinoma of the prostate. *J. Endocrinol.*, **71**, 99

Habib, F. K., Rafati, G., Robinson, M. R. G. and Stitch, S. R. (1979). Effect of tamoxifen on the binding and metabolism of testosterone by human prostatic tissue and plasma *in vitro*. *J. Endocrinol.*, **83**, 369

Haltmeyer, G. C. and Eik-Nes, K. B. (1972). Production and secretion of 5α-dihydrotestosterone by the canine prostate. *Acta Endocrinol.*, **69**, 394

Harper, M. E., Pierrepoint, C. G., Fahmy, A. H. and Griffiths, K. (1971). The metabolism of steroids in the canine prostate and testis. *J. Endocrinol.*, **49**, 213

Harper, M. E., Pike, A., Peeling, W. B. and Griffiths, K. (1974). Steroid of adrenal origin metabolised by human prostatic tissue both *in vivo* and *in vitro*. *J. Endocrinol.*, **60**, 117

Holmes, W. N. (1956). The distribution of C^{14} in mice after a subcutaneous injection of testosterone-4-C^{14}. *Acta Endocrinol.*, **68**, 79

Huggins, C. (1945). The physiology of the prostate gland. *Physiol. Rev.*, **25**, 281

Hussein, K. A. and Kochakian, C. D. (1968). DPN- and TPN-17β-hydroxy-C_{19}-steroid dehydrogenases; intra cellular localization in dog prostate. *Acta Endocrinol.*, **59**, 459

Isaacs, J. T., McDermott, I. R. and Coffey, D. S. (1979). The identification and characterization of a new $C_{19}O_3$ steroid metabolite in the rat ventral prostate: 5α-androstane-3β, 6α, 17β-triol. *Steroids.*, **33**, 639

Jacobi, G. H., Moore, R. J. and Wilson, J. D. (1978a). Studies on the mechanism of 3α-androstanediol induced growth of the dog prostate. *Endocrinology.*, **102**, 1748

Jacobi, G. H. and Wilson, J. D. (1977). Formation of 5α-androstane-3α,17β-diol by normal and hypertrophic human prostate. *J. Clin. Endocrinol. Metab.*, **44**, 107

Jenkins, J. S. and McCaffery, V. M. (1974). Effect of oestradiol-17β and progesterone on the metabolism of testosterone by human prostatic tissue. *J. Endocrinol.*, **63**, 517

Jensen, E. V. and Jacobson, H. T. (1962). Basic guides to the mechanism of oestrogen action. *Recent Prog. Horm. Res.*, **18**, 387

Kliman, B., Prout, jr., G. R., Maclaughlin, R. A., Daly, J. J. and Griffin, P. P. (1978). Altered androgen metabolism in metastatic prostate cancer. *J. Urol.*, **119**, 623

Krieg, M., Bartsch, W. Janssen, W. and Voigt, K. D. (1979). A comparative study of binding, metabolism and endogenous level of androgens in normal, hyperplastic and carcinomatous human prostate. *J. Steroid Biochem.*, **11**, 615

Krieg, M., Grobe, I. and Voigt, K. D. (1978). Human prostatic carcinoma: significant differences in its androgen binding and metabolism compared to the human benign prostatic hypertrophy. *Acta Endocrinol.*, **88**, 397

Krieg, M., Horst, H. J. and Sterba, M. L. (1975). Binding and metabolism of 5α-androstane-3α,17β-diol and of 5α-androstane-3β,17β-diol in the prostate, seminal vesicles and plasma of male rats: studies *in vivo* and *in vitro*. *J. Endocrinol.*, **64**, 529

Lasnitzki, I. (1970). The rat prostate gland in organ culture. In Williams, D. C., Briggs, M. A. and Stainford, M. (eds.) *Advances in the Study of the Prostate*. pp. 65–72. (London: Heineman)

Lasnitzki, I. (1979). Metabolism and action of steroid hormones on human benign prostatic hyperplasia and prostatic carcinoma grown in organ culture. *J. Steroid Biochem.*, **11**, 625

Lasnitzki, I. and Franklin, H. R. (1972). The influence of serum on uptake, conversion and action of testosterone in rat prostate glands in organ culture. *J. Endocrinol.*, **54**, 333

Lee, D. K. H., Bird, C. E. and Clark, A. F. (1973). *In vitro* effects of estrogens on rat prostatic 5α-reduction of testosterone. *Steroids*, **22**, 677

Lee, D. K. H., Bird, C. E. and Clark, A. F. (1975). *In vivo* metabolism of ^{3}H testosterone in adult male rats: effect of estrogen administration. *Steroids*, **26**, 137

Lemon, H. M., Wotiz, H. H. and Robitscher, T. (1953). Metabolism of testosterone by neoplastic human prostate. *J. Clin. Endocrinol.*, **13**, 948

Mabin, T. A., McMahon, M. J. and Thomas, G. H. (1970). The interconversion of oestrone and oestradiol by human endometrium and human benign prostatic hyperplasia in organ culture. *Biochem. J.*, **118**, 8

Mainwaring, W. I. P. and Milroy, E. J. G. (1973). Characterization of the specific androgen receptors in the human prostate gland. *J. Endocrinol.*, **57**, 371

Malathi, K. and Gurpide, E. (1977). Metabolism of 5α-dihydrotestosterone in human benign hyperplastic prostate. *J. Steroid Biochem.*, **8**, 141

Moore, R. A. (1944). Benign hypertrophy and carcinoma of the prostate. Occurrence and experimental production in animals. *Surgery*, **16**, 152

Moore, R. J. and Wilson, J. (1973). Effect of androgenic hormones on reduced nicotinamide adenine dinucleotide phosphate: Δ^4-3-ketosteroid 5α-oxidoreductase of rat ventral prostate. *Endocrinology*, **93**, 581

Moore, R. J. and Wilson, J. D. (1976). Androgen transport and metabolism in the prostate. In Grayhack, J. T., Wilson, J. D. and Scherbenske, M. J. (eds.) *Benign Prostatic Hyperplasia*. pp. 21–30. (Bethesda: DHEW Publication)

Morfin, R. F., Alliapoulios, M. A., Chamberlain, J. and Ofner, P. (1970). Metabolism of testosterone 4-^{14}C by the canine prostate and urinary bladder *in vivo*. *Endocrinology*, **87**, 394

Morfin, R. F., Bercovici, J. P., Charles, J. F., and Floch, H. H. (1975). Testosterone and progesterone metabolism and their interaction in the human hyperplastic prostate. *J. Steroid Biochem.*, **6**, 1347

Morfin, R. F., Distefano, S., Bercovici, J. P. and Floch, H. H. (1978). Comparison of testosterone, 5α-dihydrotestosterone and 5α-androstane-3α, 17β-diol metabolism in human normal and hyperplastic prostates. *J. Steroid Biochem.*, **9**, 245

Morfin, R. F., Distefano, S., Charles, J. F. and Floch, H. H. (1980). 5α-androstane-3β-diol and 5α-androstane-3β, 7α, 17β-triol in the hyperplastic prostate. *J. Steroid Biochem.*, **12**, 529

Morfin, R. F., Leave, I., Charles, J. F., Cavazos, L. F., Ofner, P. and Floch, H. H. (1977). Correlative study of the morphology and C_{19}-steroid metabolism of benign and cancerous human prostatic tissue. *Cancer*, **39**, 1517

Morgan, M. D. and Wilson, J. D. (1970). Intranuclear metabolism of progesterone-1, 2-^{3}H in the hen oviduct. *J. Biol. Chem.*, **245**, 3781

Neumann, F., Von Berswordt-Wallrabe, R., Richter, K. D. and Senge, T. H. (1975). The action of cyproterone acetate on the prostate and heterotransplanted human prostatic adenoma. In Goland, M. (ed.) *Normal and Abnormal Growth of the Prostate*. pp. 395–416. (Springfield: Charles C. Thomas)

Nozu, K. and Tamaoki, B. I. (1973). Testosterone metabolism in subcellular fractions of rat prostate. *Acta Endocrinol.*, **73**, 585

Nozu, K. and Tamaoki, B. I. (1974). Characteristics of the nuclear and microsomal steroid Δ^4-5-hydrogenase of the rat prostate. *Acta Endocrinol.*, **76**, 608

Ofner, P., Morfin, R. F., Vena, R. H. and Aliapoulios, M. A. (1970). Androgen metabolism in the human prostate. In Griffiths, K. and Pierrepoint, C. G. (eds.) *Some Aspects of the Aetiology and Biochemistry of Prostatic Cancer*, pp. 55–62. (Cardiff: Alpha Omega Alpha)

Ofner, P., Vena, R. L., Leav, I. and Hamilton, D. W. (1979). Metabolism of C_{19}-radiosteroids by explants of canine prostate and epididymis with disposition as hydroxylated products: a possible mechanism for androgen inactivation. *J. Steroid Biochem.*, **11**, 1367

Ofner, P., Vena, R. L., Morfin, R. F., Aliapoulios, M. A. and Leav, I. (1975). *In vivo* metabolism of C_{19}-steroids in prostatic tissue. In Goland, M. (ed.) *Normal and Abnormal Growth of the Prostate*. pp. 111–124. (Springfield: Charles C. Thomas)

Orestano, F., Klose, K., Rubin, A., Knapstein, P. and Altwein, J. E. (1974). Testosterone metabolism in benign prostatic hypertrophy: suppression by diethylstilboestrol and gestonorone capronate. *Invest. Urol.*, **12**, 151

Pearlman, W. H. and Pearlman, M. R. J. (1961). The metabolism of in vivo of Δ^4 androstene-3, 17-dione-7-H^3; its localization in the ventral prostate and other tissues of the rat. *J. Biol. Chem.*, **236**, 1321

Reel, J. R., van Dewarck, S. D., Shi, Y., Callatine, M. R. (1971). Macromolecular binding and metabolism of progesterone in the decidual and pseudopregnant rat and rabbit uterus. *Steroids*, **18**, 441

Rennie, P. and Bruchovsky, N. (1973). Studies on the relationship between androgen receptor and the transport of androgens in the rat prostate. *J. Biol. Chem.*, **248**, 3288

Robel, P., Lasnitzki, I. and Baulieu, E. E. (1971). Hormone metabolism and action: testosterone and metabolites in prostate organ culture. *Biochimie.*, **53**, 81

Robel, P., Roy, A. K., Levy, C. and Baulieu, E. E. (1975). Metabolism of androgen in rat prostatic tissues: superfusion and tissue culture. In Goland, M. (ed.) *Normal and Abnormal Growth of the Prostate.* pp. 144–155. (Springfield: Charles C. Thomas)

Romijn, J. C., Oishi, K., Bolt-de Vries, J., Schweikert, H. U., Mulder, E. and Schroder, F. H. (1980). Androgen metabolism and androgen receptors in separated epithelium and stroma of the human prostate. In Schroder, F. H. and deVoogt, H. J. (eds.) *Steroid Receptors, Metabolism and Prostatic Cancer.* pp. 134–143. (Amsterdam: Excerpta Medica)

Roy, A. K., Robel, P. and Baulieu, E. E. (1972). Hormone metabolism: III. Metabolism of 3α-hydroxy and 3β-hydroxy C_{19}-steroids in prostate organ culture. *Endocrinology*, **91**, 404

Schweikert, H. U. (1979). Conversion of androstenedione to estrone in human fibroblasts cultured from prostate, genital and nongenital skin. *Horm. Metab. Res.*, **11**, 635

Schweikert, H. U., Hein, H. J. and Schroder, F. H. (1980). Androgen metabolism in fibroblasts from human benign prostatic hyperplasia, prostatic carcinoma and nongenital skin. In Schroder, F. H. and de Voogt, H. J. (eds.) *Steroid Receptors, Metabolism and Prostatic Cancer.* pp. 126–133. (Amsterdam: Excerpta Medica)

Shida, K., Shimazaki, J., Ito, Y., Yamanaka, H. and Nagai-Yuasa, H. (1975). 3α-reduction of dihydrotestosterone in human normal and hypertrophic prostatic tissue. *Invest. Urol.*, **13**, 241

Shimazaki, J., Kurihara, H., Ito, Y. and Shida, K. (1965a). Testosterone metabolism in prostate; formation of androstan-4-ene-3, 17-one and inhibitory effect of natural and synthetic estrogens. *Gumma J. Med. Sci.*, **14**, 313

Shimazaki, J., Kurihara, H., Ito, Y. and Shida, K. (1965b). Metabolism of testosterone in muscular tissue. *Gumma J. Med. Sci.*, **14**, 326

Shimazaki, J., Kato, N., Nagai, H., Yamanaka, H. and Shida, K. (1972). 3α-reduction of 5α-dihydrotestosterone by rat ventral prostate. *Endocrinol. Jpn.*, **19**, 97

Shimazaki, J., Matsushita, I., Furuya, N., Yamanaka, H. and Shida, K. (1969). Reduction of 5α-position of testosterone in the rat ventral prostate. *Endocrinol. Jpn.*, **16**, 453

Smith, C. B., Ghanadian, R. and Chisholm, G. D. (1978a). A soluble androgen receptor in the cytoplasm of the *Mastomys* prostate. *Urol. Res.*, **6**, 29

Smith, C. B., Ghanadian, R. and Chisholm, G. D. (1978b). Inhibition of the nuclear dihydrotestosterone receptor complex from rat ventral prostate by antiandrogens and stilboestrol. *Mol. Cell. Endocrinol.*, **10**, 13

Smith, C. B., Ghanadian, R. and Chisholm, G. D. (1979). Nuclear androgen receptors in the prostate of the male *Praomys (Mastomys) natalensis. Urol. Res.*, **7**, 243

Smith, C. B., Masters, J. R. B. and Ghanadian, R. (1980). Differential androgen metabolism in prostatic tumours. *J. Endocrinol.*, **85**, 5

Thomas, J. A. and Manandhar, M. (1975). Effects of prolactin and/or testosterone on nucleic acid levels in prostatic glands of normal and castrated rats. *J. Endocrinol.*, **65**, 149

Tveter, K. J. and Aakvaag, A. (1969). Uptake and metabolism *in vivo* of testosterone-1, 2-^{3}H by accessory sex organs of male rats; influence of some hormonal compounds. *Endocrinology*, **85**, 683

Unhjem, O. (1970). Partial separation of a 3α-ketosteroid oxidoreductase and an androgen binding substance present in rat ventral prostate cytoplasm. *Acta Endocrinol.*, **65**, 525

Wilson, J. D. and Gloyna, R. E. (1970). The intranuclear metabolism of testosterone in the accessory organs of reproduction. *Recent Prog. Horm. Res.*, **26,** 309

Wilson, J. D. and Lasnitzki, I. (1971). Dihydrotestosterone formation in the fetal tissue of the rabbit and rat. *Endocrinology*, **89,** 659

Wotiz, H. H. and Lemon, H. M. (1954). Metabolism of testosterone by human prostatic tissue slices. *J. Biol. Chem.*, **206,** 525

7
Mechanism of action of androgens in the prostate

S. LIAO AND C. CHEN

In this chapter the current views on the biochemical processes that may be involved in the action of androgens in the rat ventral prostate are summarized. The action of other steroid hormones is also discussed, since this may be helpful for a general understanding of the mechanism of action of steroid hormones at the molecular level. The reader may also consult relevant symposium books (Schimke *et al.*, 1975; Pasqualini, 1976; Liao, 1977; O'Malley and Birnbaumer, 1977; Kurtz and Feigelson, 1978; Roy, 1979; Liao *et al.*, 1980; Roy and Clark, 1980) and review articles (Liao, 1975a; Gorski and Gannon,

1976; Liao, 1977; Jensen, 1979; Katzenellenbogen, 1980) on the mechanism of action of steroids.

7.1 RECEPTOR MECHANISM

7.1.1 Isolation and characterization of androgen receptor

The existence of receptors for steroid hormones was first indicated in the classic study by Jensen and his co-workers (1962), who showed that radioactive oestrogens can be retained by oestrogen sensitive organs for a prolonged length of time. Several years later, Toft and Gorski (1966) were able to show, by gradient centrifugation, that the cytosol of rat uteri contained a protein that can form a complex with radioactive oestradiol.

Unlike oestradiol, which is not metabolized to any significant extent in the rat uterus, testosterone, the major androgen produced in the testis and circulating in the blood, is transformed into several metabolites. It was, therefore, important to determine which metabolite of testosterone was the active androgen. Since the RNA synthesis in the prostate nuclei could be very rapidly enhanced by androgen (Liao et al., 1975), we assumed that the active androgen metabolite was very likely to be found in the nuclei. Therefore, we injected [^{3}H]testosterone into castrated rats, and identified the radioactive steroid selectively retained by prostate cell nuclei. Our study (Anderson and Liao, 1968) and that of Bruchovsky and Wilson (1968) revealed that the major androgen retained by prostate nuclei was 5α-dihydrotestosterone, DHT (Figure 7.1). Since the selective retention of DHT by cell nuclei of target tissues can be demonstrated by incubation of minced prostate and radioactive testosterone (Anderson and Liao, 1968; Fang et al., 1969), testosterone must be taken up by prostate cells, reduced to DHT and retained by the cell nuclei. The enzyme that catalyses this reaction is a NADPH-dependent Δ^4-3-ketosteroid-5α-oxidoreductase (5α-reductase) that appears to associate with the cytoplasmic membrane fraction of the prostate (Shimazaki et al., 1965; Moore and Wilson, 1972).

After the selective retention of DHT had been reported, specific binding of DHT to cytosol and nuclear proteins was demonstrated (Fang et al., 1969; Mainwaring, 1969a, 1969b; Baulieu and Jung, 1970; Fang and Liao, 1971). The biological significance of nuclear and protein binding was underlined by the observation that antiandrogens, such as cyproterone acetate, could inhibit these binding processes both in vivo and in vitro (Fang and Liao, 1969). The discovery of specific androgen binding proteins which behaved very much like the uterine oestrogen receptor considerably strengthened the contention that such receptor proteins exist in all target cells for steroid hormones. Soon after these studies, the receptors for progestins and adrenal corticosteroids were found in their target organs.

Since it has not been possible to assay steroid receptors by analysing their biochemical activity, steroid receptors have been characterized by measurements of their apparent physical properties such as sedimentation behaviour and steroid binding specificity and affinity. Different forms of radioactive

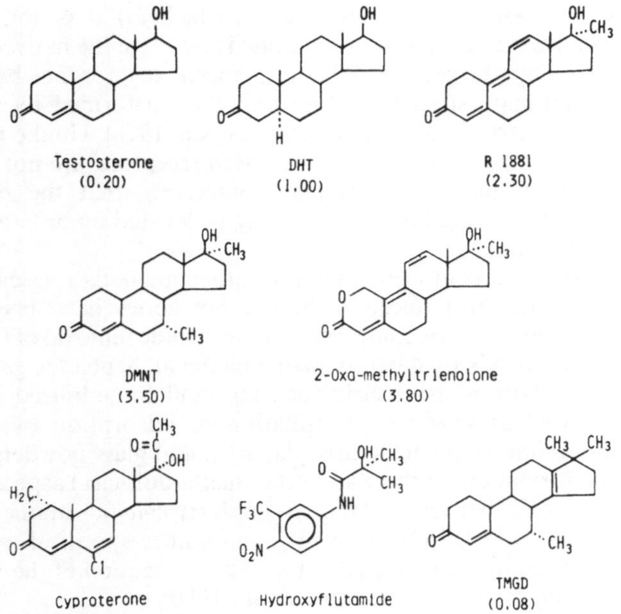

Figure 7.1 Chemical structures of androgens and antiandrogens. The numbers in the parentheses represent the relative affinities for the steroids to bind to the receptor protein of rat ventral prostate. The abbreviations are: R 1881, 17α-methyl-17β-hydroxyoestra-4,9,11-trien-3-one; DMNT, 7α-,17α-dimethyl-19-nortestosterone; TMGD, 7α-17,17-trimethylgona-4,13-dien-3-one

steroid receptor complexes have often been identified according to their rates of sedimentation in sucrose gradients (Liao *et al.*, 1975; and Blondeau *et al.*, 1975). Steroid receptor complexes including the DHT receptor complex of rat ventral prostate have been found to sediment in a gradient with low ionic strength as two forms which are usually designated as 8 ± 2S and 4 ± 1S. The cytosol 8S form can dissociate into a 4S form in a gradient containing 0.4 mol/l or higher concentrations of KCl whereas the nuclear steroid receptor complex can be extracted from nuclei by a medium with high ionic strength (0.4 mol/l KCl) and sediment as a 3 − 5S component in the high ionic strength medium.

The chemical nature of different forms of the receptor complexes is not clear. They may be the aggregated forms of monomers, but association of heteromacromolecules is also possible. Since the quantity of the receptor protein in the cytosol fractions is very small (of the order of about 0.002 % of total cytosol proteins), fortuitous interactions of the steroid receptor complex with other cellular components in the tissue extracts can occur. Thus, androgen receptor complexes have been seen to sediment differently (3 to 10S) depending on the pH of the medium (Liao *et al.*, 1975).

Since proteases in the tissue extracts may hydrolyse the receptor proteins without damaging the steroid binding capabilities of the receptors, including the receptor for androgens (Wilson and French, 1979), it is not possible to determine whether any of the forms identified so far are the native forms that function in the intact target cells. The term 'mero receptor' has been used to designate the ultimate steroid binding unit (< 3S) formed by proteolytic degradation of a cytosol receptor (Sherman *et al.*, 1978). Unlike the nuclear binding receptor complexes, some of the 'mero receptors' are not capable of binding tightly to nuclear components suggesting that the nuclear (or chromatin) and the steroid binding sites may be located on different parts of the receptor proteins.

Besides sucrose gradient centrifugation, other methods for separation of unbound hormones from receptor bound hormones have been used to characterize steroid-receptor complexes. These include removal of free or non-receptor bound steroids by dextran coated charcoal, Sephadex gel filtration, agar gel electrophoresis, isoelectric focusing, and immobilized antisteroid antibodies as well as selective precipitation or adsorption by protamine sulphate, ammonium sulphate, hydroxylapatite, and glass powders or beads. For detailed information on these and other methodological aspects, Chapter 8 in this book and articles in *Methods in Enzymology* volume 36 (1975) (Academic Press), are helpful. Recently, antibodies specific for oestrogen receptors have been raised and used in the characterization of these hormone receptors (Greene *et al.*, 1977; Greene *et al.*, 1980).

Purification of steroid receptor proteins has not been easy because their concentrations in tissue extracts are only of the order of 2–100 fmol/mg of protein (about 0.1 mg to 5 mg receptor protein per 1 kg fresh tissue). In addition, the purification process is usually followed by assaying of the bound radioactive ligands (steroids) rather than of the receptors themselves; this makes it difficult to determine whether the receptor proteins have been adversely altered during the isolation. One technique that is suitable for the purification of steroid receptors is affinity chromatography. A receptor-specific steroid covalently attached to an insoluble support is used to trap the receptor and separate it from other proteins in the crude extract. Affinity chromatography as well as the more traditional techniques such as DEAE-cellulose and DNA-cellulose chromatography have been employed success-fully for the purification of uterine oestrogen receptor (Greene *et al.*, 1977; Puca *et al.*, 1979; Greene *et al.*, 1980), oviduct progestin receptor (Vedeckis *et al.*, 1980), and hepatic glucocorticoid receptor (Wrange *et al.*, 1979).

Many of these techniques have been used in the partial purification of the prostate androgen receptor. Large scale purification of androgen receptor, however, has not been possible because the target tissues rich in the receptor have not been readily obtainable in large quantities and from convenient sources.

7.1.2 Androgen-receptor interaction

The androgenicity and the receptor binding affinity of many steroids tested are closely correlated. For receptor binding, the bulkiness and flatness of the steroid molecule, especially in the ring A area, appear to play a more important role than the detailed electronic structure of the steroid nucleus. Not only are the steroids with an A/B cis structure, such as the inactive (in rat prostate) 5β isomer of DHT, not bound by the prostate receptor, but other relatively flat steroids with rings A/B in the trans structure also differ in their receptor binding affinity according to their bulkiness in the ring A/B area (Liao et al., (1973a).

According to the results of competition (Liao et al., 1973a) and antisteroid antibody assays (see below), testosterone binds less firmly to the prostate receptor than does DHT. This is apparently due to the more rapid rate of dissociation of testosterone (compared to DHT) from the receptor. Since other Δ^4-3-ketosteroids can bind tightly to the receptor, the difference in the dissociation rates may be mainly due to the steric property at the ring A/B area, rather than to the presence of the Δ^4 double bond. This is best shown by the fact that potent androgens like 7α,17α-dimethyl-19-nortestosterone (DMNT), and 2-oxa-17α-methyl-17β-hydroxyestra-4,9,11-trien-3-one (Figure 7.1) are capable of binding to the androgen receptor more tightly than DHT. Because they have conjugated double bonds which extend from rings A and B to C, the 2-oxatriene and other androgenic estratrienes are indeed very flat molecules. The removal of the angular methyl group between ring A and ring B also makes the area less bulky, and it may facilitate tight binding of these androgens to the receptor. This view is supported by the fact that A-nor-17β-acetoxyestra-4,9,11-trien-3-one, with five carbons in ring A, is a very potent androgen, whereas A-homotestosterone and A-homo-DHT, each with seven carbons in ring A, are virtually inactive. An additional carbon ring B or D does not distort the gross geometry of androstanes. Thus, B-homo-DHT and D-homo-DHT are potent androgens which probably can bind to the prostate receptor protein (Liao et al., 1973a).

If a methyl group is substituted in the 7α-position on 19-nortestosterone, the receptor binding affinity increases significantly (Liao et al., 1973a). It appears that the receptor protein has a specific (M) site for binding the 7α-methyl group, and that both the binding affinity and the androgenicity are enhanced many-fold. Alternatively the 7α-methyl group may strain the nuclear structure of the steroid and make it bind more tightly to the receptor protein. If the 7-methyl substitution is made at the 7β position, both the receptor binding affinity and the androgenicity are reduced by more than 90 %. This appears to be due to the peripheral enlargement of the steroid molecule by the 7β-methyl group, which cannot be accommodated into the receptor binding cavity.

A unique structural aspect of natural steroid hormones is that they contain an oxygen function at the C-3 position. Whether this group is absolutely required for androgen action is not clear, for many synthetic steroids without this oxygen group have been shown to be androgenically active (Liao and Fang, 1969). These deoxy steroids generally have very low binding affinity toward the prostate androgen receptor and have relatively low androgenicity compared to that of natural androgens. It is entirely possible that some of the 3-deoxy androgens are oxygenated and become androgenic, or that various 3-oxygenated androgens have different affinities toward different receptors and exhibit diverse biological responses.

The 17β-hydroxy group appears to be important for high affinity binding to the receptor and for androgen action (Liao et al., 1973a; Chan et al., 1979). It is not clear, however, whether the 17β-hydroxy group is needed only for the formation of a tight androgen receptor complex or for the triggering process itself. Certain 7α-methyl-19-norandrostenes that have no hydroxy group on ring D can compete with DHT for binding to the prostate androgen receptor. For example, 7α,17,17-trimethylgona-4,13-dien-3-one (TMGD) has a moderate receptor binding affinity in the cell free system (Chan *et al.*, 1979). However, this deoxy steroid does not appear to penetrate into the target cells and interact with the receptor proteins. Without an oxygen function on ring D, TMGD may behave like a monopolar lipid and intercalate with membrane lipids. Thus, two oxygen atoms at two ends of a natural steroid molecule may pay an important role in preventing a tight association of the hormone with cellular membranes.

The way in which the receptor protein recognizes the androgen structures suggests that, during interaction, the androgens are being 'enveloped' in the hydrophobic cavity of the protein (Liao *et al.*, 1973a). The localization of steroid binding sites well inside the receptor proteins may be responsible for the very slow rate of association or dissociation of steroids from the receptor proteins at low temperatures, the very high steroid binding affinity, the acceleration of the rates of exchange of unbound steroids with bound steroid by freezing and thawing, and the fact that the receptor bound androgens are rather stable in ethanol (39 %) or detergents (2 % Triton X100 or deoxycholate).

Additional support for this view came from our study on the capability of antisteroid antibodies to interact with steroids bound to various proteins Antibodies against DHT or testosterone were found to be effective in removing steroids bound to non-receptor proteins of the blood and prostate, since these proteins (steroid metabolizing enzymes or blood steroid binding globulins) generally recognize only a portion of the steroid molecule, and since the steroids dissociate much more rapidly from these non-receptor proteins than from the receptor protein. The steroids bound well inside the receptor protein have very low rates of dissociation and, therefore, are not readily removed by the antibody. In addition, the antibody does not form a tertiary complex with the androgen receptor complex (Castaneda and Liao, 1975).

7.1.3   Receptor transformation

The cytosol androgen receptor cannot be retained tightly by the prostate nuclei unless it first interacts with DHT (Fang *et al.*, 1969; Fang and Liao, 1971). Thus, the first recognizable cellular action of the androgen is to alter the cytoplasmic receptor protein (3.8S) to the form (3S) retainable by the nuclei. A similar observation has been made for oestrogen, in uterus, which is believed to cause a temperature dependent transformation of the steroid receptor complex into a form that can be retained firmly by the cell nuclei (Jensen *et al.*, 1974). The retention of DHT receptor complex by nuclear chromatin of rat ventral prostate has also been shown to occur more effectively at 20–40° C than at 0° C by autoradiography (Sar *et al.*, 1970) and by reconstruction of cellular preparations (Fang and Liao, 1971; Mainwaring and Peterken, 1971). It is not clear whether the transformation of the receptor involves a proteolytic action, a bimolecular reaction, or a simple change in receptor conformation. It is very likely, however, that steroid enveloping by a receptor is accompanied by a conformational alteration of the receptor protein.

The prostate cytosol DHT receptor complex can interact rather specifically with certain divalent metal ions (Liao et al., 1975). When the complex was incubated with a metal ion at $0°$ C or $20°$ C before being subjected to gradient centrifugation, $MnCl_2$ or $CaCl_2$, at concentrations of 1–5 mmol/l had no significant effect on the sedimentation properties of the complex in a medium containing 0.4 mol/l KCl. In contrast, $CoCl_2$ facilitated aggregation of the complex and reduced the 3.8 S peak significantly. The most striking effect was observed with $ZnCl_2$. Incubation of the complex with 3 mmol/l Zn^{2+} at $0°$ C for 20 minutes resulted in a shift of the sedimentation coefficient from 3.8 S to 4.5 S without alteration of the total amount of $[^3H]DHT$ bound to the complex. When the incubation was carried out at $20°$ C, the radioactive peak broadened (5 ± 2 S), and a considerable amount of the radioactive androgen dissociated from the receptor and remained near the top of the tube after centrifugation. It is possible that a change in the configuration of the receptor protein is induced by Zn^{2+} at a critical steroid binding site, and that this change alters the steroid affinity.

Various mononucleotides can also affect the sedimentation pattern of the cytosol DHT receptor complex. Both ATP and GTP can interact with and stabilize the DHT receptor complex. Such an effect was observed most clearly when a fresh, untransformed receptor preparation was incubated with 1–5 mmol/l of these nucleotides at $20°$ C for 20 minutes. In the absence of the mononucleotide, the incubation caused a shift in the sedimentation coefficient of the complex from the native cytoplasmic form (3.8 S) to the nuclear form (3 S). If GTP or ATP was present, a small shift in the sedimentation coefficient was observed when the mixture was maintained at $0°$ C. When the temperature was raised to $20°$ C, the nucleotide interaction appeared to retard the transformation of the receptor to the 3 S form. With CTP and UTP some effect was also demonstrated, but this was not as clear as the effect with ATP and GTP (Liao et al., 1975).

7.1.4 Nuclear acceptor and nuclear retention of androgen-receptor complex

The first indication that there might be specific acceptor molecules which interact with and retain steroid receptors was obtained in studies showing the retention of the DHT receptor complex by prostate nuclei (Liao and Fang, 1970; Fang and Liao, 1971). Soon afterwards a similar observation was made on the retention of progestin receptor complex by the chick oviduct nuclear fraction (O'Malley et al., 1972).

The acceptor molecule appears to be more abundant or more active in the cell nuclei of the androgen-sensitive tissues than in less responsive tissues such as the liver (Fang and Liao, 1971; Tymoczko and Liao, 1971). Since the nuclear receptor binding activity, under certain conditions, could be saturated with the DHT receptor complex, and since this activity was inactivated by heating to temperatures higher than $40°C$, the acceptor molecule was considered to be a specific heat-labile protein. It was suggested that the acceptor could participate actively in specifying the nuclear sites where the androgen receptor complex was to bind and exert its cellular action. Mainwaring and Irving (1973) proposed that DNA is the ultimate acceptor, and that certain proteins might act passively by restricting the receptor binding sites available on DNA.

In intact nuclei, the acceptor protein for the progestin receptor may be masked. This masking of the acceptor protein is believed to be responsible for the low progestin receptor binding capacity of nuclei in tissues that are less sensitive to progestins (Spelsberg et al., 1979). Similar masking of acceptor molecules may occur in androgen insensitive cells.

Solubilization and isolation of nuclear protein fractions that had acceptor-like activity were first achieved by Tymoczko and Liao (1971). The prostate nuclear proteins were extracted with salt solutions from the nuclei and were mixed with DNA to form a nucleoprotein aggregate. The reconstructed chromatin was then tested for its capacity to bind the prostate [³H]DHT receptor complex (i.e. for its acceptor activity). The suitability of this assay method was evaluated by a study of various properties that were characteristic of the retention of the DHT receptor complex by the intact prostate cell nuclei. Some properties employed for this purpose were receptor dependence of the DHT binding activity, tissue specificity, heat lability, the salt solubilization of the retained [³H]DHT receptor complex, and identification of the complex as a 3 S component in gradient centrifugation. Recently, Hiremath et al. (1980) also purified a salt extractable acceptor-like protein (from rat ventral prostate).

Klyzsejko-Stefanowicz and co-workers (1976) studied the chromatin acceptor molecules by sequentially removing urea-soluble chromosomal non-histone proteins, histones, and DNA-associated non-histone proteins from the chromatin of the rat ventral prostate and testis. The prostate [³H]DHT receptor complex was found to bind much more readily to the partially deproteinized chromatin, which still contains the DNA binding non-histone proteins, than to purified DNA. The receptor binding activity of rat DNA was enhanced significantly by the addition of the DNA-associated non-histone protein of the prostate or testis, but not that of the liver.

Using covalent linkage of nuclear components to Sepharose, Puca et al. (1975) studied the interaction of these components with the cytosol oestrogen receptor complex of the uterus and suggested that the nuclear acceptor molecule or molecules may be basic proteins. Mainwaring et al. (1976), who used the same technique, found that certain non-histone basic proteins in the prostate nuclei, when bound to Sepharose, could retain the prostate cytosol [³H]DHT receptor complex. Androgens present in free form or bound to the sex steroid binding globulin were not retained. The acceptor activity was higher in the nuclear preparations from the prostate than in those from the liver, spleen, or other tissues which are relatively insensitive to androgens. When various radioactive steroids were incubated with prostate cytosol as the source of steroid receptor complexes, [³H]DHT was found to be about five times more active than labelled testosterone. Dexamethasone, progesterone, and androsterone were essentially inactive.

In cell nuclei, the function of the steroid receptor complex may depend on its interaction with different forms of acceptor molecules. To explore such a possibility, we studied the interaction of the DHT receptor complex with the ribonucleoprotein (RNP) particle extracted from prostate cell nuclei (Liao *et al.*, 1973b). The tertiary complex sedimented as heterogeneous components (60–80 S) and could be analysed by gradient centrifugation. The receptor binding sites on the RNP particles could be saturated with excess DHT receptor, indicating that a limited number of binding sites exist. The apparent association constant calculated from such experiments is of the order of $10^{10} (mol/l)^{-1}$

Nyberg and Wang (1976) fractionated the androgen labelled prostate chromatin in order to identify the intranuclear localization of the acceptor sites. After a single injection of radioactive testosterone in the castrated rats, the quantity of radioactive androgen associated with a salt-soluble non-histone protein fraction was high within the first hour, but declined rapidly during the second hour. The changes in the radioactivity associated with the salt-insoluble non-histone protein and of the DNA-histone complex fractions, however, exhibited the opposite pattern. These and other studies described above suggest that some of the acceptor molecules are tightly bound to chromatin and cannot easily be solubilized by a moderate salt (1 mol/l KCl) solution.

7.1.5 Regulation of receptor activity and receptor recycling

By chasing of radioactive DHT with non-radioactive androgen during incubation of minced prostate, we have concluded that the nuclear receptor has a half-life of about 60–90 minutes (unpublished findings). During this period, the nuclear and cytoplasmic DHT receptor complex appears to maintain an equilibrium status (3000–5000 receptor molecules each in the nucleus and cytoplasm of a prostate cell); the amount of receptor newly synthesized during this time appears to be negligible. The equilibrium may be maintained by recycling of the receptor between nuclei and cytoplasm. Earlier studies on the uterus also suggested that some of the nuclear oestradiol receptor complexes could be released from the nuclei and recycled into the cytoplasm. The process was also found to be cycloheximide insensitive and therefore, independent of new protein synthesis.

Cellular energy production is known to be important in maintaining the steroid receptor levels in the target cells (Munck and Brinck-Johnsen, 1968; Liao and Fang, 1969; Ishii *et al.*, 1972; Munck *et al.*, 1972; Davies *et al.*, 1979; Liao *et al.*, 1980). In the rat ventral prostate, respiratory poisons such as NaCN or 2,4-dinitrophenol can rapidly reduce the DHT binding capacity of the cytosol receptor and the nuclear retention of androgens (Liao and Fang, 1969; Liao *et al.*, 1980). Available information indicates that the receptor molecules released from the nuclei are inactivated very rapidly, but that most of them can be reactivated by an energy-dependent process (Rossini and Liao, unpublished findings).

Pratt and his associates (Nielsen *et al.*, 1977; Sando *et al.* 1979) have suggested that the glucocorticoid receptor of L-cells or thymocytes may be inactivated by a process involving dephosphorylation. They also succeeded in reactivating the inactive form by incubating the receptor preparation with ATP, dithiothreitol, and a heat stable factor. In our laboratory, we have been able to use molybdate or ATP to stabilize the DHT binding activity of the prostate cytosol receptor in cell-free systems (Liao *et al.*, 1975; Liao *et al.*, 1980; Rossini and Liao, unpublished findings). No direct evidence is available, however, to show whether the receptor proteins or other closely related molecules are phosphorylated or dephosphorylated during the activation or inactivation processes.

If the nuclear retention of the steroid receptor complex is a key process in steroid hormone action, it is important to determine how this receptor-chromatin interaction is controlled in the target cells. Besides the acceptor molecules described above, there may be other factors that can promote or inhibit this interaction. Since tight binding of the receptor protein to the acceptor site(s) may be dependent on receptor transformation as described above, factors such as steroid structure, the presence of metal ions, and nucleotides that can affect receptor transformation may play a role in the interaction.

Besides these small molecules, macromolecules (proteins and nucleic acids) may affect receptor-nuclear acceptor interaction. In 1971, a cytosol protein (named α-protein) isolated from the rat ventral prostate by Fang and Liao, which was found to inhibit the association of the prostate androgen receptor complex with cell nuclei or chromatin. The protein inhibitor did not cause irreversible destruction of the receptor complex or damage to the nuclear binding site. Besides acting as an inhibitor, α-protein could promote the release of the androgen receptor complex already attached to chromatin. The release process occurred more readily at 20 °C than at 0 °C and was not due to dissociation of the radioactive androgen from the receptor or to inactivation of the receptor protein (Shyr and Liao, 1978).

As will be described later, α-protein has two major subunits, A and B, each with two subcomponents. We have found that only the acidic subunit (A) is active at low concentrations. A smaller subcomponent (mol. wt = 10 000; designated as component I) of subunit A is apparently responsible for the activity (Chen *et al.*, 1979). The amino acid sequence of this component (Figure 7.2) shows that a large proportion of the acidic amino acids are arranged in a unique manner. The portion of the peptide sequence that is rich in acidic amino acid may be responsible for the inhibitory action, since polyaspartic and polyglutamic acids are moderately active in inhibiting binding of the receptor complex by the prostate nuclear chromatin. Further studies are necessary to show whether the α-protein component can actually regulate the receptor-chromatin interaction in the intact prostate cells.

7.2 GENOMIC RESPONSES

7.2.1 Early studies on RNA and protein synthesis

Induction of enzymes or proteins by steroid hormones has been very useful for biochemists in the study of hormonal responses, especially since the basic

Amino acid sequence

$$\text{NH}_2\text{-}\underset{10}{}\text{Ser-Gln-Ile-Cys-Glu-Leu-Val-Ala-His-Glu-Thr-Ile-Ser-Phe-Leu-Met-Lys-Ser-Glu-Glu-Glu-Leu-}\underset{20}{}$$

10   20
NH$_2$- Ser-Gln-Ile-Cys-Glu-Leu-Val-Ala-His-Glu-Thr-Ile-Ser-Phe-Leu-Met-Lys-Ser-Glu-Glu-Glu-Leu-
          30   40
        Lys-Lys-Glu-Leu-Glu-Met-Tyr-Asn-Ala-Pro-Pro-Ala-Ala-Val-Glu-Ala-Lys-Leu-Glu-Val-Lys-Arg-
          50   60
        Cys-Val-Asp-Gln-Met-Ser-Asp-Gly-Asp-Arg-Leu-Val-Val-Ala-Glu-Thr-Leu-Val-Tyr-Ile-Phe-Leu-
          70   80   88
        Glu-Cys-Gly-Val-Lys-Gln-Trp-Val-Glu-Thr-Tyr-Tyr-Pro-Glu-Ile-Asp-Phe-Tyr-Tyr-Asp-Met-Asn-OH

Amino acid composition: Molecular weight:

Glu$_{13}$, Gln$_3$, Asp$_5$, Asn$_2$, Lys$_6$, Arg$_2$, His$_1$,   10,191

Val$_9$, Leu$_8$, Ala$_6$, Ser$_4$, Ile$_4$, Thr$_3$, Gly$_2$,

Tyr$_6$, Phe$_3$, Pro$_3$, Trp$_1$, Met$_4$, Cys$_3$

Figure 7.2   Amino acid sequence of component I of α-protein isolated from rat ventral prostate. This component inhibits the chromatin retention of the androgen-receptor complex in cell free systems (Liao et al., 1982)

steps involved in RNA and protein synthesis were elucidated in the early 1960s. Among some of the important earlier observations was the finding that ecdysone, an insect steroid hormone, injected into Drosophila larvae could cause a chromosome puff in the salivary gland (Clever and Karlson, 1960). Mueller and his associates (1961) showed that a single dose of oestradiol could cause a rapid accumulation of phospholipids, RNA, and proteins in rat uterus, and they suggested that an early protein synthesis was required for these oestrogenic responses.

In the study of the androgen effect on the protein synthesizing activity of the ribosomal particles of the rat ventral prostate, we presented the first biochemical evidence that androgen can increase the levels of mRNA associated with ribosomes (Liao and Williams-Ashman, 1962) and nuclei (Liao, 1965), and that androgen could increase RNA polymerase activity (Williams-Ashman et al., 1974). The stimulation of nuclear RNA polymerase activity of the rat uterus by oestradiol (Gorski, 1964) and of the rat ventral prostate by testosterone (Liao et al., 1965) was found to occur within 1 hour after these hormones were administered to castrated animals. Subsequently, many other steroid hormones have been found to have a rapid effect on nuclear RNA polymerase activity in their target organs.

Androgens and certain growth-promoting hormones can rapidly enhance the synthesis of nucleolar (or ribosomal) RNA (Liao and Lin, 1967; Liao, 1975). Why an early increase in rRNA synthesis is desirable for hormone action is not very clear. In some cases, however, the steroid hormone effects appear to be independent of rRNA synthesis. Examples are the effect of glucocorticoids on the induction of enzymes in the liver (Gelehrter and Tomkins, 1967), and the oestrogen-primed increase in avidin synthesis in the chick oviduct (O'Malley and McGuire, 1968).

With some exceptions (see below), many hormonal responses have been shown to depend on initial RNA synthesis and subsequent protein induction. This information came, in part, from the observation that actinomycin D (an inhibitor of RNA synthesis in nuclei) and puromycin or cycloheximide (inhibitors of protein synthesis at the ribosomal level) could suppress the hormonal responses. Some of the conclusions from these studies may need careful re-evaluations since these inhibitors may act elsewhere in the target cells. However, these and other studies in the 1960s have led to the now very popular hypothesis that steroid hormones and their receptors act in the nuclei where they influence RNA synthesis.

7.2.2   Chromatin modification and RNA synthesis

In organs such as the prostate and liver, the cell nuclei and cytosol fractions contain large quantities of chromatin-free RNA polymerase (Liao et al., 1968). Since the amounts of these 'reserved' polymerases do not respond rapidly to changes in the hormonal status of the animals (Liao and Fang, 1969), the hormonal action may not be on the polymerase core proteins, but on factors that may affect the specific association of the polymerase with DNA (Liao and Lin, 1967).

To assess whether hormones could change the chromatin in such a way that more RNA polymerase can utilize the chromatin template, several investigators prepared chromatin from hormone-deficient and from hormone-treated animals and assayed the capability of the chromatin preparations to support RNA synthesis in the presence of excess amounts of purified RNA polymerase. By this technique, enhancement of chromatin template activity was observed (including androgen effect on rat ventral prostate, Davies et al., 1979) in a matter of a few hours to several days after steroid hormones had been administered to the experimental animals. Other investigators, however, were not able to detect large changes in template activity due to the hormones (Liao and Fang, 1969; 1975a). The interpretation of the results of these studies has been very difficult, since factors such as hydrolytic enzymes that may affect template activity have not been studied carefully. It is also doubtful that the isolated chromatin represents the native state of all chromatin regions and that, under the experimental conditions, RNA is faithfully transcribed from the genomes by the added polymerase. In fact, the polymerase may transcribe pieces of RNA and DNA that are associated with the chromatin preparations (Palmiter and Lee, 1980).

By measuring the DNA sites available for actinomycin D binding in intact prostate nuclei, one could conclude that there is no androgen-induced gross unmasking of DNA. Androgen could, however, modify an RNA synthesizing activity of the prostate chromatin in the nucleolar or perinucleolar region that is highly sensitive to a low concentration of actinomycin D (Liao and Lin, 1967). This conclusion is in line with the finding that androgen can increase high affinity actinomycin D binding sites on the prostate chromatin (Mainwaring and Jones, 1975).

In the rat ventral prostate, it was found that certain nuclear proteins could be selectively labelled with radioactive phosphate within hours after rats had been treated with androgen (Ahmed et al., 1978). The nucleus-associated protein kinase reactions of the rat ventral prostate show varying androgen sensitivity. The kinase reactions involving non-histone proteins as substrates appear to be very sensitive to the androgen level of the animals. The cytosol cAMP-dependent protein kinase, however, is relatively insensitive to androgens.

The alteration of chromatin components by hormones may cause a detectable change in certain physical properties of the isolated chromatin. Thus, androgen effects on the chromatin of rat ventral prostate were detected by analysis of the thermal denaturation pattern, the circular dichroism spectrum, and the polylysine interaction of prostate chromatin (Loor *et al.*, 1977). Many of the above observations may be pertinent to, but do not prove, the view that steroid receptor complex functions by interacting with non-histone proteins to cause a specific local modification and/or decondensation of chromatin and to enhance template activity for RNA synthesis.

7.2.3 Induction of specific protein

Steroid hormones can induce or increase the production of specific proteins in many target organs. Some of these proteins may play important roles in the regulation of growth and function of the target cells, whereas others are major protein products of hormone action on the target cells. One of the earliest and most notable research achievements in this area came from the laboratories of Schimke and of O'Malley in their studies of the effect of steroid hormones on the production of chick oviduct proteins (Schimke *et al.*, 1975; O'Malley *et al.*, 1979). These and other investigators have rather clearly attributed the steroid hormone effect on the ovalbumin and on other protein synthesis in the oviduct to the hormone-induced level of specific mRNA for the proteins. Steroid hormone induction of mRNA has now been demonstrated in many other systems (see the books and reviews cited in the introduction) including oestrogen effects on the synthesis of vitellogenin in the liver and of prolactin in the pituitary, as well as glucocorticoid effects on growth hormone in cultured rat pituitary cells and on several enzymes in hepatic cells.

In the case of tyrosine aminotransferase induction by glucocorticoids in hepatoma tissue culture, Tomkins and his colleagues (1972) proposed that the inducing steroids (and receptors) act by antagonizing a labile post-transcriptional repressor which both inhibits mRNA translation and increases mRNA degradation. They devised this model to explain why actinomycin D inhibited the initial steroid hormone-dependent induction of the enzyme, but could increase the enzyme activity if the drug was added after induction had been allowed to proceed for a while. This phenomenon (called super induction) has been observed in a number of other systems, such as progesterone induction of chick oviduct proteins and hydrocortisone stimulation of glutamine synthetase in the neural retina of chick embryos. Tomkins' view, however, has not been supported by direct experimental evidence.

Glucocorticoids were also shown to stimulate the accumulation of mouse mammary tumour virus RNA in a cultured cell line of a mammary carcinoma in 15 minutes to several hours without appreciably affecting the overall rate of cellular RNA synthesis. This effect was insensitive to inhibitors of protein or

DNA synthesis and could be explained by, an increase in RNA synthesis. The possibility that the hormone action is due to the alteration of the processing of viral RNA and/or its degradation could not be excluded (Ringold et al., 1977).

The induction of several major cellular proteins has been found to be androgen-sensitive. The process studied most extensively is the induction of α_{2u} globulin (Roy and Neuhaus, 1966; Kurtz and Feigelson, 1978; Roy et al., 1977; Roy, 1979). This protein (mol. wt. = 20 000) was first found by Roy and Neuhaus (1966) in the urine of mature male rats, but was not present in the urine of female rats. It is synthesized in the liver and accounts for about 1 % of the total production of hepatic protein. The rate of production of this protein is maintained at a normal level by androgens, glucocorticoids, thyroid hormones, and pituitary growth hormones. These multiple hormonal effects on the level of mRNA for α_{2u} globulin have been investigated. Androgens and glucocorticoids appear to act by stimulating the induction of mRNA whereas thyroid hormone may modulate this induction. Growth hormone is believed to be required for maintenance of the normal α_{2u} globulin levels by post-transcriptional control. An early effect of androgen on the liver in castrated males appears to be the induction of the androgen receptor protein. Oestradiol antagonizes the androgen effect on α_{2u} globulin synthesis and this may be due to a reduction in circulating androgen levels or a decrease in the uptake and receptor binding of androgen.

Androgens are known to enhance the synthesis of abundant proteins in a number of target organs such as the mouse kidney (Toole et al., 1979) and liver (Hastie et al., 1979; Szoka et al., 1980) and the rat seminal vesicle (Ostrowski et al., 1979; Higgins and Burchell, 1978) and ventral prostate.

One of the abundant proteins in the rat ventral prostate was found and isolated more than a decade ago (Fang and Liao, 1971). During the isolation of the cytosol androgen receptor complex in the prostate, we found that the cytosol fraction contains another low affinity, high capacity steroid binding protein that can bind DHT, oestradiol and progesterone but not glucocorticoids. For convenience, we named the protein α-protein to distinguish it from a receptor protein that was called β-protein. The complexes of these proteins with DHT were named Complex I and Complex II:

α-protein + DHT → Complex I
β-protein + DHT → Complex II

The two complexes (or proteins) can be separated by ammonium sulphate fractionation or DEAE-cellulose. Complex II, but not Complex I can bind tightly to prostate nuclear chromatin.

α-Protein is apparently identical to the protein studied recently by several investigators and referred to as a steroid binding protein (Ichii, 1975), prostate binding protein (Heyns and DeMoor, 1977), prostatein (Lea et al., 1979), or oestramustine binding protein (Forsgren et al., 1979) There is general agreement that the protein has two major subunits (A and B) which are non-covalently associated with each other. Subunit A contains components I and III, whereas the subunit B has components II and III'. The components in the individual subunits are held together by disulphide linkages and can be separated from each other by β-mercaptoethanol. We have isolated the individual components and have determined their amino acid compositions and their N- and C-terminal amino acids. The complete sequence of the component I is shown in Figure 7.2. Available evidence (including the partial amino acid sequence) strongly suggests that components III and III′ are identical (Chen *et al.*, 1981).

Those mRNAs that could be translated into the components of α-protein have been partially purified in the laboratories of Parker (Parker and Scrace, 1979) and Heyns (Peeters *et al.*, 1980). Some increase in the production of these mRNAs could be observed within several hours after the injection of androgen to rats. A marked increase in mRNA production was seen in 2–3 days.

7.2.4 Mediatory proteins

Despite the extensive studies on the steroid induction of specific proteins, it has not been possible to prove that a steroid or the steroid receptor complex can act directly on the genes responsible for the synthesis of mRNA for these protein products. In fact, for several reasons some of the well studied examples may not represent the direct effect of the steroid receptor complexes on the genes being examined: (1) Steroid hormone-induced accumulation of mRNA for some of these proteins is preceded by a lag phase (one hour or more) after the hormone receptor complexes reach the nuclei. (2) A steroid can induce different proteins in different target cells and/or at different developmental stages. (3) Most proteins studied appear to be the ultimate products of hormone action in the target cells and are not likely to be the key regulatory proteins through which other responses in the same cells are mediated. (4) Cycloheximide, a protein synthesis inhibitor, can inhibit the hormonal induction of mRNA for some of the major proteins studied. (5) The number of steroid receptor complexes found in the nuclei *in vivo* greatly exceeds the number of gene sites for these major proteins.

The 'early' and 'late' effects of steroid hormones on gene expression were well illustrated many years ago. Mueller *et al.* (1961), as described above, demonstrated that, in the rat uterus, inhibition of protein synthesis by puromycin can block the early oestrogen stimulation of phospholipid and RNA synthesis and water imbibition. Also, ecdysone was shown to cause gene puffing in a defined sequence, and puromycin, a protein synthesis inhibitor, was shown to affect 'late' but not 'early' puffing (Clever and Karlson, 1960). Recently, translational inhibitors have been shown to prevent glucocorticoid induction of hepatic mRNA for tryptophan oxygenase (DeLap and Feigelson, 1978) and α_{2u}-globulin (Chen and Feigelson, 1979), oestrogen or progesterone induction of oviduct mRNA for ovalbumin and conalbumin (McKnight, 1978).

These observations were very similar to the finding that steroid hormone stimulation of ribosomal RNA synthesis could be prevented by cycloheximide or by α-amanitin, which inhibits RNA polymerase II but not RNA polymerase I (Lampert and Feigelson, 1974). For example, an androgen effect on rRNA synthesis in kidney was found to be dependent on protein synthesis (Janne *et al.*, 1976). In the study of androgen effect on nucleolar RNA synthesis in the rat ventral prostate, we have shown that manipulation of the androgen level of rats could result in an increase or decrease in nucleolar RNA synthesis within several hours but this is apparently not due to loss of the catalytic units of RNA polymerase (Liao and Fang, 1969). We proposed that specific factors are needed in steroid-hormone mediated changes in nuclear RNA polymerase activity. However no such mediating factor has been identified in any target cells.

In the search for the earliest protein(s) that might be induced by oestrogen in rat uterus, Notides and Gorski (1966) were able to demonstrate that treatment of uteri *in vivo* with oestradiol for periods of 30 minutes to 2 hours, followed by a 1 hour incubation of uteri *in vitro* with labelled amino acid, dramatically increased the incorporation of amino acids into a specific uterine cytosol protein fraction that can be detected by starch gel electrophoresis. The protein(s), referred to as 'induced protein(s)' (IP), could also be induced by incubation *in vitro* of rat uteri (Katzenellenbogen and Gorski, 1972). One of the components (mol. wt. = 45 000) was purified to homogeneity by SDS polyacrylamide gel electrophoresis (Manak *et al.*, 1980). A more recent study (Skipper *et al.*, 1980) suggested that the electrophoretic band identified as IP has at least three components. One of the components appeared to be an acidic enolase (Kaye and Reiss, 1980).

Several years ago we found that the rat ventral prostate contains a specific spermine binding protein (SBP) that is highly sensitive to androgens. The protein was discovered (Liang *et al.*, 1978) during our study of factors, such as polyamines, which could affect the androgen-sensitive initiation of protein synthesis (Liang *et al.*, 1977). At pH 7.0–8.5, the radioactive spermine was bound much more tightly than spermidine or other natural diamines by this protein. The apparent spermine binding activity of the prostate cytosol protein fraction was reduced by about 50 % within a day after the rats had been castrated. This effect could be reversed by injection of DHT. The hormonal effect was reduced when rats were injected with cycloheximide or actinomycin D (Mezzetti *et al.*, 1979).

The purified SBP has a molecular weight of about 34 000. Polyacrylamide gel electrophoresis indicated that there might be two or three forms of the protein. The stimulatory effect of androgen *in vivo* on the synthesis of an SBP-like protein was shown by incubation of minced prostate with ^{14}C or ^{3}H labelled amino acids and analysing the incorporation of labelled amino acids into the acidic protein fraction by polyacrylamide gel electrophoresis.

The production of IP in the rat uterus and of SBP in the rat ventral prostate appear to be modulated specifically by sex steroids very soon after steroid hormones enter the target cells. Since their cellular roles are not clearly understood, it is not possible to predict whether these proteins actually play key functions in mediating the later hormonal responses. Furthermore, there is some controversy as to whether IP is present in the uterus of animals other than rats (Galand *et al.*, 1978). Similarly, we have not been able to detect SBP-like proteins in dog or human prostates. Thus, one cannot suggest that these proteins are universal proteins through which sex steroids mediate their actions.

7.3 NON-GENOMIC RESPONSES

Most actions of steroid hormones appear to depend on the synthesis of RNA in the nuclei of target cells. There are experimental observations, however, suggesting that some steroid hormones act without having a direct hormonal effect on RNA synthesis.

One of the most convincing observations showing that steroid hormones can function outside the cell nucleus was made in a study on the induction of frog oocyte maturation or meiosis by progesterone and other steroid hormones (Smith and Eker, 1971; Schuetz, 1976). To analyse this induction, the breakdown of the germinal vesicle (nucleus) and the increase in protein synthesis in oocytes in culture were studied. The effect was very rapid and was actinomycin D-insensitive. Nuclear RNA synthesis was apparently not involved in the hormonal action, since many of the events associated with maturation (including the synthesis of proteins and of a maturation promoting factor) could be seen in enucleated oocytes. In fact, steroid hormones appeared to act on oocytes by interacting with the cell surface (Smith and Eker, 1971; Masui and Markert, 1971; Schuetz, 1976; O'Connor *et al.*, 1977; Robinson, 1979); a progestin linked to a polymer that could not enter the cell was shown to promote oocyte meiosis (Godeau *et al.*, 1978). The possibility that steroid hormones act on the oocyte system by calcium efflux and control the cyclic nucleotide activity has been proposed (Maller and Krebs, 1977; Cartaud *et al.*, 1980). This is in line with an earlier suggestion, by Hechter and Halkerston (1965) that steroids or steroid receptors may act at the plasma membrane. The interaction of divalent metal ions with androgen and other steroid receptors has been described by many investigators during the last 10 years (Liao, 1975a).

The insensitivity of steroid hormone action to actinomycin D has been reported for several systems besides the oocyte system. The effect of oestrogen in the rat uterus on the uptake of precursors of RNA (Billing *et al.*, 1969), the rate of peptide elongation on ribosomes (Whelly and Barker, 1974), the effects of androgens on the growth of the chick comb (Talwar *et al.*, 1965), induction of renal arginase activity (Frieden and Fisher, 1968), NAD biosynthesis (Ritter, 1966), nuclear protein phosphorylation (Ahmed and Ishida, 1971), and the very rapid increase in the activity of an initiation factor necessary for protein synthesis in the rat ventral prostate (Muldoon, 1980) were all shown to be insensitive to actinomycin D. Many of these reports, however, have not been confirmed independently or studied in detail. One can also argue that actinomycin D, at the doses employed, did not inhibit RNA synthesis completely. Nevertheless, non-genomic action of steroid hormones and their receptors is a possibility that should be pursued further. This view is in line with the recent report by Muldoon (1980) that 4-mercurioestradiol, a synthetic oestrogen, could transform the uterine cytosol receptor to a 5 S form, but that the 5 S complex was not retained by nuclei or bound to calf thymus DNA.

A clear-cut proof for the cellular site of action, however, may come only by demonstration of the effect of steroid hormones in a well-defined cell-free system. Many attempts to achieve such a proof have been made in the past, but their impact on the study of the biochemical mechanism of steroid hormone actions has been minimal. In one such study, Vesely (1979) reported recently that many sex steroid hormones, including androgens, at concentration of 1 nmol/l to 1 μmol/l, stimulated guanylate cyclase activity in cytosol prepared from liver, kidney, skeletal muscle, and ventral prostate of rats. This unusual observation has not been confirmed. Increases in uterine cyclic GMP content *in vivo* or during incubation of uteri with oestradiol and testosterone at a high concentration have also been observed (Flandroy and Galand, 1980).

7.4 CONCLUSIONS

7.4.1 Stromal-epithelial interaction

The differentiation and development of many organs are highly dependent on interaction among different types of cells in the organs. Chemical signals may be sent from one type of cell to the others to control their morphogenesis and/or cellular activity. In the study of androgens and their effect on epithelium, Cunha and his associates (1980) have found in the last few years that androgen-induced prostatic organogenesis can occur when epithelium of the urogenital sinus from a wild (androgen-sensitive)-type or Tfm/Y (androgen insensitive) embryo was combined with wild-type mesenchyme (stroma). Morphogenesis of prostatic epithelium was not observed when mesenchyme was taken from Tfm/Y animals and combined with either the wild-type or Tfm/Y epithelium. The result appears to indicate that mesenchyme can mediate androgen effects during epithelial organogenesis, although normal function of the prostate may also depend on direct and coordinated effects of androgen on both epithelial and stroma cells. Mediation of steroid hormone effects through cell–cell interaction in the same organ, as exemplified by the case just described, is probably general rather than exceptional.

7.4.2 RNA binding of receptor and post-transcriptional regulation

Very little is known about the fate of the steroid receptor complex after its interaction with chromatin. The nuclear receptor or the steroid may be modified in such a way that they do not bind to each other tightly, causing the release of the receptor from the genomic structure. Another possibility we have considered is that RNA made in nuclei may be bound to the receptor complex (and other proteins) and facilitates the release of the complex from the nuclei. The receptor complex, in turn, may play an important role in processing, stabilization, and/or utilization of RNA. Although direct evidence supporting this idea is still lacking, our studies have shown that both the oestrogen and androgen receptor complexes can bind to certain ribonucleoprotein (RNP) particles in the uterus and in the prostate (Liao *et al.*, 1972; Liao *et al.*, 1973b; Liang and Liao, 1974).

To test the possibility that certain RNA molecules promote the release of steroid receptor complex from DNA or chromatin, we employed DNA-cellulose column chromatography (Liao *et al.*, 1980). We found that ribopolymers rich in uracil and guanine are more effective than polymers rich in adenine and cytosine in dissociating the prostatic androgen receptor complex bound to DNA-cellulose. The progestin and oestrogen receptor complexes from rat uterus and the glucocorticoid receptor complex from rat liver behaved similarly to the androgen receptor complex of the rat ventral prostate. It is conceivable that certain natural RNA molecules with proper nucleotide sequences can bind to the steroid receptor complex and can exhibit high specificity toward different steroid receptor complexes.

It is plausible to suggest that the receptor protein can lose its capacity to bind to RNP at various stages of RNA processing and utilization, especially if the steroid hormone of the cell is depleted. Both the receptor proteins and the acceptor proteins may reassociate with these particles when the steroid hormone is replenished. Thus the process may be reinitiated by the steroid hormone at different points, either in the nucleus or in the cytoplasm. This implies that the importance of gene transcription (RNA synthesis) in relation to gene translation (protein synthesis) for the overall functioning of a steroid hormone in target cells may be dependent on the level of different types of RNP particles and on their RNA and protein constituents in the target cells at the time the hormone is supplied. If the target cells contain sufficient amounts of RNA and of the protein constituents of RNP, the early actions of the hormone may simply be dependent on the processing and utilization of RNP, and not upon RNA synthesis (Liao *et al.*, 1972; Liang and Liao, 1974; Puca *et al.*, 1975).

7.4.3 A hypothetical model of receptor dynamics

A hypothetical scheme for the intracellular pathway and function of an androgen receptor is summarized in Figure 7.3. To avoid confusion in terminology, we recommend the use of the term 'activation' strictly for the change in the receptor from the form that cannot bind hormones to the hormone binding form. 'Transformation' is reserved for the alteration of a steroid receptor complex to a form that has a higher affinity toward nuclear components, such as chromatin. In the rat ventral prostate, 'activation' has been shown to depend on a continuous supply of cellular energy, whereas 'transformation' has been shown, *in vitro*, to be promoted by a temperature-dependent process. Neither of these two steps is well understood at the biochemical level.

Chromatin binding of a steroid receptor complex may be regulated by protein factors that can either promote or inhibit the interaction. Early responses may result in the increased production of certain promoting factors that can enhance the synthesis of late (and ultimate) protein products. The late response may also yield a protein factor that can suppress interaction of the chromatin with the receptor complex. The imbalance between promoters and inhibitors may cause abnormal responses that result in either hypersensitivity or insensitivity phenomena.

Loss of the steroid hormone receptor has often been regarded as the reason

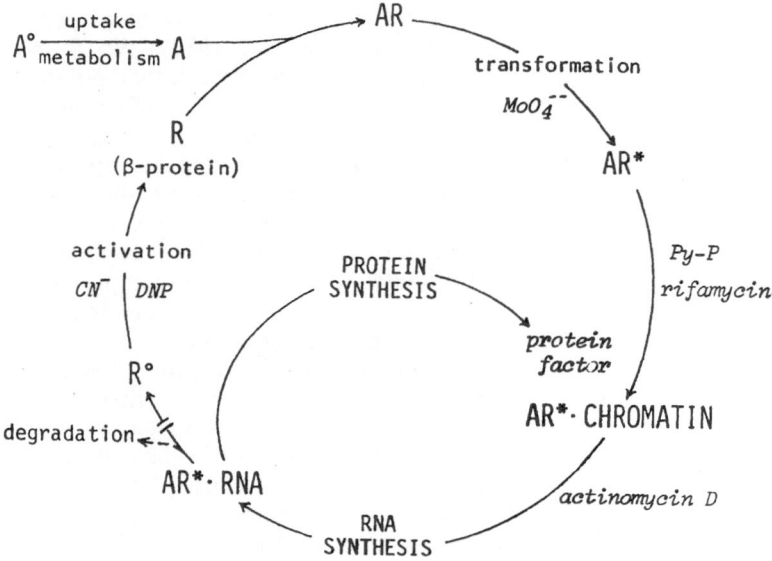

Figure 7.3 A working model for the steps involved in intracellular cycling of the androgen receptor in target cells. In this hypothetical model, the receptor protein ($R°$) is activated by an energy-dependent process that is sensitive to respiratory poisons such as CN, azide, and DNP. The activated receptor (R) then binds an active androgen (A) such as DHT that may be formed from a precursor such as testosterone ($A°$). The androgen-receptor complex (AR) is transformed in a temperature-dependent step to the form AR*, which can be retained tightly by chromatin. The stability of AR or AR* can be affected by ATP and/or MoO_4^{2-}. The nuclear retention of AR* can be inhibited by MoO_4^{2-}. The nuclear retention of AR* can be inhibited by MoO_4^{2-}, pyridoxal phosphate, rifamycins, and chloroquine. The nuclear AR* appears to have a half-life of about 70 minutes. The release of AR* may be promoted by certain RNAs, but can be inhibited by chloroquine or actinomycin D. The released AR* is recycled, inactivated, or degraded

for hormone insensitivity of target tissues. However, insensitive cells are often found to function or grow as well as sensitive cells. If the steroid receptor complex in the sensitive cells plays a vital role, it is reasonable to suggest that a protein similar to the receptor, or an altered form of the receptor, may function in the insensitive cells. Because the protein may be structurally compatible with the functional site, the protein may function without a prior interaction with steroid hormones (Liao, 1975b, Zava *et al.*, 1977).

Acknowledgement

The work from the authors' laboratory was supported by Grant BC-151 from the American Cancer Society, Research Grant AM-09461, and CA-09183 from the US National Institutes of Health.

7.5 REFERENCES

Ahmed, K. and Ishida, H. (1971). Effect of testosterone on nuclear phosphoproteins of rat ventral prostate. *Mol. Pharmacol.*, **7**, 323

Ahmed, K., Wilson, M. J., Goueli, S. A. and Williams-Ashman, H. G. (1978). Effects of polyamines on prostatic chromatin and non-histone-protein-associated protein kinase reactions. *Biochem. J.*, **176**, 739

Anderson, K. M. and Liao, S. (1968). Selective retension of dihydrotestosterone by prostatic nuclei. *Nature (London)*, **219**, 277

Baulieu, E. E. and Jung, I. (1970). A prostatic cytosol receptor. *Biochem. Biophys. Res. Commun.*, **38**, 599

Billing, R. J., Barbivoli, G. and Smellie, R. M. S. (1969). The mode of action of oestradiol. II. The synthesis of RNA. *Biochim. Biophys. Acta*, **190**, 52

Blondeau, J. P., Corpechot, C., LeGoascogne, C., Baulieu, E. E. and Robel, P. (1975). Androgen receptors in the rat ventral prostate and their hormonal control. *Vit. Horm.*, **33**, 319

Bruchovsky, N. and Wilson, J. D. (1968). The intranuclear binding of testosterone and 5-alpha-androstan-17-beta-ol-3-one by rat prostate. *J. Biol. Chem.*, **243**, 2012

Cartaud, A., Ozon, R., Walsh, M. P., Haiech, J. and Demaille, J. G. (1980). *Xenopus laevis* oocyte calmodulin in the process of meiotic maturation. *J. Biol. Chem.*, **255**, 9404

Castaneda, E. and Liao, S. (1975). The use of anti-steroid antibodies in the characterization of steroid receptors. *J. Biol. Chem.*, **250**, 883

Chan, K. M. B., Smythe, S. and Liao, S. (1979). Androgen receptor binding and androgenicity of methylated 4-ene-3-ketosteroids having no 17-hydroxy group. *J. Steroid Biochem.*, **11**, 1193

Chen, L. C. and Feigelson, P. (1979). Cycloheximidine inhibition of hormonal induction of alpha 2u-globulin mRNA. *Proc. Natl. Acad. Sci. USA*, **76**, 2669

Chen, C., Hiipakka, R. and Liao, S. (1979). Prostate alpha-protein: Subunit structure, polyamine binding and inhibition of nuclear chromatin binding of androgen-receptor complex. *J. Steroid Biochem.*, **11**, 401

Chen, C., Shilling, K., Hiipakka, R. A., Haung, I-Y. and Liao, S. (1981). *J. Biol. Chem.*, **256**,

Clever, V. and Karlson, P. (1960). Induction of puff changes in the salivary gland chromosomes of *Chironomus tetans* by ecdysone. *Exp. Cell. Res.*, **20**, 623

Cunha, G. R., Chung, L. W. K., Shannon, J. M. and Reese, B. A. (1980). Stromal-epithelial interactions in sex differentiation. *Biol. Reprod.*, **22**, 19

Davies, P., Thomas, P., Giles, M. G., Boonjawat, J. and Griffiths, K. (1979). Regulation of transcription of the prostate genome by androgens. *J. Steroid Biochem.*, **11**, 351

DeLap, L. and Feigelson, P. (1978). Effect of cycloheximide on the induction of trytophan oxygenase mRNA by hydrocortisone *in vivo*. *Biochem. Biophys. Res. Commun.*, **82**, 142

Fang, S., Anderson, K. M. and Liao, S. (1969). Receptor proteins for androgens. On the role of specific proteins in selective retension of 17-beta-hydroxy-5-alpha-androstan-3-one by rat ventral prostate *in vivo* and *in vitro*. *J. Biol. Chem.*, **244**, 6584

Fang, S. and Liao, S. (1969). Antagonistic action of anti-androgens on the formation of a specific dihydrotestosterone-receptor protein complex in rat ventral prostate. *Mol. Pharmacol.*, **5**, 428

Fang, S. and Liao, S. (1971). Androgen receptors. Steroid-and-tissue specific retention of 17-beta-hydroxy-5-alpha-androstan-3-one-protein complex by the cell nuclei of ventral prostate. *J. Biol. Chem.*, **246**, 16

Flandroy, L. and Galand, P. (1980). *In vitro* stimulation by oestrogen or quanosine 3'5'-mono phosphate accumulation in incubated rat uterus. *Endocrinology*, **106**, 1187

Forsgren, B., Bjork, P., Carlstrom, K., Gustafsson, J. A., Pousette, A. and Hogberg, B. (1979). Purification and distribution of a major protein in rat prostate that binds estramustine, a nitrogen derivative of estradiol-17-beta. *Proc. Natl. Acad. Sci. USA*, **76**, 3149

Frieden, E. H. and Fisher, S. S. (1968). Differential sensitivity of parameters of androgen action to metabolic inhibitors: arginase and beta-glucuronidase. *Biochem. Biophys. Res. Commun.*, **31**, 515

Galand, P., Flandroy, L. and Mairesse, N. (1978). Relationship between the estrogen induced protein ip and other parameters of estrogenic stimulation. *Life Sci.*, **22**, 217

Gelehrter, T. D. and Tomkins, G. M. (1967). The role of RNA in the hormonal induction of tyrosine aminotransferase in mammalian cells in tissue culture. *J. Mol. Biol.*, **29**, 59

Godeau, J. F., Schorderet-Slatkine, S., Hubert, P. and Baulieu, E. E. (1978). Induction of maturation in *Xenopus laevis* oocytes by a steroid linked to a polymer. *Proc. Natl. Acad. Sci. USA*, **75**, 2353

Gorski, J. (1964). Early estrogen effects on the activity of uterine ribonucleic acid polymerase. *J. Biol. Chem.*, **239**, 889

Gorski, J. and Gannon, F. (1976). Current models of steroid hormone action: a critique. *Annu. Rev. Physiol.*, **38**, 425

Greene, G.L., Closs, L. E., Fleming, H., DeSombre, E. R. and Jensen, E. V. (1977). Antibodies to estrogen receptor: immunochemical similarity of estrophilin from various mammalian species. *Proc. Natl. Acad. Sci. USA*, **74**, 3681

Greene, G. L., Fitch, F. W. and Jensen, E. V. (1980). Monoclonal antibodies to estrophilin: probes for the study of oestrogen receptors. *Proc. Natl. Acad. Sci. USA*, **77**, 157

Hastie, N. D., Held, W. A. and Toole, J. J. (1979). Multiple genes coding for the androgen-regulated major urinary proteins of the mouse. *Cell*, **17**, 449

Hechter, O. and Halkerston, I. D. K. (1965). Effects of steroid hormones on gene regulation and cell metabolism. *Annu. Rev. Physiol.*, **27**, 133

Heyns, W. and DeMoor, P. (1977). Prostatic binding protein. A steroid-binding protein secreted by rat prostate. *Eur. J. Biochem.*, **78**, 221

Higgins, S. J. and Burchell, J. M. (1978). Effects of testosterone on messenger ribonucleic acid and protein synthesis in rat seminal vesicle. *Biochem. J.*, **174**, 543

Hiremath, S. T., Loor, R. M. and Wang, T. Y. (1980). Isolation of an androgen receptor from salt extract of rat prostatic chromatin. *Biochem. Biophys. Res. Commun.*, **97**, 981

Ichii, S. (1975). 5-alpha-dihydrotestosterone binding protein in rat ventral prostate; purification, nuclear incorporation and subnuclear localization. *Endocrinol. Jpn.*, **22**, 433

Ishii, D. N., Pratt, W. B. and Aronow, L. (1972). Steady-state level of the specific gluco-corticoid binding component in mouse fibroblasts. *Biochemistry*, **11**, 3896

Janne, O., Bullock, L. P., Bardin, C. W. and Jacob, S. T. (1976). Early androgen action in kidney of normal and androgen-insensitive (tfm/y) mice. Changes in RNA polymerase and chromatin template activities. *Biochim. Biophys. Acta*, **418**, 388

Jensen, E. V. (1979). Interaction of steroid hormones with the nucleus. *Pharmacol. Rev.*, **30**, 477

Jensen, E. V. and Jacobson, H. I. (1962). Basic guides to the mechanism of oestrogen action. *Recent Progr. Horm. Res.*, **18**, 387

Jensen, E. V., Mohla, S., Gorell, T. A. and DeSombre, E. R. (1974). The role of estrophilin in estrogen action. *Vit. Horm.*, **32**, 89

Katzenellenbogen, B. S. (1980). Dynamics of steroid hormone receptor action. *Ann. Rev. Physiol.*, **42**, 17

Katzenellenbogen, B. S. and Gorski, J. (1972). Estrogen action *in vitro*. Induction of the synthesis of a specific uterine protein. *J. Biol. Chem.*, **247**, 1299

Kaye, A. M. and Reiss (1980). The uterine 'estrogen induced protein' (ip): Purification, distribution and possible function. In Beato, M. (ed.) *Steroid Induced Uterine Proteins*. pp. 3—19. (New York: North Holland/Elsevier)

Klyzsejko-Stefanowicz, L., Chiu, J. F., Tsai, Y. H. and Hnilica, L. S. (1976). Acceptor proteins in rat androgenic tissue chromatin. *Proc. Acad. Sci. USA*, **73**, 1954

Kurtz, D. T. and Feigelson, P. (1978). Multi-hormonal control of the messenger RNA for the hepatic protein globulin. In Litwack, G. (ed.) *Biochemical Actions of Hormones*. vol. 5, pp. 433—455. (New York: Academic Press)

Lampert, A. and Feigelson, P. (1974). A short lived polypeptide component of one of two discrete functional pools of hepatic nuclear alpha-amanitin resistant RNA polymerases. *Biochem. Biophys. Res. Commun.*, **58**, 1030

Lea, O. A., Petrusz, P. and French, F. S. (1979). Prostatein. A major secretory protein of the rat ventral prostate. *J. Biol. Chem.*, **254**, 6196

Liang, T., Castaneda, E. and Liao, S. (1977). Androgen and initiation of protein synthesis in the prostate. Binding of met-tRNAfMet to cytosol initiation factor and ribosomal subunit particles. *J. Biol. Chem.*, **252**, 5692

Liang, T. and Liao, S. (1974). Association of the uterine 17-beta-estradiol receptor complex with ribonucleoprotein *in vitro* and *in vivo*. *J. Biol. Chem.*, **249**, 4671

Liang, T., Mezzetti, G., Chen, C. and Liao, S. (1978). Selective polyamine-binding proteins. Spermine binding by an androgen-sensitive phosphoprotein. *Biochim. Biophys. Acta*, **542**, 430

Liao, S. (1965). Influence of testosterone on template activity of prostatic ribonucleic acids. *J. Biol. Chem.*, **240**, 1236

Liao, S. (1975a). Cellular receptors and mechanisms of action of steroid hormones. *Int. Rev. Cytol.*, **41**, 817

Liao, S. (1975b). In Goland, M. (ed.) *Normal and Abnormal Growth of the Prostate*. p. 894. (Springfield: Charles C. Thomas)

Liao, S. (1977). Molecular action of androgens. In Litwack, G. (ed.) *Biochemical Action of Hormones*. Vol. 4, pp. 351—406. (New York: Academic Press)

Liao, S., Chen, C. and Huang, I. Y. (1982). α-Protein: Complete amino acid sequence of the component that inhibits nuclear retention of the androgen receptor complex. *J. Biol. Chem.*, **257**, 122

Liao, S. and Fang, S. (1969). Receptor-proteins for androgens and the mode of action of androgens on gene transcription in ventral prostate. *Vit. Horm.*, **27**, 17

Liao, S. and Fang, S. (1970). Factors and specificities involved in the formation of 5α-dihydrotestosterone nuclear receptor protein complex in rat ventral prostate. In Griffiths, K. and Pierrepoint, C. G. (eds.) *Some Aspects of Aetiology and Biochemistry of Prostate Cancer*. pp. 105—108. (Cardiff: Alpha Omega Alpha)

Liao, S., Leininger, K. R., Sagher, D. and Barton, R. W. (1965). Rapid effects of testosterone on ribonucleic acid polymerase activity of rat ventral prostate. *Endocrinology*, **77**, 763

Liao, S., Liang, T., Fang, S., Castaneda, E. and Shao, T. C. (1973a). Steroid structure and androgenic activity. Specificities involved in the receptor binding and nuclear retension of various androgens. *J. Biol. Chem.*, **248**, 6154

Liao, S., Liang, T. and Tymoczko, J. L. (1973b). Ribonucleoprotein binding of steroid – 'receptor' complexes. *Nature (New Biol.)*, **241**, 211

Liao, S. and Lin, A. H. (1967). Prostatic nuclear chromatin: an effect of testosterone on the synthesis of ribonucleic acid rich in cytidylyl (3'5') guanosine. *Proc. Natl. Acad. Sci. USA*, **57**, 379

Liao, S., Rossini, G. P., Hiipakka, R. A. and Chen, C. (1980). Factors that can control the interaction of androgen receptor complex with the genomic structure in the rat prostate. In Bresciani, F. (ed.) *Perspective in Steroid Receptor Research.* pp. 99–112. (New York: Academic Press)

Liao, S., Sagher, D. and Fang, S. (1968). Isolation of chromatin free RNA polymerase from mammalian cell nuclei. *Nature (London)*, **220**, 1336

Liao, S., Smythe, S., Tymoczko, J. L., Rossini, G. P., Chen, C. and Hiipakka, R. A. (1981). RNA-dependent release of androgen and other steroid receptor complexes of DNA. *J. Biol. Chem.*, **255**, 5545

Liao, S., Tymoczko, J. L., Castaneda, E. and Liang, T. (1975). Androgen receptors and androgen-dependent initiation of protein synthesis in the prostate. *Vit. Horm.*, **33**, 297

Liao, S., Tymoczko, J. L., Howell, D. K., Lin, A. H., Shao, T. C. and Liang, T. (1972). RNA dependent release of androgen and other steroid receptor complexes from DNA. In *Proceeding of the 4th Internation Congress of Endocrinology*. Ser. No. *273*, p. 404. (Amsterdam: Excerpta Medica)

Liao, S. and Williams-Ashman, H. G. (1962). An effect of testosterone on amino acid incorporation by prostatic ribonucleoprotein particles. *Proc. Natl. Acad. Sci. USA*, **48**, 1956

Loor, R. M., Hu, A. L. and Wang, T. Y. (1977). Structurally altered and transcriptionally activated rat prostate chromatin induced by androgens. *Biochim. Biophys. Acta*, **477**, 312

Mainwaring, W. I. (1969a). The binding of $(1, 2-^3H)$ testosterone within nuclei of the rat prostate. *J. Endocrinol.*, **44**, 323

Mainwaring, W. I. (1969b). A soluble androgen receptor in the cytoplasm of rat prostate. *J. Endocrinol.*, **45**, 531

Mainwaring, W. I. and Irving, R. (1973). The use of deoxyribonucleic acid–cellulose chromatography and isoelectric focussing for the characterization and partial purification of steroid-receptor complexes. *Biochem. J.*, **134**, 113

Mainwaring, W. I. and Jones, D. M. (1975). Influence of receptor complexes on the properties of prostate chromatin, including its transcription by RNA polymerase. *J. Steroid Biochem.*, **6**, 475

Mainwaring, W. I. and Peterken, B. M. (1971). A reconstituted cell-free system for the specific transfer of steroid receptor complexes into nuclear chromatin isolated from the rat ventral prostate gland. *Biochem. J.*, **125**, 285

Mainwaring, W. I., Symes, E. K. and Higgins, S. J. (1976). Nuclear components responsible for the retension of steroid-receptor complexes, especially from the standpoint of the specificity of hormonal responses. *Biochem. J.*, **156**, 129

Maller, J. L. and Krebs, E. G. (1977). Progesterone-stimulated meiotic cell-division in *Xenopus* oocytes. Induction by regulatory subunit and inhibiton by catalytic subunit of adenosine 3'5'-monophosphate-dependent protein kinase. *J. Biol. Chem.*, **252**, 1712

Manak, R., Wertz, N., Slabaugh, M., Denari, H., Wang, S. and Gorski, J. (1980). Purification and characterization of the estrogen-induced protein (1P) of rat uterus. *Mol. Cell. Endocrinol.*, **17**, 119

Masui, Y. and Markert, C. (1971). Cytoplasmic control of nuclear behaviour during meiotic maturation of frog oocytes. *J. Exp. Zool.*, **177**, 129

McKnight, G. S. (1978). The induction of ovalbumine and conalbumin mRNA by estrogen and progesterone in chick oviduct explant cultures. *Cell*, **14**, 403

Mezzetti, G., Loor, R. and Liao, S. (1979). Androgen-sensitive spermine-binding protein of rat ventral prostate. Purification of the protein and characterization of hormonal effect. *Biochem. J.*, **184**, 431

Moore, R. J. and Wilson, J. D. (1972). Localization of the reduced nicotinamide adenine dinucleotide phosphate: 4-3-keto steroid 5-oxidoreductase in the nuclear membrane of the rat ventral prostate. *J. Biol. Chem.*, **247**, 958

Muldoon, T. G. (1980). Molecular and functional anomalies in the mechanism of the estrogenic action of 4-mercuri-17 beta estradiol. *J. Biol. Chem.*, **255**, 1358

Mueller, G. C., Gorski, J. and Aizawa, Y. (1961). The role of protein synthesis in early estrogen action. *Proc. Natl. Acad. Sci. USA*, **47**, 164

Munck, A. and Brinck-Johnsen, T. (1968). Specific and non-specific physiochemical interactions of glucocorticoids and related steroids with rat thymus cells *in vitro. J. Biol. Chem.* **243**, 5556

Munck, A., Wira, C., Young, D. A., Mosher, K. M., Hallahan, C. and Bell, P. A. (1972). Glucocorticoid-receptor complexes and the earliest steps in the action of glucocorticoids in thymus cells. *J. Steroid Biochem.*, **3**, 567

Nielson, C. J., Sando, J. J., Vogel, W. M. and Pratt, W. B. (1977). Glucocorticoid receptor inactivation under cell-free conditions. *J. Biol. Chem.*, **252**, 7568

Notides, A. and Gorski, J. (1966). Estrogen-induced synthesis of a specific uterine protein. *Proc. Natl. Acad. Sci. USA*, **56**, 230

Nyberg, L. M. and Wang, T. Y. (1976). The role of androgen-binding nonhistone proteins in the transcriptions of prostatic chromatin. *J. Steroid Biochem.*, **7**, 267

O'Connor, C. M., Robinson, K. R. and Smith, L. D. (1977). Calcium, potassium and sodium exchange by full-grown and maturing *Xenopus laevis* oocytes, *Dev. Biol.*, **61**, 28

O'Malley, B. W. and Birnbaumer, L. (1977). *Receptors and Hormone Action.* (New York: Academic Press)

O'Malley, B. W. and McGuire, W. L. (1968). Studies on the mechanism of estrogen mediated tissue differentiation: regulation of nuclear transcription and induction of new RNA species. *Proc. Natl. Acad. Sci. USA*, **60**, 1527

O'Malley, B. W., Roop, D. R., Lai, E. C., Nordstrom, J. L., Catterall, J. F., Swaneck, G. E., Colbert, D. A., Tsai, M. J., Dugaiczyk, A. and Woo, S. L. C. (1979). The ovalbumin gene: organization, structure, transcription and regulation, *Recent Progr. Horm. Res.*, **35**, 1

O'Malley, B. W., Spelsberg, T. C., Schrader, W. T., Chytil, F. and Steggles, A. W. (1972). Mechanisms of interaction of a hormone-receptor complex with the genome of a eukaryotic target cell. *Nature (London)*, **235**, 141

Ostrowski, M. C., Kistler, M. K. and Kistler, W. S. (1979). Purification and cell-free synthesis of a major protein from rat seminal vesicle secretion. A potential marker for androgen action. *J. Biol. Chem.*, **254**, 383

Palmiter, R. D. and Lee, D. C. (1980). Regulation of gene transcription by estrogen and progesterone. Lack of hormonal effects on transcription by *Escherichia coli* RNA polymerase. *J. Biol. Chem.*, **255**, 9693

Parker, M. G. and Scrace, G. T. (1979). Regulation of protein synthesis in rat ventral prostate: cell-free translation of mRNA. *Proc. Natl. Acad. Sci. USA*, **76**, 1580

Pasqualini, J. R. (1976). *Receptors and Mechanism of Action of Steroid Hormones.* (New York: Marcel Dekker)

Peeters, B. L., Mous, J. M., Rombauts, W. A. and Heyns, W. J. (1980). Androgen induced messenger RNA in rat ventral prostate: translation, partial purification and preliminary characterization of the mRNAs encoding the components of prostatic binding protein. *J. Biol. Chem.*, **255**, 7017

Puca, G. A., Nola, E., Hibner, V., Cicala, G. and Sica, V. (1975). Interaction of the estradiol receptor from calf uterus with its nuclear acceptor sites. *J. Biol. Chem.*, **250**, 6452

Puca, G. A., Sica, V., Nola, E. and Bresciani, F. (1979). Purification and properties of native oestradiol receptor. *J. Steroid Biochem.*, **11**, 301

Ringold, G. M., Yamamoto, K. R., Bishop, J. M. and Varmus, H. E. (1977).

Glucocorticoid-stimulated accumulation of mouse mammary tumour virus RNA increased rate of synthesis of vital RNA. *Proc. Natl. Acad. Sci. USA*, **74**, 2879

Ritter, C. (1966). NAD biosynthesis as an early part of androgen action. *Mol. Pharmacol.*, **2**, 125

Robinson, K. R. (1979). Electrical currents through full-grown and maturing *Xenopus* oocytes. *Proc. Natl. Acad. Sci. USA*, **76**, 837

Roy, A. K. (1979). In Litwack, G. (ed.) *Biochemical Actions of Hormones*. vol. 6, pp. 481–517. (New York: Academic Press)

Roy, A. K. and Clark, J. H. (1980). *Gene Regulation by Steroid Hormones* (New York: Springer-Verlag)

Roy, A. K., Dowbenko, D. J. and Schiop, M. J. (1977). Studies on the mode of oestrogenic inhibition of hepatic synthesis of alpha 2u-globulin and its corresponding messenger ribonucleic acid in rat liver. *Biochem. J.*, **164**, 91

Roy, A. K. and Neuhaus, O. W. (1966). Proof of the hepatic synthesis of a sex-dependent protein in the rat. *Biochim. Biophys. Acta*, **127**, 82

Sando, J. J., Hammond, N. D., Stratford, C. A. and Pratt, W. B. (1979). Activation of thymocyte glucocorticoid receptors to the steroid binding form. The roles of reduction agents ATP, and heat-stable factors. *J. Biol. Chem.*, **254**, 4779

Sar, M., Liao, S. and Stumpf, W. E. (1970). Nuclear concentration of androgens in rat seminal vesicles and prostate demonstrated by dry-mount autoradiography. *Endocrinology*, **86**, 1008

Schimke, R. T., McKnight, G. S. and Shapiro, D. J. (1975). Nucleic acid probes in analysis of hormone action in oviducts. In Litwack, G. (ed.) *Biochemical Actions of Hormones*. vol. 3, pp. 245–269. (New York: Academic Press)

Schuetz, A. W. (1976). Induction of oocytic maturation and differentiation: mode of progesterone action. *Ann. NY Acad. Sci.*, **286**, 408

Sherman, M. R., Pickering, L. A., Rollwagen, F. M. and Miller, L. K. (1978). Mero-receptors: proteolytic fragments of receptors containing the steroid binding site. *Fed. Am. Soc. Expt. Biol.*, **37**, 167

Shimazaki, J., Kurihara, H., Ito, Y. and Shida, K. (1965). Metabolism of testosterone in muscular tissue. *Gumma. J. Med. Sci.*, **14**, 313

Shyr, C. and Liao, S. (1978). Protein factor that inhibits binding and promotes release of androgen-receptor complex from nuclear chromatin. *Proc. Natl. Acad. Sci. USA*, **75**, 5969

Skipper, J. K., Eakle, S. A. and Hamilton, T. H. (1980). Modulation of oestrogen of synthesis of specific uterim proteins. *Cell*, **22**, 69

Smith, L. D. and Eker, R. E. (1971). The interaction of steroids with *Rana pipiens* oocytes in the induction of maturation. *Dev. Biol.*, **25**, 232

Spelsberg, T. C., Knowler, J., Boyd, P. A., Thrall, C. and Martin-Dani, G. (1979). Support for chromatin acidic proteins as receptors for progesterone in the chick oviduct. *J. Steroid Biochem.*, **11**, 373

Szoka, P. R., Gallagher, J. F. and Held, W. A. (1980). *In vitro* synthesis and characterization of precursors to the mouse major urinary proteins. *J. Biol. Chem.*, **255**, 1367

Talwar, G. P., Modi, S. and Rao, K. N. (1965). DNA-dependent synthesis of RNA is not implicated in growth response of chick comb to androgens. *Science*, **150**, 1315

Toft, D. and Gorski, J. (1966). A receptor molecule for oestrogens: isolation from the rat uterus and preliminary characterization. *Proc. Natl. Acad. Sci. USA*, **55**, 1574

Tomkins, G. M., Levinson, B. B., Baxter, J. D. and Dethlefsen, L. (1972). Further evidence for post transcriptional control of inducible tyrosine aminotransferase synthesis in cultured hepatoma cells. *Nature (New Biol.)*, **239**, 9

Toole, J. J., Hastie, N. D. and Held, W. A. (1979). An abundant androgen regulated mRNA in the mouse kidney. *Cell*, **17**, 441

Tymoczko, J. L. and Liao, S. (1971). Detention of androgen-protein complex by nuclear chromatin aggregates: heat labile factors. *Biochem. Biophys. Acta*, **252**, 607

Vedeckis, W. V., Schrader, W. T. and O'Malley, B. W. (1980). Progesterone-binding components of chick oviduct: analysis of receptor structure by limited proteolysis. *Biochemistry*, **19**, 343

Vesely, D. L. (1979). Testosterone and its precursors and metabolites enhance guanylate cyclase activity. *Proc. Natl. Acad. Sci. USA*, **76**, 3491

Whelly, S. M. and Barker, K. L. (1974). Early effect of oestradiol on the peptide elongation rate by uterine ribosomes. *Biochemistry*, **13**, 341

Williams-Ashman, H. G., Liao, S., Hancock, R. L., Kurkowitz, L. and Silverman, D. A. (1974). Testicular hormones and the synthesis of ribonucleic acids and proteins in the prostate gland. *Recent Progr. Horm. Res.*, **20**, 247

Wilson, E. M. and French, F. S. (1979). Effects of proteases and protease inhibitors on the 4.5s and 8s androgen receptor, *J. Biol. Chem.*, **254,** 6310

Wrange, O., Carlstedt-Duke, J. and Gustafsson, J-A. (1979). Purification of the glucocorticoid receptor from rat liver cytosol. *J. Biol. Chem.*, **254**, 9284

Zava, D. T., Chamness, G. C., Horwitz, K. B. and McGuire, W. L. (1977). Human breast cancer: biologically active estrogen receptor in the absence of estrogen? *Science*, **196,** 663

8
Analysis of steroid receptors in the prostate

R. GHANADIAN AND G. AUF

Steroid receptor proteins are generally characterized by their ability to bind to their respective steroids with high affinity and limited capacity. The binding of steroid to the receptor is a highly specific event with respect to both the tissue and the ligand. Thus a steroid receptor can be demonstrated by its binding to a specific radioligand and the subsequent separation of the radiolabelled steroid receptor complex from other non-receptor binding components. In order to detect the receptor, it is, therefore, essential to use a specific radioligand which exhibits high affinity towards the receptor and to employ appropriate techniques to separate the receptor from the other non-receptor components. The initial qualitative demonstration of a steroid receptor encompasses several criteria which include tissue and ligand specificity of the receptor, the binding affinity and saturability of the receptor to the radioligand, and finally the physicochemical characters of the receptor protein such as molecular weight, sedimentation constant, precipitability with polycations such as protamine sulphate, thermolability and isoelectric point. Having established these criteria, the quantitative evaluation of the receptor content in the tissue can then be made. The quantitation of the receptor, particularly in some malignant tumours, is of great importance as a diagnostic tool in distinguishing a hormone responsive tumour from a non-responsive one. With regard to the prostate, as the growth and functional activity of this gland is dependent upon testicular hormones, the qualitative and quantitative assessment of steroid receptors and, in particular, those for androgens has attracted the attention of several research laboratories. Although the fundamental approach in terms of methodological requirements for steroid receptor analysis in this gland has followed the same path as that used for other target organs, progress with regard to the human prostate and its tumours has proved to be exceedingly slow. This has been mainly due to the complex nature of the tissue, the presence of high levels of enzymic activity and the existence of other high affinity steroid binding components which interfered with the detection of receptors in this gland. It is therefore essential that techniques which are to be used for the characterization and quantitation of steroid receptors in this gland are capable of resolving these problems. This chapter examines the suitability of a number of available techniques which have been used for the analysis of steroid receptors and their potential application to the characterization and measurement of steroid receptors in the normal prostate and its tumours.

8.1 EVALUATION OF METHODS FOR STEROID RECEPTOR ANALYSIS IN THE PROSTATE

8.1.1 Density gradient centrifugation

Although sucrose gradient centrifugation had been used for the separation of particles of high molecular weight (Britten and Roberts, 1960) its application for the separation of proteins with different molecular weights and shapes was originally suggested by Martin and Ames (1961). Subsequently this technique has been employed for the characterization and measurement of steroid receptors (Toft and Gorski, 1966). The technique has been particularly popular in the study of steroid receptors because of its ability to separate receptors from other steroid binding components such as sex hormone binding globulin (SHBG) as well as smaller molecules such as albumin and free steroids. In principle, the technique consists of layering the radiolabelled sample on a linear gradient made of 5–20% sucrose or 5–35% glycerol in buffered media and subjecting the gradient to ultracentrifugation. The centrifugation has generally been carried out with a swing out rotor for periods of 7–20 h, although a vertical rotor head which requires a shorter running time of 2–3 h to achieve a satisfactory separation can also be used. The latter rotor head has been shown to be more advantageous in that the shorter period of centrifugation prevents receptor degradation and ligand dissociation, thus enhancing the yield of the radiolabelled receptor (Olsson et al., 1979).

Both sucrose and glycerol density gradients have been used in the study of cytoplasmic and nuclear androgen receptors from the prostate of experimental animals and man. In density gradient centrifugation, the receptor protein migrates down the gradient a certain distance depending upon its molecular weight and shape and the force applied. The sedimentation coefficient (s) of the receptor can then be determined by comparing the distance travelled by the receptor with that of a standard protein of known sedimentation constant centrifuged under the same experimental conditions. Alternatively, the sedimentation constant ($S_{T,m}$) can be determined by the equation:

$$S_{T,m} = \frac{dx/dt}{w^2 x},$$

where T is temperature, m is medium, w represents the angular velocity of the rotor in radians per second, x is the distance from the rotor centre to the boundary and dx/dt is the velocity of the movement of the boundary. This equation should be considered in conjunction with the density of the protein in solution, the density of the medium at the temperature of centrifugation and the density of water at 20° C (Martin and Ames, 1961). The determination of the sedimentation constant requires the use of an analytical ultracentrifuge whereas the sedimentation coefficient can be accomplished with a high speed preparative ultracentrifuge. The latter comparative technique has been widely applied in the studies of steroid receptors.

There are several factors which influence the sedimentation pattern of steroid receptors. These include the temperature of incubation for radiolabelling the receptor, pH of the medium, ionic strength of the medium and the degree of purification of the receptor (Ghanadian, 1976). A classical example of the effect of these factors can be observed in the analysis of androgen receptors in the rat ventral prostate. When the cytoplasmic fraction of the ventral prostate of the castrated rat is labelled with DHT, the androgen receptor sediments at an 8–10S region. (Mainwaring, 1969a; Unjhem et al., 1969; Baulieu and Jung, 1970). However, at higher temperatures ranging between 20 and 37°C the 8S form is transformed into smaller units of 3–5S (Liao et al., 1975). Similarly the ionic strength of the media could also alter the sedimentation pattern. The inclusion of 0.4 mol/l KCl to the incubation media transforms the 8S receptor into a 3–4S unit depending on the concentration of KCl (Mainwaring, 1970; Baulieu and Jung, 1970). The pH of the medium also influences the sedimentation pattern of the androgen receptor. In a media of 0.1 mol/l KCl and a pH lower than 7.5 the 8S receptor aggregates to a larger form. However, if the pH of the media is raised to 9 the amount of aggregate decreases and the 8S form reappears (Liao et al., 1975). In addition to these factors, the purification of the receptor can also influence the gradient profile (Liao and Liang, 1974).

Density gradient centrifugation has been successfully applied in the identification and characterization of cytoplasmic androgen receptors, not only for the rat ventral prostate but also in a number of other experimental animals such as dog (Dube et al., 1979), male mastomys (Smith et al., 1978a) and the prostate of female mastomys (Ghanadian et al., 1977c). Most of these investigations have been performed on prostatic tissues obtained from the castrated animals. The reduction of circulating androgens following castration reduces the level of endogenous tissue steroids, hence increasing the number of unoccupied (free) receptors. This would, therefore, facilitate the labelling of the receptor with radioactive steroid. In earlier studies the demonstration of cytoplasmic androgen receptors in the human prostate by gradient centrifugation has not always been possible. Whilst the presence of an 8S cytoplasmic androgen receptor was reported in approximately 50% by Mainwaring and Milroy (1973), 30% by Davies and Griffiths (1975) and 77% by Menon et al. (1978) of BPH tissues, others were unable to demonstrate the existence of androgen receptors by this technique (Steins et al., 1974; Nijs et al., 1976). This apparent inconsistency may be attributed partly to incomplete labelling and in part to difficulties in homogenization of the tissue which could destroy the receptor by heat generated during this step. In addition, the conditions used for the labelling of the receptor, i.e. 2 h incubation at 0–4°C would label the unoccupied receptor sites which constitute only a small fraction of the total receptor concentration (Rosen et al., 1975; Ghanadian et al., 1978a, b). The problem related to homogenization can be resolved by homogenizing the frozen samples in a microdismembrator (Braun Melsungen) which not only overcomes the problems associated with heat, but is also extremely efficient in breaking the fibromuscular elements and thus enhancing receptor recovery. With regard to the labelling of this receptor, the extension of the incubation period to 16–20 h could increase the number of labelled receptors by allowing the radiolabelled steroid to exchange with the endogenous androgen bound to the receptor. Although the modifications should theoretically yield a more consistent result, this, however, has not been the case in practice. In our laboratory when cytosol labelled at 0–4° C for 16–20 hours with tritiated synthetic androgen (R1881) was analysed on a 5–35 % glycerol gradient, evidence of polydispersed aggregates with no distinct receptor peak at the 8 S region was apparent. This initial failure may be attributed to factors such as proteolytic enzymes which may have cleaved the receptor protein into polydisperse units (Wilson and French, 1979). This problem can be resolved by the inclusion of sodium molybdate in the homogenization buffer. This compound has been shown to exert a stabilizing effect on both oestrogen and progesterone receptors (Krozowski and Murphy, 1981; Bevins and Bashirelahi, 1980). In our studies, the introduction of 10 mmol/l sodium molybdate in the homogenization media led to a consistent recovery of a 7-8 S androgen receptor (Figure 8.1).

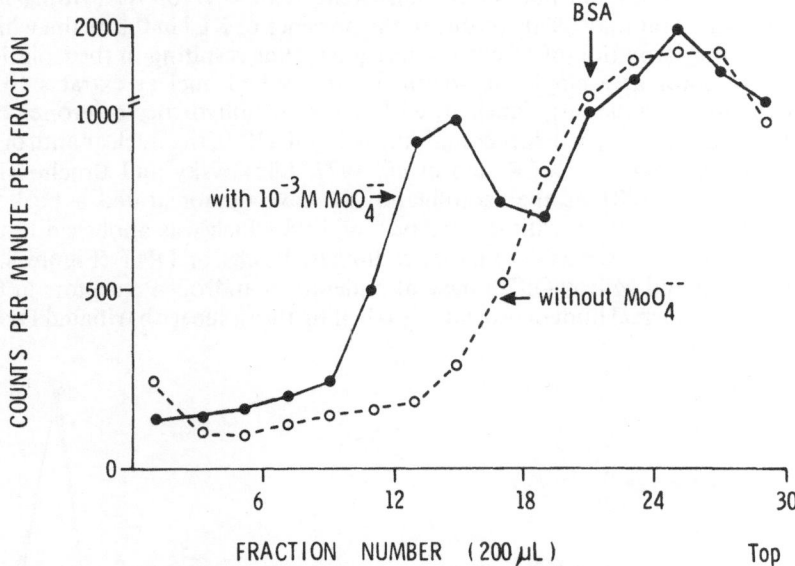

Figure 8.1 Glycerol density gradient centrifugation of BPH cytosol labelled with 30 nmol/l tritiated R1881 in the presence and absence of 10^{-3} mol/l sodium molybdate. Data from author's laboratory

It is therefore, apparent that density gradient centrifugation can be used for the isolation and the possible quantitation of cytoplasmic androgen receptors in the human prostate provided that appropriate measures with regard to the homogenization of the tissue, labelling of the receptor and its stabilization are considered. Density gradient centrifugation has also been successfully applied to the isolation of the nuclear androgen receptor. For these studies the radiolabelled receptors can be prepared by whole tissue incubation with radiolabelled steroid and subsequent tissue fractionation and extraction of the nuclear receptors with 0.4–0.5 mol/l KCl. An alternative method is to equilibrate the nuclear pellets with radiolabelled steroid under conditions which allow exchange between the endogenous steroid bound to the receptor with the radioligand (Anderson *et al.*, 1972). Finally a more efficient procedure to label the nuclear receptor is to extract the receptor initially with 0.4 mol/l KCl and then directly incubate the nuclear extract with radiolabelled ligand. Analysis of the 0.4 mol/l KCl nuclear extract of rat ventral prostate on sucrose gradient has revealed the presence of a receptor with a sedimentation coefficient of 3.0 S (Fang *et al.*, 1969; Smith *et al.*, 1978b). A similar sedimentation coefficient has also been demonstrated for the nuclear androgen receptors in the prostate of the male (Smith *et al.*, 1979) and female mastomys (Ghanadian *et al.*, 1978c). A higher sedimentation coefficient (4.6S) for the nuclear androgen receptors of rat ventral prostate has been reported by Mainwaring (1969b). This difference in the reported *s* value may be attributed to variations in experimental procedures.

The isolation of nuclear androgen receptors from the human prostate has been less troublesome and more consistent than that of its cytoplasmic counterpart. This may partly be due to the presence of KCl in the media which prevents the formation of receptor aggregates, thus resulting in the isolation of the receptor as a single well-defined peak. When nuclear extracts from human BPH tissue are labelled with tritiated dihydrotestosterone and analysed on sucrose gradients containing 0.4 mol/l KCl, the nuclear androgen receptor sediments at 3S (Menon *et al.*, 1977; Lieskovsky and Bruchovsky, 1979). Using R1881 as the radioligand, we have demonstrated a peak of radioactivity associated with the receptor of 3.0S which was abolished in the presence of 100-fold excess of either radioinert R1881 or DHT (Figure 8.2). Mainwaring and Milroy (1973) have also identified androgen receptors in the nuclei of the normal human prostate by labelling the tissue with tritiated DHT.

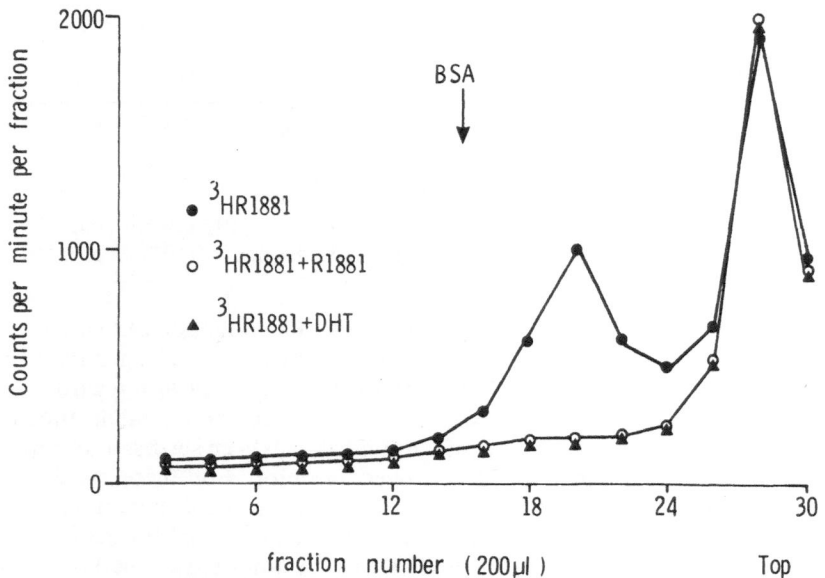

Figure 8.2 Glycerol density gradient centrifugation profile of nuclear extract labelled with 20 nmol/l tritiated R1881. Data from author's laboratory

The analysis of nuclear extract was carried out on high ionic strength sucrose gradient. The sedimentation pattern in their studies revealed 4.2–4.4 S peak corresponding to the androgen receptor.

8.1.2 Gel exclusion chromatography

Gel exclusion chromatography has been widely used for the isolation of steroid receptors. This type of chromatography is mostly carried out on a column packed with beads made of either polymerized dextran, agarose or polyacrylamide. The choice of matrices depends on the type of separation required. Essentially two types of separation can be achieved with this system. These are either the separation of small molecules down to about 5000 daltons from the heavier steroid binding components or the fractionation of steroid bound proteins with similar molecular weights from other protein components. The first type, which is generally referred to as a desalting column, is used for the separation of free steroids from protein bound steroids. In this case, the gel should be chosen where the steroid binding components are eluted at the void volume and which will give minimum zone broadening and dilution, and allow minimum time during which the binding proteins are on the column.

The most commonly used commercial preparations for this type of separation are Sephadex G-25 or Biogel P2 and Sephadex G-50 or Biogel P6. Sephadex type matrices are made of dextran whereas the corresponding Biogel series are polyacrylamide. Both G-25 and P2 separate material with molecular weight ranging from 100 to 5000 daltons, whilst G-50 and P6 are suitable for the separation of proteins ranging from 1000 to 10 000 daltons. Because of the fast elution rate and low dilution of the recovered sample, these columns have been utilized for the separation of free from protein bound steroids with the view to quantitate the saturable binding components. Such a procedure is acceptable provided the sample contains a single saturable binding entity. This separation procedure has been utilized for quantitating the effect of drugs on the cytoplasmic (Ghanadian et al., 1977b) and nuclear (Smith et al., 1978b) androgen receptors in rat ventral prostate. Because of the inability of G-25 and G-50 type columns to separate SHBG which also binds with high affinity to DHT from the human cytoplasmic androgen receptor, such a technique cannot be used either for the quantitative or qualitative evaluation of the androgen receptors in the human prostate.

Another important application of gel exclusion chromatography has been in the isolation and characterization of the receptor. The materials used in this type of chromatography are similar to those utilized for desalting columns but have different pore sizes which make it possible to separate different protein binding components from one another. An example of materials used for this application are Sephadex G-100, G-150, G-200 or Biogel P100, P150 and P200 which can resolve proteins with molecular weights of 5×10^3–10×10^4, $15 \times 10^3 - 15 \times 10^4$ and $30 \times 10^3 - 20 \times 10^4$ daltons respectively. Neither Sephadex G-100 nor G-150 are appropriate for characterization of the receptor, as the latter is not retained by this range of columns due to its high molecular size. On the other hand, the G-200 column, which has a better resolving power, has been used for the characterization of cytoplasmic (Unjhem *et al.*, 1969; Mainwaring, 1969a) and nuclear (Mainwaring, 1969b) androgen receptors in the rat ventral prostate. However, in this system the receptor is eluted near the void volume of the column and therefore G-200 cannot be considered a favourite choice for the isolation and molecular weight determination. Indeed the application of this column for the characterization of androgen receptors in the human prostate does not provide reliable results as the receptor is not well separated from SHBG (Hansson *et al.*, 1975). A similar shortcoming is also encountered with the use of a duo-gel column of Sephadex G-50 over Biogel A 1.5 m (Geller *et al.*, 1975).

The shortcomings of the gel exclusion chromatography based on matrices made of dextran beads can be surmounted by using gels prepared from agarose. This matrix has an extremely open gel structure and therefore extends the range of separation to include proteins with heavier molecular weights. In its natural form agarose occurs as part of the complex mixture of charged and neutral polysaccharides referred to as agar. The agarose used for gel exclusion chromatography is obtained by a purification process which removes the charged polysaccharides to give a gel with only a small number of residual charged groups. The commonly employed commercial agaroses are Sepharose and the Biogel A series, which have a protein fractionation range between 1×10^4 and 15×10^7 daltons. The main advantages of the agarose over the dextran bead gel-types lies in its more rigid structure, which allows a higher flow rate with minimum loss of resolution and in that the molecular weight of proteins may be determined directly from a linear correlation between the logarithm of the molecular weight and the elution volume on the gel (Lehmann, 1970). By contrast, the dextran series of matrices such as Sephadex G-200 does not provide a linear logarithmic relationship between the molecular weight and elution volume. In addition Sephadex G-200 has a slower elution rate and the gel bed has a tendency to compact (Andrews, 1965). Amongst the available agarose series, Sepharose 6B, which has a resolving power ranging from 10^4 to 10^6 daltons, has been shown to be the most appropriate choice for the isolation and molecular weight determination of the androgen receptor. Using this gel matrix the isolation and molecular weight determination of the cytoplasmic androgen receptors has been successfully performed in the rat ventral prostate (Smith, 1977), the prostate of the Rhesus monkey (Ghanadian *et al.*, 1977a; Ghanadian 1981) and the human benign hypertrophied prostate (Ghanadian *et al.*, 1978a). Analysis of cytosol from benign hypertrophied prostates labelled with the potent synthetic androgen methyltrienolone (R 1881) on a calibrated column of Sepharose 6B gives three peaks of radioactivity. The first peak which is associated with material taken up by the gel matrix is inhibited with an excess of radioinert R1881 and DHT but not progesterone (Figure 8.3a). This peak is destroyed with the sulphydryl blocking agent parachloromercuriobenzoate (PCMB) which has been shown by Jensen *et al.* (1976) to destroy irreversibly the receptor proteins. The other two peaks corresponding to non-specific proteins and free steroid are unaffected by unlabelled competitors or PCMB. By comparing the elution volume of the receptor peak with that of proteins with known molecular weight, the androgen receptor is found to have a molecular weight of 2.78×10^5 daltons (Figure 8.3b). A similar molecular weight (2.8

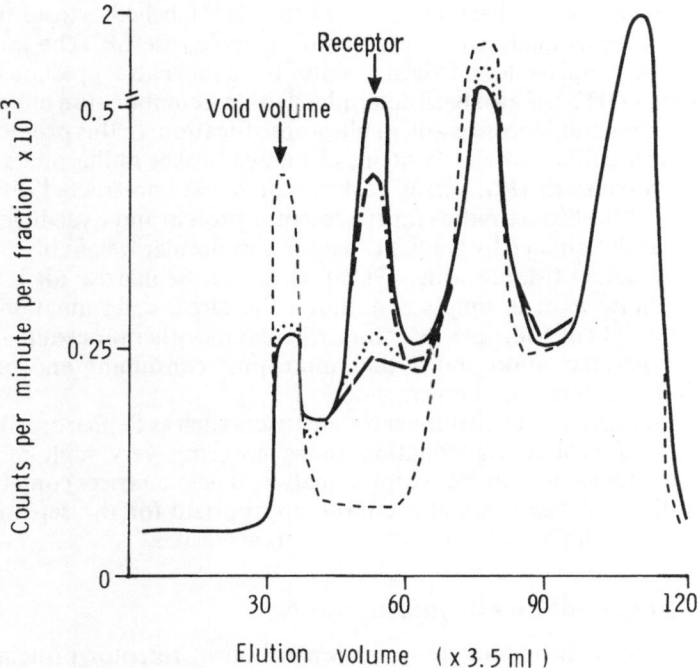

Figure 8.3a Chromatography on Sepharose 6B of BPH cytosol labelled with 30 nmol/l ³H R 1881 ——; ³H R 1881 + R 1881 ———; ³H R 1881 + DHT . . . . . ; ³H R 1881 + PCMB---; ³H R 1881 + progesterone — —. Data from author's laboratory

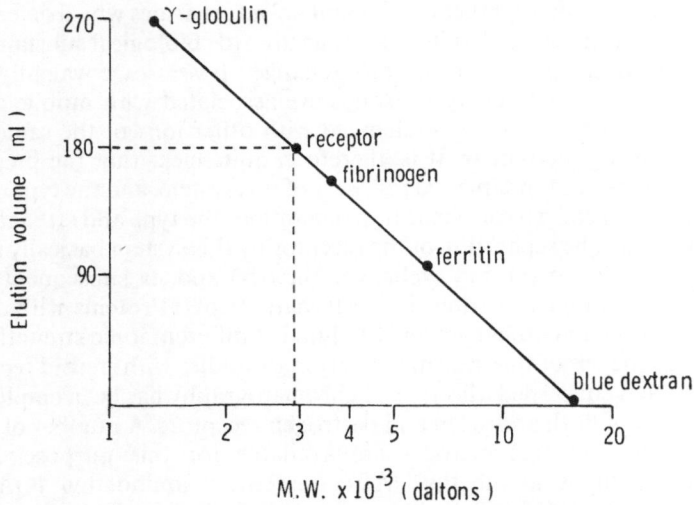

Figure 8.3b Determination of the molecular weight of the cytoplasmic DHT receptor complex by Sepharose 6B column chromatography. Data from author's laboratory

$\times 10^5$ daltons) has also been obtained when DHT labelled cytosol from rat ventral prostate is analysed on a column of Sepharose 6B. The molecular weight of the cytoplasmic androgen receptor from rat ventral prostate labelled with tritiated DHT has also been determined using a combination of Sephadex G-200 columns and sucrose gradient ultracentrifugation. In this procedure the columns were calibrated with proteins of known Stokes radius and a plot of dissociation constant (K_d) versus Stokes radius was constructed. From the knowledge of the Stokes radius for the receptor protein and its sedimentation coefficient as determined by gradient analysis, a molecular weight of 2.74×10^5 was also obtained (Mainwaring, 1969a). However, Sepharose 6B is a more desirable choice as it is simple and allows the direct determination of the molecular weight of androgen receptors, whereas the other procedure involves multiple experimentation and is thus more time consuming and prone to accumulative experimental error.

Other commercially available agarose matrices such as Sepharose 4B or 2B, which have a protein fractionation range covering very high molecular weights, are not as suitable for receptor analysis. These matrices contain lower concentrations of agarose and are more appropriate for the separation of substances with high molecular weights such as viruses.

8.1.3 Ion exchange chromatography

In ion exchange chromatography the separation of receptor proteins from other binding components is based upon the charge carried by solute proteins. Thus molecules with small differences in charge can be effectively separated from each other. In this type of chromatography separation is obtained by the reversible adsorption of the receptor onto the matrix and its subsequent elution with a suitable buffer. The matrix may be based on a number of compounds including synthetic resins and polysaccharides which determine its physical properties as well as its behaviour towards biological substances. The matrix which is referred to as ion-exchanger possesses covalently bound charged groups. These charged groups are associated with mobile counter-ions which can be reversibly exchanged with other ions of the same charge without altering the matrix. It is, therefore, quite clear that the presence of charged groups is a fundamental property of this system, and the type of group which has been chosen for separation determines the type and strength of the ion exchanger. The separation of the receptor by this system basically involves its adsorption onto the ion exchanger (matrix) and its subsequent elution employing solutions of various ionic strength or pH. Proteins with different affinities for the ion exchanger will be eluted at different ionic strength or pH.

As far as the use of this system in relation to studies with steroid receptor in the prostate is concerned, this type of chromatography has been employed for the isolation of both androgen and oestrogen receptors. A number of anionic and cationic exchange matrices are available for this purpose. Anionic groupings such as aminoethyl (AE), quaternary aminoethyl (QAE) and diethylaminoethyl (DEAE) can be covalently linked to insoluble matrices such as Sephadex, Sepharose or cellulose. Using DEAE-cellulose column chromatography, Hsu et al. (1975) isolated the cytoplasmic androgen receptor from the normal human prostate. The authors showed that although DEAE-cellulose retained both androgen receptors and SHBG, the former complex could only be eluted with 0.4 mol/l phosphate buffer whereas SHBG was easily eluted with 0.04 mol/l buffer. The separation of the receptor from SHBG in this procedure was extremely good. DEAE-cellulose column chromatography has also been used for the identification of oestrogen receptors in human BPH tissues (Bashirelahi et al., 1979). In this system a gradient of phosphate buffer from 0.0175 to 0.4 mol/l was used to elute the adsorbed oestradiol binding complex. A cationic exchanger such as phosphocellulose can also be used for the purification of steroid receptors. Atger and Milgrom (1976) have utilized this type of ion exchanger for the purification of glucocorticoid receptors.

Ion exchange chromatography has been mainly used in the qualitative analysis of steroid receptors in prostatic tissues. Although this system has a great potential for purification of the receptor, its usage for quantitation is limited, since prior purification steps are desirable before utilizing this type of matrix and additionally quantitative recovery of receptor is rarely achieved. The losses incurred during these purification steps would be a major disadvantage that makes this method unsuitable for receptor quantitation.

In addition to DEAE-cellulose, it is also possible to use a natural exchanger such as DNA linked to cellulose. Mainwaring and Mangan (1971) studied the interaction of tritiated steroid receptor complexes to DNA cellulose, and subsequently Mainwaring and Irving (1973) used columns of DNA-cellulose as a specific matrix for the isolation of cytoplasmic androgen receptors from the rat ventral prostate. In this system the androgen receptor complex was retained to a very significant degree, whereas tritiated steroids either in the free state or in complex with SHBG or albumin were not retained. The advantages of the DNA-cellulose system is said to be that any non-specific protein will not be retained by the column and that the matrix will only bind to the steroid receptor complex which is eluted as a single sharp peak with 0.5 mol/l KCl. However, this procedure requires a lengthy preparative stage for obtaining a fairly purified native form (double stranded) DNA and its subsequent immobilization by adsorption to cellulose.

In addition to these matrices, heparin coupled to CN-Br activated agarose has been used for the characterization and partial purification of androgen receptors. Mulder et al. (1979) have compared the use of heparin agarose and DNA cellulose for the isolation of cytoplasmic and nuclear androgen receptors from the rat ventral prostate. This study suggested that, whilst heparin agarose retained cytoplasmic as well as nuclear androgen receptors, the DNA cellulose system was only capable of retaining cytoplasmic androgen receptors. The heparin cellulose system also had the advantage of avoiding the formation of receptor aggregates. Apart from the above mentioned types of ion-exchange chromatography, the use of calcium phosphate notably in the form of hydroxylapatite has been suggested for studying steroid receptors. This material possesses adsorption as well as ion exchange properties. However, the elution of substances from this material is not solely dependent upon the ionic strength, but also requires that the eluting agent should have an affinity for calcium or phosphate sites in the cytosols. The use of spheroidal hydroxylapatite chromatography for the purification of the progesterone receptor of the guinea-pig uterus has been suggested by Dyer and Faber (1980) who obtained a fivefold purification of the receptor by this system. The main advantage of this procedure is that it is capable of rapid fractionation of the cytosol and results in a reasonably high yield of the partially purified receptor. The application of this system for the purification of androgen receptors, however, has yet to be investigated.

8.1.4 Affinity chromatography

In affinity chromatography the molecule which is to be purified is specifically and reversibly adsorbed by a complementary binding substance, i.e. ligand which is immobilized on an insoluble matrix. Ligand immobilization can be achieved by its covalent attachment to a chromatographic matrix such as agarose bead. In this type of adsorption chromatography purification as well as recovery is extremely high and the technique, which has a concentrating effect, enables a large volume of sample to be processed. It is important that the ligand should have chemically modifiable groups which allow it to be attached to the matrix without destroying its binding activity and that the immobilized ligand retains its specific binding affinity for the substance to be purified. Moreover, a suitable method must be available for desorbing the bound receptor once the unbound materials are washed away.

Receptor proteins for steroids are ideally suited for purification by affinity chromatography due to the reversible nature of the steroid receptor interaction, the stereochemical specificity of the binding and the high affinity of the complex (K_d 10^{-9} to 10^{-10} mol/l). The use of this technique for the purification of oestrogen receptors was first reported by Jensen et al. (1967) who linked the phenolic ring of oestradiol to para-aminobenzyl cellulose by coupling of the diazonium derivative. Despite partial success, the elution of specific oestrogen binding protein from these columns was found to be difficult. Two problems were encountered with this technique. Firstly, the release of the proportion of free oestradiol, which does not covalently bind to the matrix, can lead to the 'inactivation' or apparent removal of the oestrogen binding activity from the sample. Secondly, the irreversible denaturation of the receptor, which occurs when the very tightly bound receptor on the adsorbant is eluted as the conditions necessary to dissociate the receptor complex are somewhat extreme, such as presence of guanidine HCl or urea or changes in the pH of the buffer. These problems have been highlighted by Sica et al. (1973) who have successfully managed to overcome these difficulties, by combining the use of native oestradiol as a specific competing ligand with the selection of experimental conditions which enhance the rate of dissociation of the gel-bound oestradiol receptor complex, thus permitting the effective exchange of the intact receptor from an insoluble to a soluble ligand bound state. The most effective affinity adsorbants were prepared by attaching oestradiol-17-hemi-succinate to agarose derivatives containing albumin or the branched copolymer of poly L-lysine (backbone) and poly DL-alanine (side arms). These macromolecular leashes possess numerous functional groups which permit a high degree of ligand substitution and the attached ligand is very distant from the agarose back bone. Using such an adsorbant matrix, the 4.5s uterine oestradiol receptor from crude supernatant was purified between 10^4 and 10^5 fold in overall yields of 30–50% in a single step. The comprehensive studies by Sica *et al.* (1973) on the usage of affinity columns for the purification of oestradiol receptors has paved the way for the utilization of this technique for other steroid receptors. Kuhn *et al.* (1975) have used the affinity resin, deoxycorticosterone-bovine serum albumin-sepharose, which binds with high affinity (K_d 8–10^{-10} mol/l) the cytoplasmic progesterone receptor of chick oviduct. In this system the receptor was purified greater than 2000 fold in a single step. Although affinity chromatography has provided an excellent means for the single step purification of oestrogen and progesterone receptors, its application in the studies of androgen receptor is yet to be investigated.

8.1.5 Gel electrophoretic separations

Electrophoretic separation processes utilize the ability of the charged protein to migrate in an electrical field. The separation of a mixture of proteins is based upon differences between their net charge, size and shape. In gel electrophoresis a stabilizing medium such as agar or polyacrylamide serves as a matrix for the buffer in which the proteins travel and as a structure to which proteins become attached. One of the most popular matrices used for the electrophoretic separation of steroid receptors is agar, as the separation of protein in this gel is rather rapid and relatively complete. Furthermore, the large pore size of this gel matrix does not hinder particle migration. The use of agar gel electrophoresis for the separation of steroid receptors was first introduced by Wagner (1972). In a comprehensive study, he demonstrated the separation of androgen receptors from other interfering proteins and in particular SHBG (Wagner *et al.*, 1975). In this system the receptor which electrophoretically behaves like α-globulin migrates towards the anode whereas SHBG which is a β-globulin moves towards the cathode.

A major factor which may interfere with this separation technique and possibly jeopardize the potential application of this technique is the presence of protein binding components of similar electrophoretic mobility, molecular weight and binding specificity as the receptor. Such a problem, however, can be resolved by exercising certain precautionary measures as reviewed by Wagner (1977). The inclusion of an excess of radioinert steroid which binds selectively to the interfering protein and not the receptor would saturate the binding sites on the protein contaminant, thus preventing the radioligand from binding to it. A good example of this approach is the inclusion of excess radioinert cortisol to saturate the corticosteroid binding globulin (CBG) and prevent tritiated progesterone from binding to it. Both CBG and progesterone receptors are α-proteins and possess similar electrophoretic mobilities. However, this approach does not always produce a reliable estimate of the receptor as the extent by which CBG is suppressed by cortisol cannot be accurately assessed. Furthermore, complexes between α_1-acid-globulins and progesterone can also contribute to the measured binding, since they cannot be abolished by cortisol. This approach, however, cannot be applied for the removal of some other interfering proteins when considering other classes of steroid receptors. For instance, α-fetoprotein (AFP), which binds oestrogens with high affinity and has a similar electrophoretic mobility to that of the oestradiol receptor, may interfere with the quantitative analysis of the latter.

The use of synthetic steroids which bind specifically to a given class of receptor protein can considerably enhance the reliability of this technique for both identification and quantitation of the receptor. However, in the case of synthetic androgen which is specific for the receptor, the need for the application of a physical purification step such as agar gel electrophoresis becomes unnecessary. A more appropriate approach to improve the separation ability of this technique when natural steroids are used to label the receptor is to introduce neuraminidase in the sample preparation. This compound is able to remove the terminal neuraminic acidic residues from the interfering binding proteins such as CBG, SHBG and AFP without altering the molecule's binding characteristics. The cleavage of this charge contributing carbohydrate decreases the electrophoretic mobility of these interfering proteins without affecting that of the receptor (Wagner and Jungblut, 1976). The effect of neuraminidase is such that it can shift CBG which is an α-globulin into a β-globulin position.

In virtually all the studies in which agar gel electrophoresis has been employed, the receptor has been labelled with dihydrotestosterone for a short incubation period at 0–4°C. As previously described, this procedure does not label the whole receptor population. In order to improve the labelling conditions it is essential to prolong the period of incubation, thus allowing the steroid endogenously bound to the receptor to exchange with the radioligand. However, this is not possible when tritiated DHT is used as it is metabolized to androstanediols. The substitution of methyltrienolone (R1881) for DHT could resolve this shortcoming. However, if R1881 is to be used for labelling the receptor, there would be no need for a further separation step such as agar gel electrophoresis. It can therefore be concluded that although agar gel electrophoresis provides adequate separation of androgen receptors from SHBG, the overall conditions in which the receptor is labelled and analysed severely underestimates the number of binding sites. This can be clearly demonstrated by comparing the values for the cytoplasmic androgen receptor obtained by this technique to others in which exchange conditions were used. Using agar gel electrophoresis a mean concentration of 23 fmol/mg protein (Wagner, 1977), 12.3 fmol/mg protein (Krieg et al., 1979), 8.0 fmol/mg protein (de Voogt and Dingjan, 1980) have been reported. The latter group, however, could only demonstrate DHT receptors in 27% of the BPH samples. When these values are compared with those reported by others who have used R1881 under exchange conditions, significant differences can be observed. The mean values obtained by the latter techniques are 80.3 fmol/mg protein (Ghanadian et al., 1978a) and 51.7 fmol/mg protein (Shain et al., 1978).

Despite the aforementioned limitation of agar gel electrophoresis in the quantitative evaluation of androgen receptors, this technique can nevertheless be of value for qualitative analysis. Polyacrylamide agar gel electrophoresis has also been used in the analysis of steroid receptors. Although this gel matrix has been utilized in the analysis of progesterone receptor in the cytoplasmic fraction of the chick oviduct (Miller *et al.*, 1975), the use of a buffer system at pH 10.2 reported in this method makes it unfavourable for the analysis of androgen and oestrogen receptors.

8.1.6 Isoelectric focusing

The separation of steroid receptor proteins by the technique of isoelectric focusing is based upon the movement of the receptor protein on a pH gradient formed on a supporting media under the influence of electric current. In conventional electrophoresis protein separation occurs in a buffer solution of constant pH and ionic strength and the proteins will migrate to the anode or cathode according to their overall net charge. However, in isoelectric focusing the separation occurs in a continuous, stable and linear pH gradient. The formation of a linear pH gradient in an electrical field is achieved by carrier ampholytes which are essentially a complex mixture of synthetic copolymerized amino and carboxylic acids. These ampholytes possess properties such as good conducting and buffering capacity which are essential for the formation of natural pH gradients.

Receptor proteins like other proteins or amino acids are amphoteric compounds which can have no net charge, a negative charge or a positive charge depending upon the pH of the surrounding medium. The charge depends on the amine and carboxyl groups of the receptor protein. When the charge of the amine groups (+) is equal to that of the carboxyl groups (−) the overall charge of the protein becomes zero. When this is achieved a protein is said to be at its isoelectric point (pI) in which the solubility, swelling and viscosity are reduced and the protein does not migrate in an electrical field. The pI of a protein depends solely upon its composition and is, therefore, a physicochemical constant. Because every protein is composed of different numbers and ratios of amino acids, these differences are reflected in their pI values.

In the earlier studies, columns of sucrose gradients containing ampholytes were utilized for determining the isoelectric point of oestrogen and androgen receptors (de Sombre *et al.*, 1969; Puca *et al.*, 1971; Mainwaring and Irving, 1973). In these procedures focusing was accomplished following 16 h of isoelectrophoresis at 4 °C, but the extended period of running may result in some dissociation of the radioligand from the receptor protein. Another disadvantage of this method is the possible precipitation of contaminating proteins at their pI values prior to the receptor reaching its own. This may result in receptor loss as well as difficulty in ascertaining the true pI of the receptor. Finally, the limitation of this technique in handling more than one sample at a time makes this particular procedure unsuitable for application to receptor analysis. The introduction of isoelectric focusing on a flat bed (thin layer) of polyacrylamide has allieviated most of the disadvantages associated with the column technique. In this procedure the sample is applied to a flat bed of polyacrylamide gel containing carrier ampholytes. The sample may be applied at pH regions in which the receptor is more stable and problems associated with formation of precipitates by contaminating proteins may be avoided. When a current is applied a linear pH gradient is formed and the receptor moves towards the electrode of the opposite charge to that carried by the protein at the relevant pH. Finally as the receptor migrates through the pH gradient its charge gradually diminishes until eventually it ceases to migrate further when its net charge is zero. Additionally, the flat bed system allows the concurrent analysis of several samples for each plate and can be utilized as a microanalytical technique. This procedure was initially applied for the analysis of the cytoplasmic oestradiol receptor in human mammary carcinoma (Wrange *et al.*, 1978) and subsequently applied to the analysis of cytoplasmic and nuclear androgen and oestrogen receptors (Auf and Ghanadian, 1981, 1982) in human BPH tissues. In this system, we found that the cytoplasmic androgen receptor which was labelled with R1881 at 15°C for 16 h had a pI of 6.2 (Figure 8.4). A similar profile was also obtained when the receptor was labelled with DHT and subsequently precipitated with 33 % ammonium sulphate prior to analysis. The addition of heparin caused a slight shift in the pI of the cytoplasmic receptor from 6.2 to 6.0, whilst the heparin extracted nuclear androgen receptor also focused with a pI of 6.0 (Figure 8.5) (Auf and Ghanadian, 1981). The isoelectric focusing technique also provided opportunities to investigate the steroid specificity of the receptor. The receptor was found to be thermolabile and specific for DHT and R1881 but not progesterone or oestradiol (Figures 8.4, 8.5).

Polyacrylamide gel isoelectropheresis is also potentially applicable for receptor quantitation, but it is less suited for purification purposes. This is because of the limitation on the amount of each sample that can be applied to the plate. An alternative to polyacrylamide for purification purposes may be the use of granulated flat gel beds which utilize polymerized dextran such as Sephadex G-75 as the gel matrix and ampholytes for the formation of pH gradients. This technique has been applied to the analysis of oestradiol receptors (Coffer and King, 1974). It can be concluded that, whilst isoelectric focusing on flat beds of polyacrylamide is most suited for analytical and quantitative aspects of the receptor studies, focusing on a column of sucrose or a granulated flat bed gel is more appropriate for preparative purposes and receptor purification. Preparative electrofocusing in granulated gels appears, however, to be more advantageous than the column technique. This is because the former procedure not only allows full accessability to the gel bed during the run, but also the contaminating precipitated proteins that are trapped within the gel do not affect the separation of the receptor.

8.1.7   Receptor separation by precipitation

The separation of steroid receptor proteins by precipitation techniques encompasses two major procedures, namely ammonium sulphate precipitation and protamine sulphate precipitation.

8.1.7.1   Ammonium sulphate precipitation

Precipitation of steroid receptors can be performed using salts such as ammonium sulphate. Androgen receptors from the rat ventral prostate have

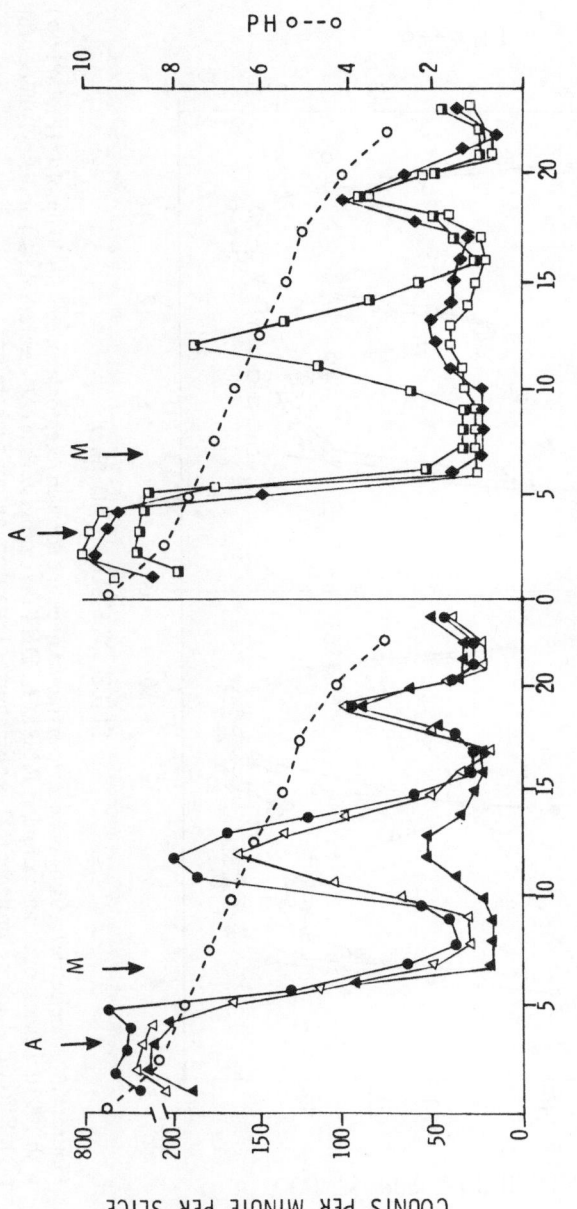

Figure 8.4 Isoelectric focusing of BPH cytosol labelled with 30 nmol/l ^{3}H R1881 (●) with 100 fold excess of either radioinert R1881 (▲), DHT (◆), progesterone (△) or oestradiol (■), or with heating at 45°C for 15 min (□). Data from author's laboratory

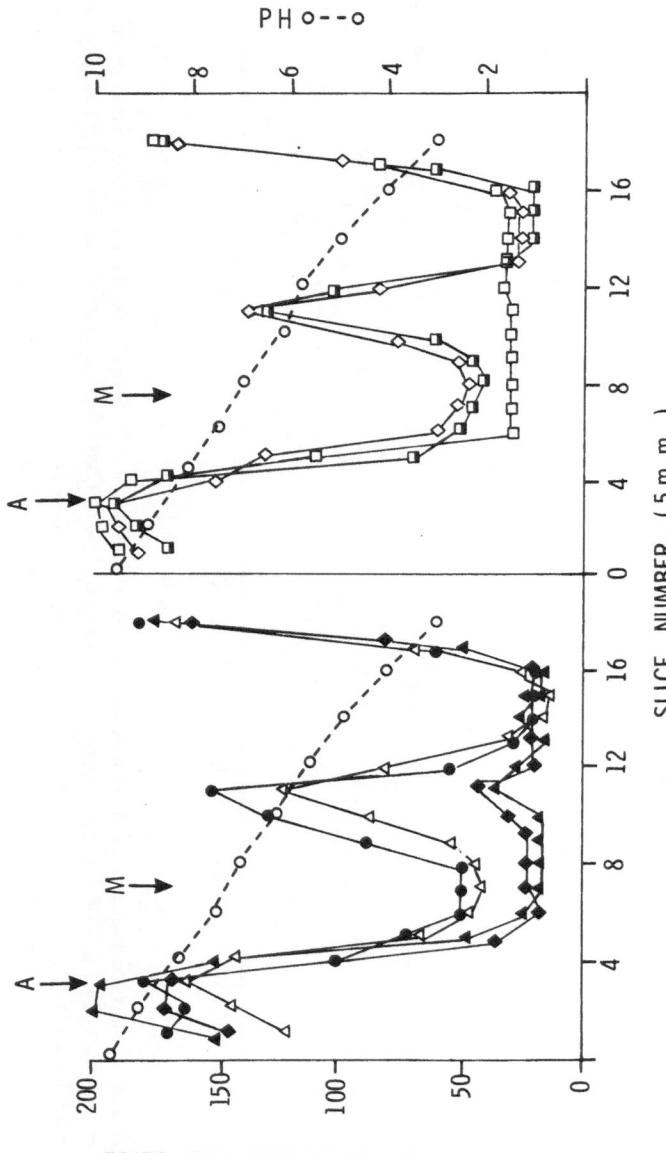

Figure 8.5 Isoelectric focusing of heparin extracted nuclear androgen receptor labelled with 30 nmol/l ^{3}H R1881 (●) with 100 fold excess of either radioinert R1881 (▲), DHT (◆), progesterone (△), oestradiol (■) or diethylstilboestrol (◇). Effect of 1 mg/ml protease (□) is also shown. Data from author's laboratory

been shown to precipitate at a concentration of 0–40% of ammonium sulphate (Fang and Liao, 1971; Mainwaring and Peterken, 1971). The precipitation of the receptor can be achieved by the gradual addition of either solid ammonium sulphate to the required concentration, or an appropriate volume of the saturated salt solution. In this procedure proteins with lower molecular weight than the receptor, such as SHBG, ABP or albumin, will not form precipitable complexes and thus they could be separated from the fractionated receptor. Because of the ability of this procedure to separate the receptor from the other contaminating binding proteins, this technique has also been used for the quantitation of cytoplasmic androgen receptors of the rat ventral prostate (Verhoeven et al., 1975). However, the method involves two precipitation steps, and the possibility of receptor losses during these steps may limit the use of this technique for quantitative purposes.

Ammonium sulphate precipitation has also been applied to the partial purification of steroid receptors in human prostate. The cytoplasmic androgen receptor of human BPH has been reported to precipitate in the 0–35% fraction of ammonium sulphate (Davies and Griffiths, 1975). However, Hsu et al. (1975) have reported that the receptor is recovered in the 30–50% fraction. Although the reason for the discrepancy between these two reports is not clear, the recent study by Auf and Ghanadian (1981) appears to have confirmed the results reported by Davies and Griffiths (1975).

Despite the ability of ammonium sulphate precipitation to provide a reasonably simple means of separating the receptor from other protein binding components, this procedure is not sufficiently accurate for the quantitative analysis of the receptor. Its application will be to remain primarily as a tool for qualitative analysis and, in particular, as the initial step in the partial purification of the receptor.

8.1.7.2 Protamine sulphate precipitation

The ability of protamine sulphate to interact with certain acidic proteins and cause their precipitation has been known for many years. Although the precise mechanism by which this compound interacts with some proteins is not clear, it is generally assumed that this highly basic compound interacts with acidic proteins, thus forming a precipitable complex. In 1970, Steggles and King made the important observation that both the 4–6s and 8s forms of oestradiol receptor from rat uterus are precipitated with protamine sulphate. These authors also observed that SHBG, which displays high affinity for oestradiol, does not form precipitable complexes with protamine. This property of protamine was subsequently put to use by several research groups for both qualitative and quantitative evaluation of oestrogen and androgen receptors in human mammary tumours (Chamness et al., 1975; Lippman and Huff, 1976). The use of protamine sulphate for quantitation of androgen receptors in rat ventral prostate has also been reported by Davies et al. (1977). In a comprehensive study these authors precipitated both cytoplasmic and nuclear receptor proteins by protamine sulphate and incubated the precipitate with tritiated DHT either for a short period at 0–4°C or under the exchange condition of 15°C for 16 h. They suggested that protamine sulphate precipitation conferred stability on the receptor complex, thus allowing application of exchange conditions for the measurement of the total binding sites. Furthermore, this procedure rendered steroids refractory to enzymic action.

Protamine sulphate precipitation has also been applied for the quantitative (Menon *et al.*, 1977; Mobbs *et al.*, 1978), and qualitative (Ghanadian *et al.*, 1978b) evaluation of androgen receptors in human benign hypertrophied prostate. For the quantitative evaluation, the receptor was labelled either prior to (Mobbs *et al.*, 1978) or after precipitation (Menon *et al.*, 1977). Whilst the former labelling procedure is best suited for the measurement of low concentrations of binding sites such as unoccupied receptor, the latter technique is more appropriate for the assay of total sites by exchange.

Although protamine sulphate precipitation provides an excellent means by which the receptor can be separated from other contaminating binding proteins and in particular SHBG, which is present in high concentration in human prostate, this technique suffers from two main disadvantages. Firstly, the experimental design of this method generates a high background of non-specific radioactivity which can be removed only by multiple washing of the precipitates; such a procedure is not only tedious but may also result in losses and inconsistency of the duplicate or triplicate samples. Secondly, because protamine sulphate does not completely precipitate the total androgen receptor content of the cytoplasmic preparation (Menon *et al.*, 1977), this could lead to under-estimation of the receptor content of the tumour.

8.1.8 Antisteroid antibodies

The use of antisteroid antibodies to separate the free and non-specifically bound steroids from that of the receptor was originally suggested by Castaneda and Liao (1975). They observed that various antibodies against DHT and testosterone were effective in removing steroid bound to non-receptor proteins of blood and prostate but not the DHT bound to the receptor. This finding is based on the relative binding affinities of proteins to DHT. In this system the receptor has a higher affinity for DHT than the antibody, which in turn has a higher binding affinity to this steroid than other non-receptor binding proteins. Based on this model, these authors devised a method for the qualitative and quantitative evaluation of androgen receptors in the rat and human prostate. They suggested that the antibody can be coupled to a solid phase such as Sepharose which can be used to remove free steroid and steroid bound to non-receptor protein. Kliman *et al.* (1979) subsequently utilized this procedure for the quantitation of androgen receptors in BPH tissue. In their technique tritiated DHT was used as radioligand for labelling the receptor. As previously discussed, the use of DHT would only allow incubation to be carried out at a low temperature, thus resulting in the underestimation of the receptor population. This can be illustrated from the work by Kliman *et al.* (1979) who reported a mean concentration of 8.89 fmol/mg protein for the cytoplasmic androgen receptors in BPH tissues. This value is substantially lower than those reported for this tissue by others (Table 8.1).

8.1.9 Antibodies to steroid receptor

An extremely important approach which could be of considerable value both in the quantitative and qualitative analysis of steroid receptors, including processes involved in the receptor activation, nuclear uptake and biosynthesis, would be the generation of antibodies to steroid receptors. If a highly specific antibody to a steroid receptor is raised, it can be used to provide information concerning structural and conformational changes that accompany receptor activation. In addition, such antibodies could be utilized both for the localization and quantitation of steroid receptors in tissues and target cells using methods such as immunohistological techniques or simple radioimmunoassay for the receptor.

The pioneering work from Jensen's laboratory (Greene *et al.*, 1977; Jensen *et al.*, 1979; Greene *et al.*, 1980) in this field has led them to produce specific antibodies to oestrophilin as a probe for the study of the oestrogen receptors. An important precondition for generating a specific antibody would be the preparation of a highly purified receptor protein, which could then be used as the antigen. This successful approach in the study of the oestrogen receptor has provided excellent opportunities to extend our present knowledge regarding the mechanism of action of steroid hormones for this class of receptor. The generation of antibodies to androgen receptors would undoubtedly be a step forward in the future studies of receptor mediated events in the prostate.

8.1.10 Separation by dextran coated charcoal adsorption

The ability of activated charcoal with molecules of appropriate molecular size and configuration to separate free steroid from the same steroid bound to a protein has been known for many years. In theory, the proper molecular sieve coat for the charcoal would be a molecule with a molecular weight and configuration such that the free steroid could pass between the adjacent molecule into the charcoal, but the steroid bound to the protein would be excluded. An appropriate coating material which allows free steroids to pass, but rejects steroid bound to the protein, is dextran with average molecular weights of $7 \times 10^4 - 8 \times 10^4$ daltons. Apart from dextran, other compounds such as gamma globulin, fibrinogen, albumin and Ficoll could also be utilized (Herbert *et al.*, 1965).

Dextran coated charcoal as a separation technique is influenced by a number of factors, including the sample protein concentration, the pH and ionic strength of the media, the type and percentage of charcoal and dextran and the duration of incubation. Any alteration in these parameters may cause significant changes in the efficiency of the technique to separate free steroid from steroid bound to protein. In most studies, the separation of free and loosely bound steroids from the steroid bound to high affinity proteins has been achieved following the incubation of labelled samples with an appropriate volume of dextran coated charcoal suspension. This procedure is followed by centrifugation in order to separate the free steroid adsorbed to the charcoal from the protein bound steroid which remains in the supernatant. The radioactivity remaining in the supernatant represents both the binding of steroids to specific high affinity, low capacity binding sites and, to a great extent, the low affinity and high capacity binding components. A popular approach to distinguish the two classes of binding proteins is to measure the binding of the labelled steroid in the presence and absence of an excess of radioinert steroid. The labelled steroid is displaced from the high affinity, low capacity binding sites by the competing radioinert competitor, whereas the low affinity, high capacity sites (non-saturable) are unaffected. The difference between the two sets is a measure of the high affinity, low capacity binding components.

This technique has been widely used for the determination of equilibrium constant (K) and the number of binding sites. In addition to this, the dextran coated charcoal technique has been most popular in the studies of steroid specificity of the receptor. A variety of procedures are available, when the equilibrium constants (K) and the number of binding sites (n) are to be evaluated. The data obtained by the dextran coated charcoal technique can be analysed either by Scatchard plot, graphical method of Rosenthal, double reciprocal plot and finally single point analysis (simple method).

8.1.10.1 Scatchard plot

Analysis of the results by Scatchard plot (Scatchard, 1949) is the most widely used method for the determination of dissociation constant (K_d) and the number of binding sites (n). In this procedure data is generated following the incubation of samples with increasing amounts of radiolabelled steroid in the presence and absence of an excess of radioinert steroid. After incubation and subsequent treatment with dextran coated charcoal, aliquots of supernatant containing steroid bound to the high affinity binding sites are counted. In Scatchard plot analysis, the estimation of dissociation constant and the number of binding sites are obtained by plotting the steroid bound to the receptor (bound) versus the ratio of the bound to the free steroid. At least three methods are available for the calculation of the bound and free steroid.

(1) In this procedure the bound is plotted against bound/free and in this case Bound = $(B_T - B_{NS})$ and Free = $[T - (B_T - B_{NS})]$, where B_T corresponds to total bound steroid, B_{NS} is non-specifically bound steroid and T is the total amount of the radioactivity added. All these parameters are expressed in molar concentration. This method of calculation has been utilized for the analysis of steroid receptors by most laboratories.

(2) The equation used for this type of calculation is similar to the previous one. However, in this case free is derived from $T - B_T$.

(3) In this type of calculation B_{NS} (non-specifically bound) is plotted against T (total activity added) and a straight line fitted, giving an intercept (a) and slope (b) for the equation $B_{NS} = a + bt$. Using this formula, the theoretical values for B_{NS} at each ligand concentration can be obtained. Having determined the value for B_{NS} the specific binding can be calculated by subtracting the corrected B_{NS} from B_T. Once the corrected

values for B_T are obtained Scatchard plot can be constructed by the method outlined in (1) or (2).

Scatchard plot analysis is meant to provide a linear relationship between the bound receptor and the ratio of the bound over free steroid. The intercept at the X axis gives the number of binding sites, whereas the negative reciprocal of the gradient gives the dissociation constant (K_d). A comparison of these three types of calculation was made by Braunsberg and Hammond (1979) who analysed cytoplasmic progesterone receptors in human endometrium using these and other types of calculation. They suggested that the arbitrary rejection of experimental results is a major cause of variation, irrespective of the method of calculation used. Based on type 1, calculations in which the free steroid is estimated as $T - (B_T - B_{NS})$ could lead to flattening of the curve and overestimation of the number of binding sites, particularly at low receptor concentration and in conditions where there is a high background of non-specific binding. This method, however, has been used by most laboratories and could produce relatively reliable results provided the upper range of radioactive steroid added is not greater than approximately ten times the dissociation constant (Chamness and McGuire, 1975). From the theoretical point of view calculations based on type 2 and 3 do not appear to be correct, since B_T and B_{NS} which are used to calculate specific binding are not in equilibrium with the same concentration of unbound ligand.

It can, therefore, be concluded that, although the use of Scatchard plot for receptor analysis provides a reasonably simple means for the determination of K_d and the number of binding sites, the method does not always provide a linear regression line relationship between bound and bound/free steroid. Because of the occasional curvature in the Scatchard plot, there is a strong tendency in some cases to eliminate one or more points which do not fit on the straight line. This has been clearly demonstrated by studies carried out by Braunsberg and Hammond (1979). The common approach in estimating the amount of steroid bound to the receptor by subtracting non-specific binding (B_{NS}) from total binding (B_T) is not theoretically correct. This is because the separation procedure of dextran coated charcoal does not allow the complete separation of B_{NS} from B_T. This may be responsible for the curvature seen with Scatchard plot. This problem has been studied by Blondeau and Robel (1975), who suggested the application of a mathematically derived correction factor which can be subsequently used for the estimation of the true specifically bound ligand concentration.

8.1.10.2 Graphical method of Rosenthal

In the case of imperfect Scatchard plot, i.e. curvature, a more accurate analysis of the results can be performed by the application of the graphical method suggested by Rosenthal (1967). This method does not make any assumptions about the shape of the curve and it can be widely applied. In the method of Rosenthal, a plot of B_T against B_T/F and B_{NS}/F is constructed. Using the graphical procedure outlined by Rosenthal the amount of specific binding at each ligand concentration can then be accurately determined. In the comparative study by Braunsberg and Hammond (1979) this method was found to be superior to that of Scatchard plot when applied for the analysis of progesterone receptor.

8.1.10.3 Reciprocal plot

Reciprocal plots have been used in the analysis of steroid receptors mainly with the view to determine the steroid specificity of the receptor (Liao et al., 1973). The method can also be applied for the determination of the dissociation constant (K_d) and the number of binding sites (n). In this procedure a single concentration of the radioactive ligand is equilibrated with an increasing concentration of radioinert competitors. In general the concentration of the radioligand is approximately ten times greater than the dissociation constant. The choice of the radioligand concentration is governed by the amount required to saturate the high affinity binding sites and give minimal contribution from the non-specific binding components. In addition, the concentration should not be more than tenfold the concentration of radioligand. This would prevent the oversaturation of the receptor, hence avoiding curvature of the reciprocal plot and subsequent inaccuracy in the receptor estimation. The reciprocal plot is generated by plotting the reciprocal of the free steroid competitor against the reciprocal of the bound radioactive steroid. The disadvantage of this method is that the values calculated for the bound steroid at high concentrations of radioinert competitor tend to cluster near the axis and hence the presence of any secondary binding sites can easily be missed. This method of analysis has been applied by Boesel et al. (1977) for the analysis of androgen receptors. Reciprocal plots, however, do not appear to offer any advantages over Scatchard plots.

8.1.10.4 Single point analysis

This is the simplest approach for the quantitative analysis of steroid receptors. The procedure is based on the use of a single concentration of radioligand steroid, high enough to saturate the total number of binding sites. An estimate of the amount of radiolabelled steroid specifically bound to the receptor can be obtained by the inclusion of 100 fold excess of radioinert steroid in a separate set of tubes. The difference between the two readings is taken as a measure of the receptor content of the sample. This extremely simple approach requires minimal amounts of tissue and allows several samples to be analysed simultaneously. However, it does not provide information with regard to the dissociation constant and thus the affinity of the binding component to the steroid will remain unknown. In addition, on theoretical grounds, the technique is subject to errors such as contribution from secondary binding components which could lead to gross receptor overestimation. Conversely, if the concentration of radioligand has not been sufficient to saturate the binding sites, it could lead to gross underestimation. Despite these shortcomings, this type of analysis has been applied for the measurement of both oestrogen (King et al., 1980) and androgen (Hicks and Walsh, 1979) receptors. The latter group have shown that this method provides comparable results to that of corrected Scatchard plot analysis.

8.2 QUANTITATION OF ANDROGEN RECEPTORS

Despite numerous reports on the isolation and characterization of androgen receptors in normal prostate and its tumours, the development of reliable methods for the quantitation of this receptor has been exceedingly slow. With the exception of protamine sulphate, which separates the receptor from SHBG and allows the quantitation of the total receptor population by labelling the precipitated receptor with tritiated DHT under exchange conditions, results with the other techniques have not been consistent. This inconsistency is basically related to the use of DHT as radioligand rather than the techniques themselves. At least three major factors should be considered for the quantitative analysis of androgen receptors in the prostate, namely the choice of ligand, considerations regarding the receptor occupancy by androgenic hormones and, finally, the interference by other non-receptor binding components.

8.2.1 The choice of ligand

The choice of ligand is the most important consideration in the studies of androgen receptors in the prostate. Indeed, problems related to the interfering proteins as well as those associated with receptor occupancy govern the choice of the radioligand.

Early attempts to quantitate androgen receptors in the human prostate involved the use of natural androgens, mainly testosterone or DHT. In these studies the tissues were either incubated with tritiated testosterone which subsequently undergoes reduction to DHT and then binds to the receptor or the tissue extracts were directly labelled with tritiated DHT. In either case, it soon became apparent that there are some serious shortcomings associated with the use of tritiated natural steroid in the quantitation of androgen receptors. The main problems were found to be the binding of DHT to SHBG and the metabolism of DHT to androstanediols. The latter problem prohibited the use of exchange conditions for the labelling of the total binding sites by DHT. Some of these problems have been encountered for other classes of steroid hormones when natural tritiated steroids were used for labelling the receptors. The introduction of synthetic steroids, which exhibit high affinity towards their corresponding receptors with minimal or no binding to the non-receptor binding components and reasonably high stability against enzymic degradation, have made significant contributions towards resolving some of the above mentioned problems. In the case of androgen receptors the use of the synthetic androgen (17β-hydroxy-17α-methylestra-4,9.11-trien-3-one; R1881) has been most useful. This compound was originally introduced by Bonne and Raynaud (1975) for the measurement of androgen receptors in the rat ventral prostate and human BPH (Bonne and Raynaud, 1976). They demonstrated that R1881 was specifically bound to androgen receptors and, unlike DHT, it did not undergo metabolism. Indeed, because of these two properties this compound exhibited some stabilizing effect on androgen receptors. In addition, these authors also showed that R1881 did not bind to SHBG. These properties indicated that R1881 should be a suitable probe for the quantitation of total androgen receptors. Subsequently, the usefulness of this compound for the analysis of androgen receptors was substantiated by a number of laboratories (Ghanadian *et al.*, 1977a; Snochowski *et al.*, 1977; Ghanadian *et al.*, 1978a,b; Shain *et al.*, 1978; Hicks and Walsh, 1979; Asselin *et al.*, 1979). However, despite these advantages, the main concern in the use of R1881 in the studies of androgen receptors is its crossreactivity with other classes of receptors. Earlier reports by Asselin *et al.* (1976) and Dube *et al.* (1976) suggested that R 1881 crossreacts with progesterone receptors. This, therefore, raised the problem that in those tissues which also contain progesterone receptors, the use of this radioligand would lead to overestimation of the androgen receptors. Their conclusion was based on experiments where R1881 was shown to bind the progesterone receptor of the oestrogen primed rat uterus. At the same time, these authors also showed that the specificity of R1881 for human BPH cytosol is different to that of rat ventral prostate. Both studies, which were carried out at 4 °C, showed that progesterone and the synthetic progestin R5020 (17α, 21-dimethyl-19-norpregna-4, 9-diene-3, 20-dione) were strong competitors of the binding of R1881 in human BPH cytosol, but not the rat ventral prostate. In addition R5020 was also found to bind with high affinity only to BPH cytosol (Asselin *et al.*, 1976; Gustafsson *et al.*, 1978). Therefore, it was concluded that at 4 °C R1881 binds to both androgen and progesterone receptors in human BPH cytosol.

It has been suggested that the inclusion of an excess amount of triamcinolone acetonide (TMA) could eliminate the binding of R1881 to the progesterone receptor (Asselin et al., 1979; Zava *et al.*, 1979). At a temperature of 0 °C this compound is known to bind sufficiently to progesterone receptors but not to androgen receptors. Thus its presence in the incubation media could block the binding of R1881 to the progesterone receptors. The relative binding affinity of TMA for progesterone and androgen receptors at this temperature is reported to be 12 % and less than 0.1 % respectively (Raynaud and Bouton, 1980). However, it has been reported that at a higher temperature of incubation the binding of R1881 to the androgen receptor may be inhibited to some extent by TMA (Shain *et al.*, 1980). However, this inhibition has been found to be insignificant (Geller and Albert, 1979).

The specificity of the binding of R1881 to androgen receptors in the cytoplasmic fraction of human BPH has also been investigated at 15 °C by Shain and Boesel (1978a) and Ghanadian and Auf (1980). At this temperature the endogenously bound DHT is exchanged for the radiolabelled R1881, thus allowing the labelling of the total androgen binding sites. Under these conditions, these authors clearly demonstrated that neither progesterone nor R5020 were able to compete for the binding of R1881. Furthermore they showed that whilst at 0–4 °C DHT was a relatively poor competitor for R1881, at 15 °C DHT was a stronger competitor. In addition, the former authors demonstrated that radiolabelled R5020 is unable to bind saturable binding components in BPH cytosol. It was, therefore, suggested that at this temperature, the steroid specificity of the cytoplasmic R1881 binding component is consistent with its identification as an androgen receptor. Further evidence that at this temperature R1881 does not crossreact with progesterone receptors is also provided from the analysis of R1881 labelled human BPH cytosol on columns of Sepharose 6B (Figure 8.3a) and by isoelectric focusing in polyacrylamide gel plate (Figure 8.4).

The suitability of R1881 for the measurement of androgen receptors in the nuclear extracts of prostatic tumours has also been studied by Menon *et al.* (1978), Shain and Boesel (1978a) and Ghanadian and Auf (1980). These studies have demonstrated that in nuclear extract, the binding specificities of R1881 at both 0–4 °C and 15 °C were comparable and were characteristic of binding to androgen receptors. The relative effectiveness of R1881, DHT, R5020 and oestradiol-17β as inhibitors of R1881 binding to nuclear receptors at 15 °C are reported to be 100%, 74%, 0.5% and 2.5% respectively (Shain and Boesel, 1978a). Similarly, at 4 °C the relative binding affinities for R1881, DHT and progesterone are reported to be 100%, 90% and 0% respectively (Walsh and Hicks, 1979). All these studies strongly support the view that in the nuclear extract of the human BPH the binding of R1881 at either 0–4 °C or 15 °C is to an androgen receptor.

It can be concluded that as far as the choice of radioligand for the quantitative measurement of androgen receptors is concerned, R1881 is a more suitable radioligand in terms of stability to enzymic degradation, binding affinity and specificity at 15 °C than are natural steroid ligands such as DHT.

8.2.2 Receptor occupancy by endogenous hormone

It is now well established that the human prostate contains a high level of endogenous androgens (see Chapters 3 and 4). Consequently most of the androgen receptor proteins are present in an occupied form (bound), and only a limited number of the binding sites are unoccupied (free) by the endogenous androgens. In a preliminary study, Rosen *et al.* (1975) found that the ratio of the bound to free androgen receptor in the cytosol fraction from human BPH tissue was approximately 9:1. It became apparent, therefore, that the ideal condition for the receptor assay should allow the dissociation of the endogenously bound hormone and its replacement (exchange) by the radioligand. This approach had already been adopted in the quantitation of oestrogen receptors in the rat uterus (Katzenellenbogen *et al.*, 1973), and for the measurement of the occupied androgen receptor in the rat ventral prostate (Bonne and Raynaud, 1976). At least three basic requirements are essential for the development of an exchange assay.

Firstly, the employed radioligand should not undergo metabolism during the duration of exchange. As previously discussed DHT does not fulfil this requirement, as it undergoes metabolism in the prostate. Studies by Bonne and Raynaud (1976) have demonstrated that as much as 60% of the radiolabelled DHT in the cytosol of rat ventral prostate undergoes metabolism within the first 6 h of incubation at the low temperature of 0 °C. The rate of metabolism approaches approximately 80% when the incubation is carried out at 25 °C for 16 h. By contrast R1881 does not undergo metabolism and remains stable under these incubation conditions.

Secondly, the receptor should be stable under the exchange conditions. In their studies Bonne and Raynaud (1976) demonstrated that optimal exchange was achieved at a temperature of 15 °C following an incubation period of 16 h. Within the first 16 h of incubation the loss of receptor was found to be approximately 16 % whereas under similar experimental conditions the loss of receptor labelled with DHT was about 87 %. This clearly shows that DHT is not a suitable radioligand for the measurement of androgen receptor under exchange conditions.

Thirdly, the exchange conditions should allow rapid dissociation of the endogenously bound hormone from the receptor sites. In the rat ventral prostate, the dissociation of DHT from the cytoplasmic androgen receptors has been shown to be 100 % following 16 h incubation at 15 °C (Bonne and Raynaud, 1976). These investigators suggested that 15 °C is the optimal temperature for the exchange between the radiolabelled R1881 and the endogenously bound DHT to the receptor.

It is quite apparent that the exchange conditions for the measurement of total androgen receptors could be applied in human prostatic tissues provided a stable ligand such as R1881 is used. Indeed, these incubation conditions have been applied for the measurement of cytoplasmic androgen receptors in human prostatic tumours (Ghanadian et al., 1978a; Shain and Boesel, 1978a; Geller and Albert, 1979; Ghanadian and Auf, 1980) as well as monkey prostate (Ghanadian et al., 1977a) and dog prostate (Shain and Boesel, 1978b). In addition to receptor analysis at 15 °C, the measurement of androgen receptors has also been carried out following 16 h incubation at 0–4 °C (Snochowski et al., 1977; Walsh and Hicks, 1979). However, as previously stated, at this temperature care should be exercised to eliminate the binding of R1881 to the progesterone binding components.

The exchange conditions of 15 °C for 16 h have also been extended to the measurement of androgen receptors in the nuclear extracts of the human prostatic tumours (Shain and Boesel, 1978a; Sirett and Grant, 1978; Ghanadian and Auf, 1980). This measurement has also been performed following incubation at 0–4 °C for a period of 16–20 h (Walsh and Hicks, 1979). Studies in our laboratory have shown that the dissociation of steroid from the nuclear receptors proceeds at a fast rate at either 0–4 °C or 15 °C, thus facilitating the exchange of radiolabelled R1881 with the DHT bound endogenously to the receptor. It would therefore appear that both temperatures may be equally used for the measurement of the occupied nuclear androgen receptor.

8.2.3 The interference of non-receptor binding components

The presence of non-receptor high affinity, low capacity androgen binding components in human prostatic tissues constitutes a major problem in the quantitative analysis of androgen receptors. The main interfering component is that of sex hormone binding globulin (SHBG). This protein is not only a serum contaminant, but it is also present in significant quantities in human prostatic tissues (Cowan et al., 1976). As discussed previously, this high affinity, binding protein could be eliminated either by employing a purification step or by using a radioligand which does not bind to it. The latter approach has formed the basis for the use of R1881 as this compound does not bind to

SHBG (Bonne and Raynaud, 1975; Snochowski *et al.*, 1977). Further evidence for the inability of R1881 to bind to SHBG was obtained when the isoelectric focusing profile of DHT and R1881 labelled human BPH cytosol were compared (Auf and Ghanadian, 1981).

As far as the quantitation of androgen receptors is concerned the use of the synthetic androgen R1881 appears to satisfy most of the required criteria for this assay in the cytoplasmic and nuclear fractions of human prostatic tissues. However, due to the absence of SHBG in the nuclear fraction (Foekens *et al.*, 1980) radiolabelled DHT has also been used for the quantitative measurement of androgen receptors in this compartment without application of a purification step (Sirett and Grant, 1978).

8.3 FACTORS AFFECTING VARIABILITY IN RECEPTOR ANALYSIS

Apart from the above mentioned factors which are of prime importance in the quantitation of androgen receptors, i.e. type and stability of radioligand, time and temperature of incubation, interference of non-receptor binding components, receptor occupancy by endogenous hormone and ligand receptor dissociation, there are several other factors which influence the quantitation of receptors and are responsible for the interlaboratory variations. These factors can be summarized as follows: (1) tissue sampling, (2) homogenization procedure, (3) removal of the free endogenous steroid, (4) range of steroid ligand concentration, (5) the amount of dextran coated charcoal, (6) sample protein concentration and (7) tissue storage.

8.3.1 Tissue sampling

An important consideration in the analysis of androgen receptors in prostatic tumours is the type of operation by which the tissue is obtained. In most cases the tissue is removed either by transurethral resection (TUR) or by retropubic prostatectomy (RPP). Differences in the biochemical composition of the two types of tissues are discussed in Chapter 4. As far as the receptor evaluation is concerned, special care should be exercised when TUR materials are used. In this case large TUR chips must be selected and the burnt portion must be removed prior to the analysis. Small chips must be discarded as they contain a high proportion of damaged tissue and this could lead to unreliable results.

8.3.2 Homogenization procedure

Because of the heterogenous nature of human prostatic tissues and the presence of considerable quantities of fibromuscular elements, the need for an efficient homogenization procedure is most desirable. At least three types of homogenization instruments have been used in the studies of steroid receptors. These included the use of an ultraturrax, all glass pot homogenizer and microdismembrator. A comparative study on the percentage yield of receptor following the use of these three instruments has been conducted by Wagner

(1977). This study clearly favoured the use of a microdismembrator which was found to provide the highest yield of receptor. Homogenization by the microdismembrator technique involves freezing the tissue specimen in liquid nitrogen together with a precooled tungsten carbide ball and the subsequent pulverization of the tissue by vibration for two cycles of 45 s at 50 Hz. The resulting frozen powdered tissue is immediately mixed with buffer and used for preparation of cytoplasmic and nuclear fractions. This procedure has the advantage of being able to disrupt the cell efficiently without damaging the cell nuclei or generating heat.

8.3.3   Removal of the free endogenous steroid

This is an important consideration, since the prostate contains a high level of endogenous androgens, some of which are bound to the receptor and the remainder are present in a free or loosely bound form. As far as the binding of hormone to the receptor is concerned, the problem can be overcome by the application of exchange conditions. With regard to the free and loosely bound steroids, their presence could exert an isotopic dilution effect, thus leading to underestimation of the receptor content of the tissue. This problem can be resolved by the use of a primary step employing dextran coated charcoal to strip the cytosol of its free and loosely bound hormones. In our experience the addition of 1:10 (v/v) of dextran (0.5%) coated charcoal (5%) to cytosol is sufficient to remove the free and loosely bound androgens from human prostatic cytosol.

8.3.4   Range of steroid ligand concentration

In order to accurately estimate the number of binding sites, it is essential to use a broad range of radioligand concentration and this should include a sufficient number of points below the saturation level. It is generally accepted that the upper limit of the concentration range should not exceed tenfold the value for the dissociation constant (K_d). On the other hand, the concentration for the lower limit should be enough to stabilize the receptor and prevent its degradation (Chamness and McGuire, 1975).

8.3.5   The concentration of dextran coated charcoal

Dextran coated charcoal (DCC) is used in the quantitation of the androgen receptors to separate the free and loosely bound radioligand from the radioligand bound to the receptor. It is necessary to use conditions in which DCC could remove most of the free and loosely bound steroids without affecting the specific binding components. In general, long term exposure could lead to the inactivation of the specific binding components, whereas short term exposure may partially remove the radioligand bound to non-specific binding sites. At least two concentrations of DCC suspension appear to fulfil the aforementioned criteria. The first one contains 5% charcoal, 0.5% dextran and 1% human γ-globulin. In this system a 2.2 volume of DCC is added to 1 volume of cytosol and the mixture is incubated at 0–4° C for 10 min followed by the addition of 7.8 % absolute ethanol and a further incubation of 20 min (Shain *et al.*, 1975). The second procedure which is equally efficient but simpler, is to incubate cytosol for 10 min with half volume of 1.25 % charcoal, 0.625 % dextran (Bonne and Raynaud, 1975).

In the case of nuclear androgen receptors, which are extracted with 0.4 mol/l KCl, the removal of the free radioligand by DCC requires special care. This is due to the fact that the high salt media interferes with the adsorption of steroid to charcoal. This problem can be resolved by diluting the nuclear extract with a salt free media in order to reduce the ionic strength of the solution.

8.3.6 Sample protein concentration

The protein concentration of the cytosol and nuclear extract can influence the efficiency of DCC adsorption in removing the free and loosely bound steroids. For this reason, it is essential to investigate the linearity of the assay over a wide range of the sample protein concentration with the particular DCC suspension used. In our experience using a DCC suspension containing 1.25 % charcoal to 0.625 % dextran gives a linear assay over a protein concentration range of 1–10 mg/ml. Similar results have also been reported by Shain *et al.* (1975).

8.3.7 Tissue storage

The last but not the least concern in the quantitation of androgen receptors is the temperature and duration of the storage of the tissue prior to the assay. Although it is generally accepted that the activity of steroid receptors could be significantly diminished by frequent freezing and thawing of the tissue, it is possible to preserve the receptor activity provided certain precautions are taken. The tissue should be cooled immediately after surgery, adequately cleaned, placed in a sterile airtight container and snap frozen in liquid nitrogen prior to storage at least at − 35° C or preferably at − 70 °C. Using this protocol we found that the cytoplasmic and nuclear receptors in the human prostate are stable for a period of up to 12 months storage at − 35 °C. The loss of receptor during this period was not statistically significant. In a similar study Shain *et al.*(1980) have indicated that storage of the whole tissue at − 70 °C for up to 20 weeks, which was the longest interval evaluated, does not result in significant loss of the tissues content of androgen receptor. It should be emphasized that in these studies the tissues were not exposed to frequent freezing and thawing. For practical purposes, tissue should be aliquoted into a number of separate containers prior to the freezing step.

8.4 QUANTITATION OF ANDROGEN RECEPTORS USING DIFFERENT TECHNIQUES

The preceding sections in this chapter have dealt with the current available methodology concerning the analysis of androgen receptors in the prostate. In this regard, we have adopted a critical view in order to highlight the advantages and disadvantages of each method for the analysis of androgen receptors with particular emphasis on the quantitative aspects. This section deals with the comparison of the data available on the concentration of the cytoplasmic and nuclear androgen receptors in human BPH. At the same time an attempt has been made to discuss this data in relation to the relevant method of quantitation.

A summary of the most commonly used techniques for the quantitation of androgen receptors together with data obtained by these methods are shown in Tables 8.1 and 8.2. In general, the data obtained in Table 8.1 can be classified into two major groups.

Firstly, in those methods in which tritiated DHT is used as radioligand, a purification step to separate SHBG from the receptor has been a mandatory requirement. However, an exception is the use of the antisteroid antibody technique. In addition, because of the metabolism of DHT, most of the incubation procedures with this natural steroid have been confined to a low temperature and a short duration. When protamine sulphate precipitation technique was used, this problem did not arise. As a result of these limitations most values reported for cytoplasmic androgen receptors using these methods are generally low and in most cases represent the number of free binding sites.

Secondly, in those assays in which tritiated R1881 has been employed, the need for an elaborate separation step has not been essential and only a simple procedure involving the use of dextran coated charcoal has been used. In addition, because of the stability and specificity of this radioligand, several laboratories have been able to measure total receptor sites using exchange conditions. It is apparent that data obtained by exchange assay gives a considerably higher yield of receptor and especially if preparative aspects such as homogenization and the removal of endogenous hormone have been carefully considered. These preparative aspects could explain the higher values reported by Ghanadian et al. (1978a) and Ghanadian et al. (1980a, b), compared to that by Shain et al. (1978). Although both authors have used identical conditions, the latter group have used an all glass pot homogenizer whereas the former employed a microdismembrator (see section 8.3.2). Similarly, the lower values reported by Hicks and Walsh (1979) can be explained both in terms of isotopic dilution by endogenous androgens and the low temperature of incubation which does not allow full exchange of the radioligand with the endogenously bound DHT to the receptor. This difference is not due to the possible interference of progesterone binding components, as the incubation at 15 °C eliminates this problem and subsequently those assays performed at 15 °C do not require the inclusion of TMA. Despite some slight methodological differences, data reported by Ghanadian et al. (1978a), Shain et al. (1978) and Hicks and Walsh (1979) are generally in good agreement. In the studies by Snochowski et al. (1977) the cytosol had been prepared and stored at − 20 °C for some period of time prior to the receptor analysis. It is generally accepted that such a procedure could lead to inactivation of the receptor and this, together with the low incubation temperature used by these investigators, may have been responsible for their rather low values.

Table 8.1 Comparison of the values estimated for the content of androgen receptors in the cytosol fraction of human benign hypertrophied prostate using different methods

Method	Tritiated Steroid	No. of Samples	Surgery	Receptor content 0–4°C	Receptor content 15°C	References
Glycerol gradient centrifugation	DHT	1	RPP	43 fmol/g tissue	2600 fmol/g tissue	Rosen et al. (1975)
Sucrose gradient centrifugation	DHT	15	RPP	25–50 fmol/g tissue	—	Menon et al. (1977)
Agar gel electrophoresis	DHT	15	—	23 fmol/mg protein	—	Wagner et al. (1977)
	DHT	14	RPP	12.3 fmol/mg protein	—	Krieg et al. (1979)
	DHT	66	RPP	8 fmol/mg protein	—	de Voogt and Dingjan (1980)
Protamine sulphate precipitation	DHT	15	RPP	100–700 fmol/g tissue	—	Menon et al. (1977)
	DHT	22	RPP/TUR	210 fmol/g tissue	3600 fmol/g tissue	Mobbs et al. (1980)
	DHT	—	—	—	38–92 fmol/mg protein	Davies and Griffiths (1980)
Antisteroid antibody 20h incubation	DHT	19	RPP	8.9 fmol/mg protein	—	Kliman et al. (1979)
Dextran coated charcoal 2 h incubation at 0–4°C 16 h incubation at 15°C	R1881	15	RPP	8.4 fmol/mg protein	73.6 fmol/mg protein	Ghanadian et al. (1978)
	R1881	14	RPP/TUR	10.7 fmol/mg protein	51.7 fmol/mg protein	Shain et al. (1978)
Dextran coated charcoal 18 h incubation	R1881	9	RPP	29.2 fmol/mg protein	—	Snochowski et al. (1977)
Dextran coated charcoal 20 h incubation in the presence of TMA	R1881	10	RPP	48 fmol/mg protein	—	Hicks and Walsh (1979)
Dextran coated charcoal 16h incubation at 15°C	R1881	40	RPP/TUR	—	86 fmol/mg protein 2566 fmol/g	Ghanadian and Auf (1982, unpublished)

Table 8.2 Comparison of the values estimated for the content of androgen receptors in the nuclear extract of human benign hypertrophied prostate using different methods

Method	Tritiated steroid	No. of samples	Type of surgery	Receptor content	Reference
Sucrose gradient centrifugation Incubation at 4 °C for 18 h	DHT	15	RPP	100–150 fmol/g tissue	Menon et al. (1977)
Dual column G25/G200 chromatography Incubation at 4 °C for 18 h	DHT	11	RPP	1400 molecules per nucleus	Lieskovsky and Bruchovsky (1979)
Protamine sulphate precipitation Incubation at 4 °C for 18 h	DHT	15	RPP	10–60 fmol/g tissue	Menon et al. (1977)
Protamine sulphate precipitation Incubation at 15 °C for 16 h	DHT	—	—	412–868 fmol/mg DNA	Davies and Griffiths (1980)
Mini column of Sephadex LH20 Incubation at 15 °C for 16 h	DHT R1881	5 3	RPP RPP	765 fmol/mg DNA 360 fmol/g tissue	Sirett and Grant (1978)
Dextran coated charcoal Incubation at 15 °C for 20–24 h	R1881	3	RPP and TUR	290 fmol/mg DNA	Shain et al. (1978)
Dextran coated charcoal Incubation at 0 °C for 20 h	R1881	10	RPP	1638 fmol/g tissue 104 fmol/mg nuclear protein	Hicks and Walsh (1979)
Dextran coated charcoal Incubation at 15 °C for 16 h	R1881	15	TUR	236 fmol/mg nuclear protein	Ghanadian and Auf (1980)
Dextran coated charcoal Incubation at 15 °C for 16 h	R1881	40	RPP and TUR	149 fmol/mg nuclear protein 1237 fmol/g tissue 657 fmol/mg DNA	Ghanadian and Auf (1982, unpublished)

In conclusion the use of tritiated R1881 under conditions of exchange provides a simple and reliable method for quantitation of the total cytoplasmic androgen receptors in the human prostate. An alternative to this is the application of exchange procedures to the protamine sulphate precipitated receptor as used by Mobbs *et al.* (1978) and Davies and Griffiths (1980). Although the latter technique allows the use of tritiated DHT as radioligand, the actual procedure is rather laborious as it involves several washing steps (see section 8.1.7.2).

As far as the quantitation of nuclear androgen receptors in the human prostate is concerned, this has been less troublesome, since radiolabelled DHT can be used without major complications. With the exception of the values reported by Menon *et al.* (1977) and Lieskovsky and Bruchovsky (1979) there is a general agreement between the values reported by different laboratories whether tritiated DHT or R1881 are used at different incubation temperatures (Table 8.2). The low values reported by Menon *et al.* (1977) and Lieskovsky and Bruchovsky (1979) may have been due to the dissociation of tritiated DHT from the nuclear receptor secondary to the long period needed for gradient centrifugation or column chromatography. Furthermore, the striking differences between the reported values by Menon *et al.* (1977) and Davies and Griffiths (1980), who both employed protamine sulphate precipitation, may be due to the interference by KCl with the protamine precipitation step in the studies by the former group. The higher and more acceptable values reported by Davies and Griffiths (1980) are most probably due to the fact that these authors precipitated the nuclear receptors from whole nuclei in the absence of KCl.

8.5 COMPARISON BETWEEN THE LEVELS OF ANDROGEN RECEPTORS IN RPP AND TUR SAMPLES

As previously described, transurethral resection has now become the major type of surgery for removing prostatic tissues in both benign hypertrophy and carcinoma of the prostate. This surgical procedure could seriously damage the tissue and hence special care should be exercised to remove the burnt sections from the specimens, in order to obtain a relatively reliable result. In addition to this, small prostatic chips should be discarded as these samples might have undergone irreversible biochemical damage due to the heat generated by electroresection. It is clear that the comparison between the androgen receptor levels in TUR materials obtained in different laboratories can be justified only if these precautions have been considered. Having established these criteria we have compared the androgen receptor content in 26 samples removed by RPP with that of 14 samples which were resected by TUR procedure. The results of this study which is shown in Table 8.3, indicate that in the cytosol, the overall mean of the androgen receptors in TUR samples was lower than that for the RPP. When the results were expressed in terms of wet weight, mg protein or mg DNA, the mean value for TUR samples was 37%, 23% and 28% lower respectively. However, these changes were not statistically significant. The differences in the mean values for nuclear receptors obtained from TUR and

RPP samples were less pronounced than those for the cytoplasmic receptors (Table 8.3).

Table 8.3 Comparison between the concentration of cytoplasmic and nuclear androgen receptors obtained by transurethral resection (TUR) or retropubic prostatectomy (RPP). (Ghanadian and Auf, 1982, unpublished)

| | Total cytoplasmic androgen receptors fmol per: | | | Total nuclear androgen receptors fmol per: | | |
	g tissue	mg protein	mg DNA	g tissue	mg protein	mg DNA
RPP						
Mean ± SEM	3132 ± 297	97 ± 52	1352 ± 204	1347 ± 412	183 ± 29	682 ± 197
Range	0–6625	0–222	0–3278	0–5740	0–510	0–2568
No. of samples	(26)	(26)	(14)	(14)	(26)	(14)
TUR						
Mean ± SEM	2001 ± 564	75 ± 21	979 ± 265	1126 ± 329	115 ± 25	632 ± 174
Range	0–8470	0–308	0–3756	0–4282	0–353	0–2280
No. of samples	(14)	(14)	(13)	(13)	(14)	(13)
RPP + TUR						
Mean ± SEM	2566 ± 285	86 ± 10	1166 ± 175	1237 ± 175	149 ± 21	657 ± 130
Range	0–8470	0–308	0–3756	0–5740	0–510	0–2568
No. of samples	(40)	(40)	(27)	(27)	(40)	(27)

Androgen receptors were assayed in author's laboratory by incubating cytosol or nuclear extracts with [3]H R 1881 at 15°C for 16 h and subsequent separation by dextran coated charcoal. Data were obtained by Scatchard plot analysis.

8.6 CHARACTERIZATION AND QUANTITATION OF OESTROGEN RECEPTORS

The critical role of oestrogens in the hormonal control and development of prostatic tumours has been discussed in Chapter 4. The ability of prostatic tissues to take up and retain oestradiol-17β has been recognized for several years (Ghanadian and Fotherby, 1972). There is now good evidence to suggest that the prostate of most experimental animals contains receptor proteins for oestradiol. These include the prostate of the rat (Armstrong and Bashirelahi, 1978), dog (Chaisiri et al., 1978) and monkey (Karr et al., 1979). With regard to the presence of this receptor in human prostatic tissues data has been controversial. In an earlier report Sinha et al. (1973) have demonstrated by autoradiography the localization of tritiated oestradiol and its binding to a high affinity protein in human malignant prostates. Ekman (1980) and Murphy et al. (1980) have provided evidence for the presence of an oestradiol receptor in normal as well as malignant human prostates, but these authors reported the absence of this receptor in human BPH tissues. On the other hand Bashirelahi et al. (1976), Hawkins et al. (1976), de Voogt and Dingjan (1978), Pertshuk et al. (1979) and Krieg et al. (1981) have reported the existence of an oestradiol receptor in this tissue. Moreover, Pertshuk et al. (1979) have demonstrated the localization of fluoresceinated oestradiol in the nuclear compartment of BPH tissues. With the exception of this latter study which demonstrated the presence of oestrogen receptor in BPH tissues by a histochemical method, virtually all the available data on this receptor in BPH tissues have employed biochemical procedures. Using human BPH tissues we have demonstrated that the cytoplasmic and nuclear fractions of human BPH tissues contain high affinity saturable binding components for oestradiol which have certain physicochemical characteristics similar to those of classical oestrogen receptors (Auf and Ghanadian, 1982).

Evidence for the presence of this receptor in human BPH was based on the following observations. Firstly, the analysis of oestradiol labelled cytosol on low ionic strength glycerol gradients revealed a 4s binding component. This was clearly distinguishable from the binding of oestradiol to SHBG, since the binding of oestradiol to the 4s component was inhibited with diethylstilboestrol (DES) but not DHT. Furthermore, this binding was destroyed by preheating cytosol at 45 °C or by treatment with the sulphydryl blocking agent, parachloromercureobenzoate. Secondly, unlike SHBG, the cytoplasmic oestradiol binding component was found to precipitate with protamine sulphate. Thirdly, specificity studies revealed that this binding component has a high affinity for oestradiol and DES, but not for androgen or progesterone. Fourthly, the cytoplasmic oestradiol binding components focused with a pI of 6.3 when they were subjected to isoelectric focusing on polyacrylamide gel. This pI is similar to that of oestrogen receptors of other target organs. The analysis of the nuclear extracts also revealed the presence of an oestradiol binding component which exhibited similar steroid specificity to that of the cytoplasmic receptor and had a sedimentation coefficient of 2.8 S and an isoelectric point of 6.0 (Auf and Ghanadian, 1982).

The concentrations of cytoplasmic and nuclear oestradiol receptors in the normal and benign hypertrophied human prostates have been evaluated by several research groups (Table 8.4). In most studies receptors were labelled by overnight incubation at 0–4 °C with tritiated oestradiol in the presence and absence of excess of DES, in order to correct for the non-specific binding sites. In some studies tritiated synthetic oestrogen (R2858) has been used and in these studies the receptor was labelled by incubating samples at 30 °C for 4 h (Murphy et al., 1980). The use of this synthetic oestrogen, however, does not appear to offer any advantages over that of tritiated oestradiol (Wittliff et al., 1978). In most experiments the free steroid has been removed by dextran coated charcoal adsorption and the data analysed by Scatchard plots (Bashirelahi et al., 1980; Murphy et al., 1980; Auf and Ghanadian, 1982) or a single point assay (Krieg et al., 1981). An alternative procedure has been the electrophoretic separation of the receptor on agar gel and the subsequent calculation of the area under the peak (Wagner, 1977; de Voogt and Dingjan, 1978). The latter procedure, however, has provided less consistent results. Whilst Wagner (1977) reported a mean value of 40 fmol/mg protein for the cytoplasmic oestradiol receptor concentration in BPH, de Voogt and Dingjan (1978) obtained a mean value of 798 fmol/mg protein with an upper range of 10 000 fmol/mg protein. This extremely high value is probably due to the contamination by albumin in their system. Data obtained by dextran coated charcoal assay appears to be more consistent. Murphy *et al.* (1980) have reported a mean value of 12 fmol/mg protein for the cytoplasmic oestrogen receptors of the peripheral zone of the human normal prostate. In addition, the presence of an oestradiol receptor was also reported in some biopsy samples obtained from the periurethral zone of the normal gland. Similarly, they also detected this receptor in the nuclear extract of the normal gland. Ekman (1980) also found cytoplasmic oestradiol receptors in 5 out of 13 samples of normal human prostates. The concentration of this receptor is approximately of the same order of magnitude as that reported by Murphy *et al.* (1980). However, neither of these authors were able to detect this receptor in BPH tissues.

The concentration of oestradiol receptors in the human benign hypertrophied prostate has been evaluated by a number of research groups (Table 8.4). The level of this receptor in the cytosol appears to be in the same order of magnitude as that of the normal gland. Studies in our laboratory and those by others (Bashirelahi *et al.*, 1980; Krieg *et al.*, 1981) suggest that oestradiol receptors are mainly localized in the stromal elements of the hypertrophied gland. It is interesting that the incidence for the detection of this receptor in BPH tissues appears to increase significantly if the analysis of the receptor is carried out on the stromal fraction of the tissue (Krieg *et al.*, 1981). Whereas, Krieg *et al.* could detect oestradiol receptors in only 2 out of 19 samples in whole BPH tumours, this ratio was increased to 8 out of 19 when the analysis was performed on the stromal elements of the same tissue.

8.7 PROGESTERONE RECEPTORS IN THE HUMAN PROSTATE

The initial indication that the human prostate might possess a progestenic binding component came from the studies by Asselin *et al.* (1976) and Dube *et al.* (1976) in their evaluation of the use of R1881 for the measurement of androgen receptors in the human prostate. Asselin *et al.* showed that tritiated R1881 was capable of binding to the progesterone receptor of the oestrogen primed rat uterus, and that the steroid specificity of R1881 binding to BPH cytosol at 0–4 °C was indicative of the binding of R1881 to a progesterone binding component, or an atypical androgen receptor. Furthermore, these authors demonstrated that the synthetic progestin R5020 binds to BPH cytosol with similar specificity to that of R1881. Although Snochowski *et al.* (1977) reported that at 0 °C R1881 was bound only to androgen receptors, studies by other research groups have demonstrated that progesterone is a better competitor than DHT for the binding of R1881 in BPH cytosol (Cowan *et al.*, 1977; Gustafsson *et al.*, 1978; Menon *et al.*, 1978). In general the steroid specificity of R1881 suggests that whilst at 0–4 °C progesterone crossreacts with the binding of this compound in human BPH cytosol, at 15 °C this crossreactivity was negligible (Shain *et al.*, 1978; Ghanadian and Auf, 1980). Two explanations for this change in specificity with elevation of temperature may be offered. Firstly, it is possible to envisage the presence of at least two allosteric forms of androgen receptors, each possessing different steroid specificity. The first form which is detectable at low temperature is less specific and could undergo transconformation into a more specific form which is active

Table 8.4 Concentrations of oestradiol receptors in the cytoplasmic and nuclear fractions of human normal and benign hypertrophied prostate (BPH)

Method	Tissue	Tritiated steroid	No. of samples	Type of surgery	Receptor concentration		Reference
					Cytosol	Nuclear extract	
Dextran coated charcoal Incubation 0 °C for 16–24 h Scatchard analysis	BPH	Oe$_2$	8/29	RPP and TUR	17 fmol/mg protein	—	Bashirelahi et al. (1980)
Dextran coated charcoal Incubation at 30 °C for 4 h Scatchard analysis	BPH Normal	R2858 R2858	10 5 peripheral 4 periurethral	RPP RPP biopsy	Not detectable 12 fmol/mg protein 6 fmol/mg protein	Not detectable 187 fmol/g tissue 136 fmol/g tissue	Murphy et al. (1980)
Dexatran coated charcoal Incubation conditions not stated Scatchard analysis	BPH Normal	R2858 R2858	26 8 5	RPP total cystectomy	Not detectable Not detectable 372 fmol/mg DNA	—	Ekman (1980)
Dextran coated charcoal Incubation at 0 °C for 18 h One point assay	BPH	Oe$_2$	2 17	RPP RPP	37 fmol/mg protein Not detectable	—	Krieg et al. (1981)
Dextran coated charcoal Incubation at 4 °C for 16–18 h Scatchard analysis	BPH	Oe$_2$	10	RPP	11.7 fmol/mg protein	411 fmol/mg DNA 980 fmol/g tissue	Auf and Ghanadian (1982)
Dextran coated charcoal Incubation at 4 °C for 16–18 h Scatchard analysis	BPH		9	TUR	11.6 fmol/mg protein	276 fmol/mg DNA 555 fmol/g tissue	Auf and Ghanadian (1982)
Agar gel electrophoresis Incubation at 0 °C for 2 h	BPH	Oe$_2$	15	—	40 fmol/mg protein	—	Wagner (1977)

at a raised temperature. Such a model system has been shown to operate in the case of glucocorticoid receptors in the mouse thymocytes (Feldman *et al.*, 1972). This assumption requires further investigations into the possible changes in the conformation of the receptor at different temperatures. Secondly, it is equally plausible to suggest that the change in the specificity may be due to the presence of other binding components such as progesterone receptor which could be destroyed at the higher temperature of incubation. Evidence for the latter explanation comes from the work by Bevins and Bashirelahi (1980) who have demonstrated the presence of a saturable progesterone binding component with the sedimentation coefficient of 8S, that was only detected in the presence of molybdate ion at low temperature. Based on this finding and the instability of the progesterone receptor towards higher temperatures it is possible that the crossreactivity of progesterone with the binding of R1881 at 0–4 °C is due to the presence of a progesterone binding component.

The concentrations of progesterone binding components have been estimated in the cytosol of human BPH using tritiated R5020 as radioligand. Cowan *et al.* (1977), Bevins and Bashirelahi (1980) and Ekman (1980) have reported mean concentrations of this receptor to be 31 fmol/mg protein, 64 fmol/mg protein and 420 fmol/mg DNA respectively. The latter value when expressed in terms of protein concentration would be in the same order of magnitude as that reported by Cowan *et al.* (1977). The higher value reported by Bevins and Bashirelahi may be due to the stabilizing effect of molybdate on the progesterone binding component. The presence of saturable binding components for R5020 has also been reported in 5 out of 13 samples of normal human prostates (Ekman, 1980). The mean concentration for this was found to be 376 fmol/mg DNA.

Although the term 'progesterone receptor' has been used for the R5020 binding component by most of the above mentioned research groups, the use of this terminology is not as yet justifiable, since the biological function of this component has not been investigated. In addition, steroid specificity of R1881 binding to the nuclear extract of the human prostate indicates that progesterone is not a competitor for R1881 binding. This indicates the absence of a progesterone binding component in the nuclear extracts of the human prostate and raises the question of whether or not this cytoplasmic 'progesterone receptor' is capable of translocation into the nucleus. Therefore, the significance of this 'receptor' requires further clarification.

8.8 GLUCOCORTICOID RECEPTORS

The finding of multiple receptors for different classes of steroid hormones in target organs has become a common occurrence (Ghanadian, 1982). Steroid receptors for androgens, oestrogens, progestogens and glucocorticoids have been reported to be present in a number of steroid responsive cells such as human breast cancer cell line (Horwitz *et al.*, 1975) or oestrogen induced kidney tumour of the hamster (Li *et al.*, 1979). In the prostate much attention has been focused on the characterization and measurement of androgen, oestrogen and progesterone receptors, although a number of studies have been carried out to investigate the presence of glucocorticoid receptors in malignant prostate. Ekman (1980) has reported the presence of a glucocorticoid receptor in 62 % of samples of prostatic cancer metastases. However, this finding has not been substantiated by Teulings *et al.* (1980) who reported the absence of this receptor in six lymph node metastases obtained from six patients with prostatic cancer. There is a paucity of information with regard to the presence of a glucocorticoid binding component in normal and benign hypertrophied prostates, although studies by Ekman (1980) suggest the absence of this binding component in these tissues.

8.9 CONCLUSIONS

Although the concept of a receptor mediated mechanism has long been advocated for the action of steroid hormones in the prostate, progress in the elucidation of this concept in the human prostate has been seriously hindered due to various methodological considerations. The prominent role of androgens in this gland has been a determining factor in concentrating most efforts in resolving the mechanism by which androgens exert their biological action. In this regard the characterization and quantitation of androgen receptors have been the prime target for several research laboratories. This chapter is an attempt to outline and critically evaluate the available methods for the analysis of steroid receptors with particular emphasis on androgen receptors in the human prostate. Although the presence of androgen receptors had been demonstrated in the late 60s and early 70s, only recently has this receptor been more comprehensively characterized and its concentration determined in human prostatic tissues. This progress has been achieved partly due to the application of several improved separation techniques but mainly as a result of the introduction of synthetic androgens in this field of research.

A great part of this chapter has been devoted to the use of separation techniques and their application in relation to qualitative and quantitative assessment of androgen receptors. Factors affecting the quantitation of these receptors have been discussed and precautionary measures, which are essential in the development of reliable techniques for quantitation, have also been emphasized. The important role of synthetic androgens in the qualitative and quantitative analysis of androgen receptors has been discussed and a comparative study for the use of synthetic androgens with that of the natural steroids as radioligand has been made. Additionally the effect of surgical procedures for removing prostatic tissues on the content of androgen receptors has been evaluated. Similarly, recent advances in the analysis of receptors for other classes of steroid hormones have been critically reviewed. Special attention has been given to the qualitative and quantitative evaluation of oestradiol receptors in both cytoplasmic and nuclear fraction of the human prostatic cells and a summary of the available data on the oestrogen receptor content of normal and hypertrophied prostate has also been presented.

The current available techniques for receptor analysis in the prostate are based on the binding of specific radioligand to the receptor, and the subsequent separation of the receptor from free steroid and non-receptor proteins. Although this conventional approach has been successfully employed for the analysis of steroid receptors, this has suffered certain disadvantages which have been discussed in this chapter. No doubt, in the foreseeable future some of these shortcomings will be overcome and more refined and simplified techniques such as the radioimmunoassay of the receptors will be developed. However, the present techniques are sufficiently accurate for the qualitative and quantitative analysis of steroid receptors in prostatic tumours.

8.10   REFERENCES

Anderson, J. H., Clark, J. H. and Peck, E. J. (1972). Oestrogen and nuclear binding sites. Determination of specific sites by (^{3}H) oestradiol exchange. *Biochem. J.*, **126**, 561

Andrews, P. (1965). The gel filtration behaviour of proteins related to their molecular weights over a wide range. *Biochem. J.*, **96**, 595

Armstrong, E. G. and Bashirelahi, N. (1978). Determination of the binding properties of estradiol-17β within the cytoplasmic and nuclear fractions of rat ventral prostate. *J. Steroid Biochem.*, **9**, 507

Asselin, J., Labrie, F., Gourdeau, Y., Bonne, C. and Raynaud, J. P. (1976). Binding of ^{3}H methyltrienolone (R1881) in rat prostate and human benign prostatic hypertrophy (BPH). *Steroids*, **28**, 449

Asselin, J., Melancon, R., Gourdeau, Y., Labrie, F., Bonne, C. and Raynaud, J. B. (1979). Specific binding of ^{3}H-methyltrienolone (R1881) in the presence of progesterone receptors. *J. Steroid Biochem.*, **10**, 483

Atger, M. and Milgrom, E. (1976). Chromatographic separation on phosphocellulose of activated and non-activated forms of steroid-receptor complexes, purification of the activated complex. *Biochemistry*, **15**, 4298

Auf, G. and Ghanadian, R. (1981). Analysis of androgen receptors in the human prostate by isoelectric focusing in polyacrylamide gel. *J. Steroid Biochem.*, **14**, 1261

Auf, G. and Ghanadian, R. (1982). The characterization and measurement of cytoplasmic and nuclear oestradiol-17β receptor proteins in benign hypertrophied prostate. *J. Endocrinol.*, **93**, 305

Bashirelahi, N., Kneussl, E. J., Vassil, T. C., Young, J. D., Sanefugi, J. and Trump, B. (1979). Measurement and characterization of estrogen receptors in the human prostate. In Murphy, E. P. and Sandberg, A. A. (eds.) *Progress in Clinical and Biological Research*. Vol. 33, pp. 65–84. (New York: Alan R. Liss)

Bashirelahi, N., O'Toole, J. H. and Young, J. D. (1976). A specific 17β-estradiol in human hypertrophied prostate. *Biochem. Med.*, **15**, 254

Bashirelahi, N., Young, J. D., Sidh, S. M. and Sanefugi, J. (1980). Androgen, oestrogen, progesterone and their distribution in epithelial and stromal cells of human prostate. In Schroder, F. H. and de Voogt, H. J. (eds.) *Steroid Receptors, Metabolism and Prostatic Cancer*. pp. 240–255. (Amsterdam: Excerpta Medica)

Baulieu, E. E. and Jung, I. (1970). A prostatic cytosol receptor. *Biochem. Bioph. Res. Commun.*, **38**, 599

Bevins, C. L. and Bashirelahi, N. (1980). Stabilization of 8s progesterone receptor from the human prostate in the presence of molybdate ion. *Cancer Res.*, **40**, 2234

Blondeau, J. P. and Robel, P. (1975). Determination of protein-ligand binding constants at equilibrium in biological samples. *Eur. J. Biochem.*, **55**, 375

Boesel, R. W., Klipper, R. W. and Shain, S. A. (1977). Identification of limited capacity androgen binding components in nuclear and cytoplasmic fractions of canine prostate. *Endocrinol. Res. Commun.*, **4**, 71

Bonne, C. and Raynaud, J. P. (1975). Methyltrienolone, a specific ligand for the cellular androgen receptors. *Steroids*, **26**, 277

Bonne, C. and Raynaud, J. P. (1976). Assay of androgen binding sites by exchange with methyltrienolone R1881. *Steroids*, **27**, 497

Braunsberg, H. and Hammond, K. D. (1979). Methods of steroid receptor calculation: an interlaboratory study. *J. Steroid Biochem.*, **11**, 1561

Britten, R. J. and Roberts, R. B. (1960). High resolution density gradient sedimentation analysis. *Science*, **131**, 32

Castaneda, E. and Liao, S. (1975). The use of anti-steroid antibodies in the characterization of steroid receptors. *J. Biol. Chem.*, **250**, 883

Chaisiri, N., Volotaire, Y., Brownen, A., Evans, J. and Pierrepoint, C. G. (1978). Demonstration of a cytoplasmic receptor protein for oestrogen in the canine prostate gland. *J. Endocrinol.*, **78**, 131

Chamness, G. C., Huff, K. and McGuire, W. L. (1975). Protamine precipitated estrogen receptor – a solid phase ligand exchange assay. *Steroids*, **25**, 627

Chamness, G. C. and McGuire, W. L. (1975). Scatchard plots: common errors in correction and interpretation. *Steroids*, **26**, 538

Coffer, A. J. and King, J. B. (1974). Isoelectric focusing of [^{3}H]oestradiol-17β receptor in flat beds of Sephadex. *Biochem. Soc. Trans.*, **2**, 1269

Cowan, R. A., Cowan, S. K., Giles, C. A. and Grant, J. K. (1976). Prostatic distribution of sex hormone-binding globulin and cortisol-binding in benign hyperplasia. *J. Endocrinol.*, **71**, 121

Cowan, R. A., Cowan, S. K. and Grant, J. K. (1977). Binding of methyltrienolone (R1881) to a progesterone receptor-like component of human prostatic cytosol. *J. Endocrinol.*, **74**, 281

Davies, P. and Griffiths, K. (1975). Similarities between the 5α-dihydrotestosterone receptor complexes from human and rat prostate and their effect on RNA polymerase activity. *Mol. Cell Endocrinol.*, **31**, 113

Davies, P. and Griffiths, K. (1980). Androgen receptors in human normal, hypertrophied and carcinomatous prostates. In Wittliff, J. L. and Dapunt, O. (eds.) *Steroid Receptors and Hormone-dependent Neoplasia.* pp. 145–147. (New York: Masson publishing)

Davies, P., Thomas, P. and Griffiths, K. (1977). Measurement of free and occupied cytoplasmic and nuclear androgen receptor sites in rat ventral prostate. *J. Endocrinol.*, **74**, 393

de Sombre, E. R., Puca, G. A. and Jensen, E. V. (1969). Purification of an estrophilic protein from calf uterus. *Proc. Natl. Acad. Sci., USA*, **64**, 148

de Voogt, H. J. and Dingjan, P. (1978). Steroid receptors in human prostatic cancer. A preliminary evaluation. *Urol. Res.*, **6**, 151

de Voogt, H. J. and Dingjan, P. G. (1980). Is there a place for the assay of cytoplasmic steroid receptors in the endocrine treatment of prostatic cancer. In Schroder, F. H. and de Voogt, H. J. (eds.) *Steroid Receptors, Metabolism and Prostatic Cancer.* pp. 265–270. (Amsterdam: Excerpta Medica)

Dube, J. Y., Chapdelaine, P., Tremblay, R. R., Bonne, C. and Raynaud, J.P. (1976). Comparative binding specificity of methyltrienolone in human and rat prostate. *Horm. Res. (Basel)*, **7**, 341

Dube, J. Y., Lesage, R. and Tremblay, R. R. (1979). Estradiol and progesterone receptors in dog prostate cytosol. *J. Steroid Biochem.*, **10**, 459

Dyer, R. D. and Faber, L. E. (1980). Use of spheroidal hydroxylapatite chromatography for the purification of the 7s guinea pig uterine progestin receptor system.

Presented at *The Endocrine Society, 62 annual meeting*, June 18–20, Washington, DC

Ekman, P. (1980). Androgen receptors and treatment of prostatic cancer. In Schroder, F. H. and de Voogt, H. J. (eds.) *Steroid Receptors, Metabolism and Prostatic Cancer*. pp. 208—224. (Amsterdam: Excerpta Medica)

Fang, S., Anderson, K. M. and Liao, S. (1969). Receptor proteins for androgens. On the role of specific proteins in selective retention of 17β-hydroxy-5α-androstan-3-one by rat ventral prostate *in vivo* and *in vitro. J. Biol. Chem.*, **244**, 6584

Fang, S. and Liao, S. (1971). Steroid and tissue-specific retention of a 17β-hydroxy-5α-androstan-3-one protein complex by the cell nuclei of ventral prostate. *J. Biol. Chem.*, **246**, 16

Feldman, D., Funder, J. W. and Edelman, J. S. (1972). Subcellular mechanism in the action of adrenal steroids. *Am. J. Med.*, **53**, 545

Foekens, J. A., Bolt-de Vries, J., Romijn, J. C. and Mulder, E.(1980). The use of heparin in extracting nuclei for estimation of nuclear androgen receptors in benign prostatic hyperplastic tissue by exchange procedures. In Schroder, F. H. and de Voogt, H. J., (eds.) *Steroid Receptors, Metabolism and Prostatic Cancer*. pp. 77–85. (Amsterdam: Excerpta Medica)

Geller, J. and Albert, J. (1979). Some current problems relating to androgen receptor methodology. In Murphy, G. P. and Sandberg, A. A. (eds.) *Prostatic Cancer and Hormone Receptors*. Vol. 33, pp. 97–102. (New York: Alan R. Liss)

Geller, J., Canton, T. and Albert, J. (1975). Evidence for a specific dihydrotestosterone binding cytosol receptor in human prostate. *J. Clin. Endocrinol. Metab.*, **41**, 854

Ghanadian, R. (1976). Endocrine control of the prostate: mechanism of action of androgens. In Williams, D. L. and Chisholm, G. D. (eds.) *Scientific Foundations of Urology*. pp. 138–146. (London: Heinemann)

Ghanadian, R. (1981). Androgen regulation in the prostate of Rhesus Monkey (*Macaca mulatta*). In Hafez, E. S. E. and Spring-Mill, E. (eds.) *Prostatic Carcinoma; Biology and Diagnosis*. Vol. 6, pp. 160–166. (The Hague: Martinus Nijhoff)

Ghanadian, R. (1982). Steroid receptors in urological cancer. In Javadpour, N. (ed.) *Recent Advances in Urologic Cancer*. pp. 67–81. (Baltimore: Williams and Wilkins)

Ghanadian, R. and Auf, G. (1980). Receptor proteins for androgens in benign prostatic hypertrophy and carcinoma of the prostate. In Schroder, F. H. and de Voogt, H. J. (eds.) *Steroid Receptors, Metabolism and Prostatic Cancer*. pp. 110–123. (Amsterdam: Excerpta Medica)

Ghanadian, R., Auf, G., Chaloner, P. J. and Chisholm, G. D. (1978a). The use of methyltrienolone in the measurement of free and bound cytoplasmic receptor proteins for dihydrotestosterone in benign hypertrophied human prostate. *J. Steroid Biochem.*, **9**, 325

Ghanadian, R., Auf, G. and Chisholm, G. D. (1980a). Androgen receptors in prostatic cancer. In Pavon-Macaluso, M., Smith, P. H. and Edsmyr, F. (eds.) *Bladder Tumours and Other Topics in Urological Oncology*. pp. 453–458. (New York: Plenum Press)

Ghanadian, R., Auf, G., Chisholm, G. D. and O'Donoghue, E. P. N. (1978b). Receptor proteins for androgens in prostatic disease. *Br. J. Urol.*, **50**, 567

Ghanadian, R., Auf, G., Smith, C. B., Chisholm, G. D. and Blacklock, N. J. (1977a). Androgen receptors in the prostate of rhesus monkey. *Urol. Res.*, **5**, 169

Ghanadian, R., Auf, G., Smith, C. B. and Puah, C. M. (1980b). Androgen receptors in benign hypertrophied and malignant prostate. In Wittliff. J. L. and Dapunt, O. (eds.) *Steroid Receptors and Hormone Dependent Neoplasia*. pp. 149–150. (New York: Masson publishing)

Ghanadian, R., and Fotherby, K. (1972). Interaction between steroids in regard to their uptake by rat ventral prostate. *Steroids Lipids. Res.*, **3**, 363

Ghanadian, R., Smith, C. B. and Chisholm, G. D. (1977b). The effect of antiandrogens and stilboestrol on the dihydrotestosterone in rat ventral prostate. *Br. J. Urol.*, **49**, 695

Ghanadian, R., Smith, C. B. and Chisholm, G. D. (1977c). Identification of an androgen receptor in the cytosol of the female mastomy prostate. *Mol. Cell. Endocrinol.*, **8**, 147

Ghanadian, R., Smith, C. B. and Chisholm, G. D. (1978c). Receptor protein for dihydrotestosterone in nuclei of the female prostate of *Praomys (Mastomys) natalensis*. *Invest. Urol.*, **16**, 119

Greene, G. L., Closs, L. C., Fleming, H., De Sombre, E. R. and Jensen, E. V. (1977). Antibodies to estrogen receptor: immunochemical similarity of estrophilin from various mammalian species. *Proc. Natl. Acad. Sci., USA*, **74**, 3681

Greene, G. L., Fitch, F. W. and Jensen, E. E. (1980). Monoclonal antibodies to estrophilin: probes for the study of estrogen receptors. *Proc. Natl. Acad. Sci. USA*, **77**, 157

Gustafsson, J. A., Ekman, P., Pousette, A., Snochowski, M. and Hogberg, B. (1978). Demonstration of a progestin receptor in human benign prostatic hyperplasia and prostatic carcinoma. *Invest. Urol.*, **15**, 361

Hansson, V., Tveter, K., Unhjem, O., Djoseland, O., Attramadal, A., Reusch, E. and Torgersen, O. (1975). Androgen binding in male sex organs with special reference to human prostate. In Goland, M. (ed.) *Normal and Abnormal Growth of the Prostate*. pp. 676–711. (Springfield: Charles C. Thomas)

Hawkins, E. F., Nijs, M. and Brassine, C. (1976). Steroid receptors in the human prostate. II. Some properties of the estrophilic molecule of benign prostatic hypertrophy. *Biochem. Biophys Res. Commun.*, **70**, 854

Herbert, V., Lau, K., Gottlies, C. W. and Bleicher, S. J. (1965). Coated charcoal immunoassay of insulin. *J. Clin. Endocrinol. Metab.*, **25**, 1375

Hicks, L. L. and Walsh, P. C. (1979). A microassay for the measurement of androgen receptors in human prostatic tissue. *Steroids*, **33**, 389

Horwitz, K. B., Costlow, M. E. and McGuire, W. L. (1975). A human breast cancer cell-line with oestrogen, androgen, progesterone and glucocorticoid receptors. *Steroids*, **26**, 785

Hsu, R. S., Middleton, R. C. and Fang, S. (1975). Androgen receptors in human prostates. In Goland, M. (ed.) *Normal and Abnormal Growth of the Prostate*. pp. 676–711.(Springfield: Charles C. Thomas)

Jensen, E. V., de Sombre, E. R. and Jungblut, P. N. (1967). Interaction of oestrogens with receptor sites *in vivo* and *in vitro*. *2nd International Congress, Hormonal Steroids, Milan*. p. 492. (Amsterdam: Excerpta Medica)

Jensen, E. V., Greene, G. L., Closs, L. E. and de Sombre, E. R. (1979). The immunoendocrinology of estrophilin. In Leavitt, W. W. and Clarke, J. H. (eds.) *Steroid Hormone Receptor Systems*. pp. 1–23. (New York: Plenum Press)

Jensen, E. V., Hurst, D. J., de Sombre, E. R. and Jungblut, P. N. (1976). Sulfhydryl groups and estradiol receptor interaction. *Science*, **158**, 385

Karr, J. P., Wajsmann, Z., Madajewicz, S., Kirdani, R. Y. Murphy, G. P. and Sandberg, A. A. (1979). Steroid hormone receptors in the prostate. *J. Urol.*, **122**, 170

Katzenellenbogen, J. A., Johnson, H. J. Jr. and Carlson, K. E. (1973). Studies on the uterine cytoplasmic oestrogen binding protein..Thermal stability and ligand dissociation rate. An assay of empty and filled sites by exchange. *Biochemistry*, **12**, 4092

King, R. J. B., Hayward, J. C., Masters, J. R. W., Millis, R. R. and Robens, R. D.

(1980). Steroid receptor assays as prognostic aids in the treatment of breast cancer. In Wittliff, J. L. and Dapunt, O. (eds.) *Steroid Receptors and Hormone Dependent Neoplasia.* pp. 249–256. (New York: Masson publishing)

Kliman, B., MacLaughlin, R. A. and Prout, G. R. (1979). Measurement of androgen receptors in cytosol of human prostatic tissues with sepharose-linked antibody system. In Murphy, G. P. and Sandberg, A. A. (eds.) *Progress in Clinical and Biological Research.* Vol. 33, pp. 85–96. (New York: Alan R. Liss)

Krieg, M., Bartsch, W., Janssen, and Voigt, K. D. (1979). A comparative study of binding, metabolism and endogenous levels of androgens in normal, hypertrophied and carcinomatous human prostate. *J. Steroid Biochem.,* **11,** 615

Krieg, M., Klotel, G., Kaufmann, J. and Voigt, K. D. (1981). Stroma of human benign prostatic hyperplasia: preferential tissue for androgen metabolism and oestrogen binding. *Acta Endocrinol.,* **96,** 422

Krozowski, Z. S. and Murphy, L. C. (1981). Stabilisation of the cytoplasmic oestrogen receptor by molybdate. *J. Steroid Biochem.,* **14,** 363

Kuhn, R. W., Schrader, W. T. and O'Malley, B. W. (1975). Progestrone binding components of chick oviduct. *J. Biol. Chem.,* **250,** 4220

Lehmann, F. G. (1970). Molekulargewichtsbestimmungen durch Gel Chromatographiec on Sepharose-6β. *Clin. Chim. Acta,* **28,** 335

Li, J. J., Li, S. A. and Cuthbertson, T. L. (1979). Clear retention of all steroid hormone receptor classes in the hamster renal carcinoma. *Cancer Res.,* **39,** 2647

Liao, S. and Liang, T. (1974) Receptors and mechanisms of action of androgens in prostates. In McKerns, K. W. (ed.) *Hormones and Cancer.* pp. 229–260. (New York: Academic Press)

Liao, S., Liang, T., Fang, S., Castaneda, E. and Shao, T. C. (1973). Steroid structure and endogenic capacity: specificities involved in the receptor binding and nuclear retention of various androgens. *J. Biol. Chem.,* **248,** 6154

Liao, S., Tymoczko, J. L., Castaneda, E. and Liang, T. (1975). Androgen receptors and androgen-dependent initiation of protein synthesis in the prostate. *Vit. Horm.,* **36,** 297

Lieskovsky, G. and Bruchovsky, N. (1979). Assay of nuclear androgen receptor in human prostate. *J. Urol.,* **121,** 54

Lippman, M. and Huff, K. (1976). The demonstration of androgen and estrogen receptors in a human breast cancer using new protamine sulfate assay. *Cancer,* **38,** 868

Mainwaring, W. I. P. (1969a). A soluble androgen receptor in the cytoplasm of rat prostate. *J. Endocrinol.,* **45,** 531

Mainwaring, W. I. P. (1969b). The binding of (1, 2, -³H) testosterone within the nucleus of the rat prostate. *J. Endocrinol.,* **44,** 323

Mainwaring, W. I. P. (1970). Androgen receptors. In Griffiths, K. and Pierrepoint, C. G. (eds.) *Some Aspects of the Aetiology and Biochemistry of Prostatic Cancer.* pp. 109–114. (Cardiff: Alpha Omega Alpha)

Mainwaring, W. I. P. and Irving, R. (1973). The use of deoxyribonucleic acid-cellulose chromatography and isoelectric focusing for the characterization and partial purification of steroid-receptor complexes. *Biochem. J.,* **134,** 113

Mainwaring, W. I. P. and Mangan, F. R. (1971). The specific binding of steroid receptor complexes to DNA: evidence from androgen receptors in rat prostate. *Adv. Biosci.,* **7,** 165

Mainwaring, W. I. P. and Milroy, E. J. G. (1973). Characterization of the specific androgen receptors in the human prostate gland. *J. Endocrinol.,* **57,** 371

Mainwaring, W. I. P. and Peterken, B. M. (1971). A reconstituted cell-free system for the specific transfer of steroid-receptor complexes into nuclear chromatin isolated from rat ventral prostate. *Biochem. J.,* **125,** 285

Martin, R. G. and Ames, B. N. (1961). A method for determining the sedimentation behaviour of enzymes: application to protein mixtures. *J. Biol. Chem.*, **236**, 1372

Menon, M., Tananis, C. E., Hicks, L. L., Hawkins, E. E., McLoughlin, M. G. and Walsh, P. C. (1978). Characterization of the binding of a potent synthetic androgen, methyltrienolone to human tissues. *J. Clin. Invest.*, **61**, 150

Menon, M., Tananis, C. E., McLoughlin, M. G. and Walsh, P. C. (1977). Androgen receptors in human prostatic tissue: A review. *Cancer Treat. Rep.*, **61**, 265

Miller, L. K., Diaz, S. C. and Sherman, M. R. (1975). Steroid-receptor quantitation and characterization by electrophoresis in highly cross-linked polyacrylamide gels. *Biochemistry*, **14**, 4433

Mobbs, B. G., Johnson, I. E. and Connolly, J. G. (1980). Androgen receptors and treatment of prostatic cancer. In Schroder, F. H. and de Voogt, H. J. (eds.) *Steroid Receptors, Metabolism and Prostatic Cancer*. pp. 225–239. (Amsterdam: Excerpta Medica)

Mobbs, B. G., Johnson, I. E., Connolly, J. G. and Clark, A. F. (1978). Androgen receptor assay in human benign and malignant prostatic tumour cytosol using protamine sulphate precipitation. *J. Steroid Biochem.*, **9**, 289

Mulder, E., Foekens, J. A., Peters, M. J. and Van Der Molen, H. J. (1979). A comparison of heparin agarose and DNA cellulose for the characterization and partial purification of androgen receptors from rat prostate. *FEBS lett.*, **97**, 260

Murphy, J. B., Emmott, R. C., Hicks, L. L. and Walsh, P. C. (1980). Estrogen receptors in the human prostate, seminal vesicle, epididymis, testis and genital skin: a marker for estrogen-responsive tissues? *Clin. Endocrinol. Metab.*, **50**, 938

Nijs, M., Hawkins, F. and Coune, E. (1976). Binding of 5 alpha-dihydrotestosterone in human prostatic cancer; examination by agar gel electropheresis. *J. Endocrinol.*, **69**, 18

Olsson, C. A., White, D. R., Goldstein, I., Traish, A. M., Muller, R. E. and Wotiz (1979). Prostate cancer and hormone receptors. In Murphy, G. P. and Sandberg, A. A. (eds.) *Progress in Clinical and Biological Research*. pp. 200–221. (New York: Alan R. Liss)

Pertshuk, L. P., Zava, D. T., Tobin, E. H., Brigati, D. J., Gaetjans, E., Macchia, R. J., Wise, G. J., Wax, H. S. and Kim, D. S. (1979). Histochemical detection of steroid hormone receptors in the human prostate. In Murphy, G. P. and Sandberg, A. A. (eds.) *Progress in Clinical and Biological Research.*, pp. 113–132. (New York: Alan R. Liss)

Puca, G. A., Nola, E., Sica, V. and Bresciani, F. (1971). Estrogen-binding proteins of cell uterus. Partial purification and preliminary characterization of steroid receptor complexes. *Biochemistry*, **10**, 3769

Raynaud, J. P. and Bouton, M. M. (1980). The design of estrogens and/or anti-estrogens on the basis of receptor binding. In Raus, J., Martens, H. and Leclercq, G. (eds.) *Cytotoxic Estrogens in Hormone Receptive Tumours*. pp. 49–66 (London: Academic Press)

Rosen, V., Jung, I., Baulieu, E. E. and Robel, P. (1975). Androgen-binding proteins in human benign prostatic hypertrophy. *J. Clin. Endocrinol. Metab.*, **41**, 761

Rosenthal, H. E. (1967). A graphic method for the determination and presentation of binding parameters in a complex system. *Anal. Biochem.*, **20**, 525

Scatchard, G. (1949). The attractions of proteins for small molecules and ions. *Ann., NY Acad. Sci.*, **51**, 660

Shain, S. A. and Boesel, R. W. (1978a) Human prostate steroid hormone receptor quantitation. Current methodology and possible utility as a clinical discriminant in carcinoma. *Invest. Urol.*, **16**, 169

Shain, S. A. and Boesel, R. W. (1978b). Androgen receptor content of the normal and hyperplastic canine prostate. *J. Clin. Invest.*, **61**, 654

Shain, S. A., Boesel, R. W. and Axelrod, L. R. (1975). Aging in the rat prostate. Reduction in detectable prostate androgen receptor content. *Arch. Biochem. Biophys.*, **167**, 247

Shain, S. A., Boesel, R. W., Lamm, D. L. and Radwin, H. M. (1978). Characterization of unoccupied (R) and occupied (RA) androgen binding components of the hyperplastic human prostate. *Steroids*, **31**, 541

Shain, S. A., Boesel, R. W., Lamm, D. L. and Radwin, H. M. (1980). Cytoplasmic and nuclear androgen receptor content of normal and neoplastic human prostates and lymph node metastases of human prostatic adenocarcinoma. *J. Clin. Endocrinol. Metab.*, **50**, 704

Sica, J., Parikh, I., Nola, E., Puca, G. A. and Cuatrecass, P. (1973). Affinity chromatography and the purification of estrogen receptors. *J. Biol. Chem.*, **248**, 6543

Sinha, A. A., Blackard, C. E., Dof, R. P. and Seal, U. S. (1973). The *in vitro* localization of H_3 estrodiol in human prostatic carcinoma. *Cancer*, **31**, 682

Sirett, D. A. N. and Grant, J. K. (1978). Androgen binding in cytosols and nuclei of human benign hyperplastic tissue. *J. Endocrinol.*, **77**, 101

Smith, C. B. (1977). Effects of synthetic antiandrogens and progestogens on the prostate gland. Thesis submitted for the degree of Master of Philosophy at the University of London

Smith, C. B., Ghanadian, R., and Chisholm, G. D. (1978a). A soluble androgen receptor in the cytosol of mastomys prostate. *Urol. Res.*, **6**, 29

Smith, C. B., Ghanadian, R. and Chisholm, G. D. (1978b). Inhibition of the nuclear dihydrotestosterone receptor complex from rat ventral prostate by antiandrogens and stilboestrol. *Mol. Cell. Endocrinol.*, **10**, 13

Smith, C. B., Ghanadian, R. and Chisholm, G. D. (1979). Nuclear androgen receptors in the prostate of the male *Praomys (Mastomys) natalensis. Urol. Res.*, **7**, 243

Snochowski, M., Pousette, A., Ekman, P., Bressian, D., Anderson, L., Hogberg, B. and Gustafsson, J. A. (1977). Characterization and measurement of the androgen receptor in human benign prostatic hyperplasia and prostatic carcinoma. *J. Clin. Endocrinol. Metab.*, **45**, 920

Steggles, A. W. and King, R. J. B. (1970). The use of protamine to study (6,7 -³H) oestradiol-17β, binding in rat uterus. *Biochem. J.*, **118**, 695

Steins, P., Krieg, M., Hollmann, H. J. and Voigt, K. D. (1974). *In vitro* studies of testosterone and 5α-dihydrotestosterone binding in benign prostatic hypertrophy. *Acta Endocrinol.*, **75**, 773

Teulings, F. A. G., Figusch, J. A., Henkelman, M. S., Portengen, H. and Van Gike, H. A. (1980). Steroid receptors in metastases of prostatic cancer. In Schroder, F. H. and de Voogt, H. J. (eds.) *Steroid Receptors, Metabolism and Prostatic Cancer.* pp. 257– 264. (Amsterdam: Excerpta Medica)

Toft, O. and Gorski, J. (1966). A receptor molecule for estrogens: isolation from the rat uterus and preliminary characterization. *Proc. Natl. Acad. Sci., USA*, **55**, 1574

Unhjem, O., Tveter, K. J. and Aakvaag, A. (1969). Preliminary characterization of an androgen-macromolecular complex from the rat ventral prostate. *Acta Endocrinol.*, **62**, 153

Verhoeven, G., Heyns, W. and De Moor, P. (1975). Ammonium sulfate precipitation as a tool for the study of androgen receptor proteins in rat prostate and mouse kidney. *Steroids*, **26**, 149

Wagner, R. K. (1972). Characterization and assay of steroid hormone receptors and steroid binding serum proteins by agar gel electrophoresis at low temperature. *Hoppe-Seyler's Z. Physiol Chem.*, **353**, 1235

Wagner, R. K. (1977). Critical evaluation of receptor assays in relation to tumours. In Vermeulen, A. (ed.) *Research on Steroids*. Vol. 7, pp. 205–224. (Amsterdam: Elsevier North-Holland)

Wagner, R. K. and Jungblut, P. W. (1976). Differentiation between steroid hormone receptors CBG and SHBG in human target organ extracts by a single-step assay. *Mol. Cell. Endocr.*, **4**, 13

Wagner, R. K., Schulze, K. and Jungblut, P. W. (1975). Estrogen and androgen receptor in human prostate and prostatic tumour tissue. *Acta Endocrinol. suppl.*, **193**, 52

Walsh, P. C. and Hicks, L. L. (1979). Characterization and measurement of androgen receptors in human prostatic tissue. In Murphy, G. P. and Sandberg, A. A. (eds.) *Progress in Clinical and Biological Research*. Vol. *33*, pp. 51–63. (New York: Alan R. Liss)

Wilson, E. M. and French, F. S. (1979). Effects of protease and protease inhibitors on the 4.5s and 8s androgen receptor. *J. Biol. Chem.*, **254**, 6310

Wittliff, J. L., Lewko, W. M., Park, D. C., Kute, T. E., Baker, D. J. and Kane, L. N. (1978). Establishment of uniformity in steroid receptor determinations used in clinical studies and drugscreening programmes. In McGuire, W. L. (ed.) *Hormones, Receptors and Breast Cancer*. pp. 147–164. (New York: Raven Press)

Wrange, O., Nordenskjold, B. and Gustafsson, J. A. (1978). Cytosol estradiol receptor in human mammary carcinoma: an assay based on isoelectric focusing in polyacrylamide gel. *Anal. Biochem.*, **85**, 461

Zava, D. T., Landrum, B., Horwitz, K. B. and McGuire, W. L. (1979). Androgen receptor assay with ^{3}H methyltrienolone (R1881) in the presence of progesterone receptors. *Endocrinology*, **104**, 1007

9
Predictive role of steroid receptors in evaluating the response to endocrine therapy

R. GHANADIAN

The concept of endocrine manipulation of malignant tumours was originally suggested and examined by Beatson (1896), who found that oophorectomy can effect a striking remission of advanced carcinoma of the breast in premenopausal women. However, Huggins and Hodges (1941) were the first to employ this type of treatment in the management of patients with prostatic cancer. This concept is based on the observation that malignant tumours originating from hormone responsive tissues often retain the hormone sensitivity of their parent cells, even though the tumour may be widely dispersed throughout the body. Thus, the tumours of the reproductive tract tend to be more responsive to endocrine therapy as the growth and functional activities of these organs are dependent upon the constant presence of sex hormones. Endocrine ablation or other forms of hormone manipulation can thus influence both the organ, and also the growth and proliferation of its tumour. The two major cancers of the prostate and the breast are classical examples of malignant tumours of the male and female reproductive tracts which are considered to be hormone responsive, although a great proportion of these tumours may not respond to endocrine therapy. In the case of breast only 25–30% of tumours are of a hormone-dependent type which is responsive to endocrine manipulation (Jensen, 1981). However, of those which do elicit a response, the remission induced by endocrine therapy has been reported to be of a generally superior character, both in terms of quality and duration, than that obtained by other forms of treatment such as cytotoxic chemotherapy. In prostatic cancer hormone therapy may be considered to be the principal method of treatment for systemic disease, although the response to this treatment is variable and unpredictable. Some 30–40 % of patients may be found to be non-responsive to endocrine therapy and yet neither histological nor biochemical differences have been identified to distinguish these groups (Grayhack and Wendel, 1974). Thus the need for a tumour marker to distinguish between those patients with carcinoma of the prostate who may respond to endocrine therapy and those whose tumours are unresponsive and, therefore, should be given alternative forms of treatment, is quite apparent.

9.1   STEROID-CELL INTERACTION

The concept that biologically active substances interact with cellular receptors is an old concept in medicine and dates back to 1500, when Paracelsus stated that drugs should contain 'spicula' (barbed hooks) with which they could become fixed to the organism and so produce an effect (Van Rossum, 1968). At the end of the nineteenth century, the concept of drug receptor interaction was formulated by Paul Ehrlich and has subsequently been refined to explain many of the features of drug action. With the availability of radiolabelled steroids with high specific activity, much progress has been made in the studies on the interaction between the steroids and the cellular receptors for these hormones. As a result of the synthesis of tritiated steroids of high specific activity the quantitation of physiological amounts of steroids in the tissues became possible and this facilitated studies on the steroid cell interaction in a number of target tissues. Glascock and Hoekstra (1959) demonstrated the selective accumulation of tritiated labelled hexoestrol, a synthetic oestrogen, by the reproductive organs of immature female goats and sheep. A more significant contribution came from the studies by Jensen and Jacobson (1962) who clearly demonstrated the uptake and retention of natural oestrogen, oestradiol-17β, by the target tissues for oestrogens in laboratory animals. In parallel with these studies Folca et al. (1961) administered labelled hexoestrol to ten women shortly before undergoing adrenalectomy for advanced breast cancer and found that 2 hours later the radioactivity in the tumour as compared to skeletal muscle was higher in four patients, who received benefit from this treatment than in six patients who did not. Subsequent studies by Toft and Gorski (1966) revealed that the cytosol of rat uteri contains a binding protein that can form a complex with radiolabelled steroids. From these investigations the general model of steroid-cell interaction has evolved. In this model steroid enters the cytoplasmic compartment of the target cell and binds non-covalently with a limited number of specific receptor proteins with high affinity. Subsequently this complex enters the nucleus, interacts with the chromatin and elicits a response. As discussed in Chapters 7 and 8, with certain modifications, this general scheme has been demonstrated for all classes of steroid hormones, although the finer details of these events requires further elucidation. During the 1960s, studies on the interaction of androgens with rat ventral prostate suggested a selective uptake and retention of dihydrotestosterone, the main metabolite of testosterone in this tissue. These studies were followed by the search for cellular receptors responsible for the retention of dihydrotestosterone, and resulted in the identification and characterization of both cytoplasmic and nuclear receptors for dihydrotestosterone in this gland. Details of the physicochemical characters of these receptors are also recorded in Chapter 8.

The binding of the steroid to specific receptor proteins is an integral part of the cytoplasmic events and in the case of the prostate this binding is preceded by the metabolism of testosterone to dihydrotestosterone. Therefore, the major events in the cytoplasm are the metabolism of testosterone to dihydrotestosterone and the binding of dihydrotestosterone (Ghanadian, 1976) to the cytoplasmic receptor proteins, resulting in the formation of dihydrotestosterone receptor complex. This complex will then enter the cell nucleus. This entry or translocation is known to be an energy dependent process and is hormone and tissue specific. It has been suggested that the steroid acts to stabilize the protein or supply an essential structural requirement so that the binding protein can transfer to its specific nuclear target site. Once the steroid receptor complex is within the nucleus, it can interact with the chromatin. Although the exact manner by which this interaction occurs is not yet clear, there is evidence for the presence of specific acceptor sites which may be responsible for the retention of the steroid receptor complex. It has been suggested that the acceptor can participate actively in specifying the site at which the complex binds on the chromatin and exerts its cellular action. The ultimate results of this mechanism are the synthesis of RNA, protein and finally cell division. An important aspect of these events is that stages of androgen action within the prostate are interdependent, and both the metabolism of testosterone to dihydrotestosterone and the subsequent binding of the dihydrotestosterone to the receptor protein are prerequisites for the final nuclear events to occur. More details of these events are reported in Chapter 7, and a simplified scheme for the mechanism of action of androgens in the prostate is shown in Figure 9.1. The presence of both cytoplasmic and nuclear androgen receptors has been demonstrated in the human prostate, and these binding proteins have been identified and characterized in benign and malignant tumours of this gland (Ghanadian, 1981, 1982). Again, this aspect has been extensively reviewed in Chapter 8. In addition, the quantitation of androgen receptors in prostatic tumours has been successfully achieved and has provided a basis for the investigation into the usefulness of these receptors as a tumour marker to distinguish those prostatic tumours which respond to endocrine therapy from the non-responsive ones. This is based on the assumption that if a prostate tumour depends on androgenic stimulation for its growth, it is reasonable to expect it to possess cytoplasmic and nuclear androgen receptors which are essential requirements for the mechanism of action of androgens, whereas the non-responsive tumours might not possess the receptor since they no longer need it. A simpler assumption has been the basis for the analysis of oestrogen receptors, in predicting the response of breast tumours to endocrine manipulation.

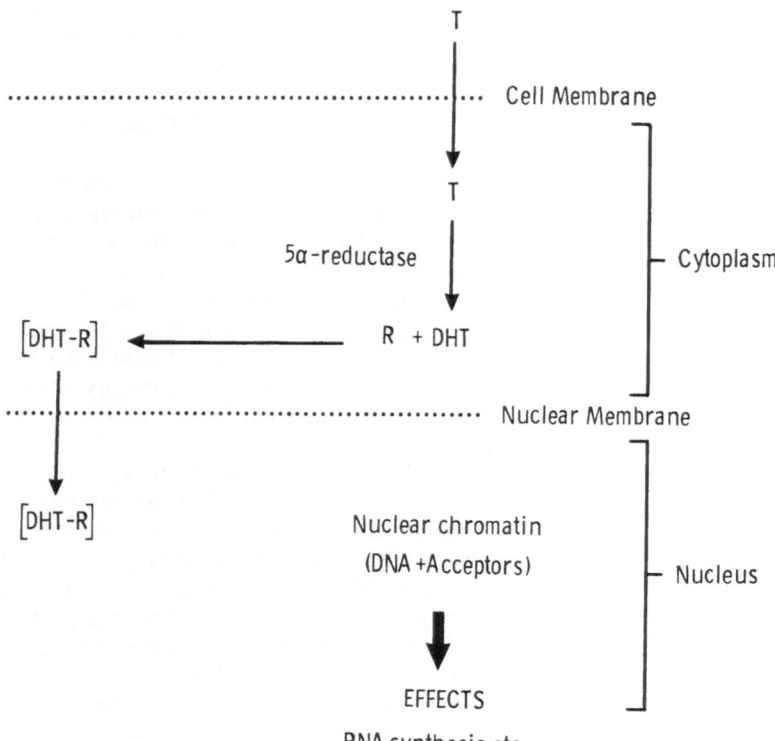

Figure 9.1 A simplified model for the action of testosterone in the prostate. Testosterone (T) enters through the cell membrane (c.m.) and metabolizes to dihydrotestosterone (DHT) which binds to a specific receptor protein (R). The steroid receptor complex (DHT-R) then translocates to the nucleus, through the nuclear membrane (N.m.) and interacts with chromatin components. This interaction leads to the biological effects of RNA synthesis, protein synthesis and finally cell division

9.2   STEROID RECEPTORS AS TUMOUR MARKERS FOR BREAST CANCER

In a report involving 42 patients with breast tumours, Jensen *et al.* (1971) reported that breast cancer showing low oestrogen binding or lacking cytoplasmic receptor rarely responded to endocrine therapy, whereas most but not all patients whose tumour contained significant amounts of receptor received objective benefits from such treatment. These findings were then confirmed and extended by reports from other research groups (Maass *et al.*,

1972; Engelsman et al., 1973; Leung et al., 1973; Savlov et al., 1974). Despite methodological differences in the analysis of oestrogen receptors in these studies, the overall conclusion was that breast tumours that lack oestrogen receptor rarely respond to endocrine therapy. This conclusion was further reinforced as the sensitivity and reliability of the techniques were increased and showed that many breast cancers, that previously would have been considered receptor negative, contained low levels of receptors (Jensen et al., 1975). In another study involving 380 patients with primary and metastatic breast cancer, McGuire et al. (1975a, b) reported that tumours that were oestrogen receptor positive responded to various forms of endocrine therapy at a rate of 55–60%, whereas tumours which were classified as receptor negative responded only at a rate of 8%. Approximately 40% of the patients with high receptor concentration in this group did not respond to endocrine therapy. De Sombre et al. (1978) have correlated the oestradiol receptor content and the response to endocrine therapy in 160 patients with metastatic breast cancer and found that, with very few exceptions, remission was not seen with tumours having low oestradiol receptor content and that the apparent 'critical level' appears to be lower in the case of patients with ovarian function, probably because they produce greater amounts of endogenous oestrogen that masks some of the receptors. Because they rarely respond to endocrine therapy, tumours with low but definite oestradiol receptor content should be classified with those lacking receptor. Jensen's group employed the terms 'receptor rich' and 'receptor poor' instead of positive and negative, with a dividing line determined empirically on the basis of clinical experience (Jensen et al., 1976). In a recent study Jensen (1981) has correlated the receptor analysis with clinical response for 117 women treated by endocrine ablation. He showed that approximately two thirds of the patients with receptor rich tumours will respond to one or another type of ablative therapy, whereas those with receptor poor cancers have little chance of benefit from endocrine manipulation and are best treated directly with cytotoxic chemotherapy. In these studies the results with additive hormone therapy were essentially similar except that the response rate seen with the receptor rich patients was slightly lower than with ablation. Jensen (1981) also reported that of more than 1300 primary and metastatic breast cancers which his group has analysed, most contain some detectable oestradiol receptor, but 60–70% can be classified as receptor poor, as defined empirically on the basis of experience with treated patients. Because of their findings, Jensen's group suggested that, since the oestradiol receptor assay predicts the clinical response correctly in approximately two thirds of the patients with receptor rich tumour and in essentially all of those belonging to the receptor poor group, its overall accuracy is between 85 and 90%. The failure of one third of patients with receptor rich cancers to respond to endocrine treatment is attributed in some cases to tumour heterogeneity and in others to the fact that receptor may be present, but non-functional. In order to identify breast tumours with non-functioning oestrogen receptors Horwitz et al. (1975) have suggested the measurement of progesterone receptor contents of the breast tumours. In normal reproductive tissues the progesterone receptor is known to be dependent on oestrogenic stimulation and thus on functioning oestrogen receptor. Studies on the relationship between oestrogen and progesterone receptors by Horwitz and McGuire (1978) have demonstrated that in human breast cancer cell lines there is a relationship between the total cytoplasmic and nuclear receptor content and the newly synthesized receptor. McGuire (1978) also reported that breast cancers with higher levels of oestrogen and progesterone receptors do show a significantly higher response rate than those containing only oestrogen receptors. Similar conclusions have been reached by King et al. (1980). Thus the measurement of both oestrogen and progesterone receptors can increase the accuracy of the predictive assay in breast tumour. There are, however, some cancers with high level of both receptors which do not respond to endocrine therapy, whilst many containing only oestrogen receptors do respond. De Sombre et al. (1979) have concluded that at the present time progesterone receptor assay can complement but not substitute for oestrogen receptor determination.

Receptor analysis of primary breast tumours is also reported to be of considerable importance. Jensen (1981) reported that of 20 patients with primary rich cancer, 15 responded favourably to endocrine therapy compared to only one response from 25 patients with receptor poor primary tumours, from which metastases appeared from 1 month to 67 months following mastectomy. Knight et al. (1977) observed that receptor analysis of the primary tumour provides valuable prognostic information concerning the probability of recurrence of metastatic disease. In addition, in patients with comparable lymph node involvement, those with receptor rich primary tumours show a low recurrence rate and a significantly longer disease free interval after mastectomy than do patients with receptor poor cancers. Jensen's group have concluded that oestrogen receptor measurement should be carried out on all primary breast cancers to provide information relevant both to the prognosis for cancer recurrence and to the selection of optimal therapy when metastases appear (De Sombre et al., 1979).

Campbell et al. (1981) have also measured cytoplasmic oestradiol receptors in the primary breast cancer of 526 patients with this tumour, 106 of whom have required hormone therapy for metastatic disease. They found the rate of response to treatment was significantly higher in patients with receptor positive primary cancers and the likelihood of response further increased in proportion to the measured receptor concentration. Preliminary analysis of this data also suggested that patients with higher receptor values in the primary tumour will enjoy a longer remission than those with low measured values. In addition to the measurement of cytoplasmic oestrogen receptors in patients with breast cancer, it has been suggested that the analysis of the receptors in the nuclei could improve the accuracy of the selection of patients for hormonal manipulation (Leake et al., 1980). This suggestion is based on the assumption that in order to promote the complete growth response in target tissue the steroid receptor complex must first bind to specific 'acceptor' sites on the chromatin. Therefore, if a biopsy from a patient contained cytosol receptors that did not translocate to the nucleus, then that patient would not be expected to respond to hormone therapy. Leake et al. (1980) measured both cytoplasmic and nuclear oestrogen receptors in biopsies from 250 patients with breast cancer and concluded that the combined measurement appears to give a more reliable guide to hormone dependence than does measurement at the cytoplasmic level alone. However, positive values at both levels do not guarantee response to hormone therapy in breast tumours.

9.3 STEROID RECEPTORS AS TUMOUR MARKERS FOR PROSTATIC CANCER

9.3.1 Androgen receptors

Despite the remarkable progress in the use of steroid receptors as a tumour marker to discriminate between the hormone responsive and non-responsive breast tumours, the progress in the utilization of androgen receptors for a similar purpose for patients with carcinoma of the prostate has been slow. This has been partly due to difficulties in establishing reliable methods for qualitative and quantitative analyses of androgen receptors and in part to the characteristics of human prostatic tumours. Initial experimental conditions were established using rat ventral prostate. Although the fundamental approach, in terms of experimental techniques for the analysis of steroid receptors in the rat and human prostates, was common, the latter presented some major obstacles. These problems are now resolved and reliable techniques for the analysis of cytoplasmic and nuclear androgen receptors developed (Ghanadian et al., 1978a; Ghanadian and Auf, 1980). A full account of the available methods for androgen receptor analysis together with a critical review of the reported techniques is given in Chapter 8, and it has been shown that some of these methods have been responsible for producing a number of unrepresentative and often erroneous results.

In addition to the methodological considerations for the receptor analysis, the subjective and objective criteria of response to endocrine manipulation is equally important and could be a major reason for the discrepancies in the reported results. These criteria are discussed in Chapter 10, and it appears that if a useful comparison is to be made, they should be carefully examined. At the present time there are a limited number of studies in which the relationship between androgen receptors in malignant prostates and the response of patients to endocrine therapy have been evaluated. Most of these studies have employed different techniques for their receptor analysis, with a short follow-up period of the patients' progress to endocrine manipulation. However, in a recent study from our laboratory we have measured both cytoplasmic and nuclear androgen receptors in prostatic tissues of 32 patients with malignant prostates and have evaluated the response to different forms of endocrine therapy for a period of up to 2 years (Ghanadian et al., 1981). In this study androgen receptors were measured by an exchange assay using radiolabelled synthetic androgen methyltrienolone ([³H]R1881) and assayed according to the procedure described previously (Ghanadian et al., 1978a; Ghanadian and Auf, 1980). In this study, patients were treated by a number of endocrine manipulations, such as bilateral orchidectomy, treatment with diethylstil-boestrol, estramustine phosphate (Estracyt) or cyproterone acetate. The clinical evaluation of the patients' response to therapy was carried out according to a protocol which was designed for this study. This protocol examined the following subjective and objective criteria of response at 6 monthly intervals.

(1) Symptoms due to primary tumour and metastases. This was based on a scoring system of either no symptoms (0), or symptomatic but improved (1), or no change (2), or worse (3). A 50 % reduction in symptoms due to either primary or metastasis was considered a positive response to treatment (regression), whilst 50 % increase was classified as non-responsive (progression). Tumours which remained stable were considered non-responsive (no change).

(2) The TMN category. Similarly this was assessed, based on 50 % changes in the size of the tumour (T), size of soft tissue metastases (M) and lymph node involvement (N).

(3) Return to normal or at least 50 % reduction in serum acid and alkaline phosphatase were considered evidence of tumour regression, while an increase or no change was classified as progression or stable.

(4) Bone scan/X-ray. Tumour regression was evident by recalcification of at least 50 % of any osteolytic metastasis while the appearance of new bony lesions was considered a sign of tumour progression.

(5) Prostatic size. An approximate evaluation was made by rectal palpation. However, this was of limited reliability. Assessment of prostatic size by this technique is questionable.

(6) Other considerations were changes in body weight and the general well-being of the patient including patient's activity. This was classified in four groups of full activity, restricted activity, confined to bed and those requiring total nursing. In addition the analgesic requirements of the patients were considered.

In this study, the tumours were classified into two groups of responsive and non-responsive. Those tumours that showed signs of progression as well as the stable tumours (no regression, no progression) were considered non-responsive. The responsive tumours were those with evidence of regression. The results demonstrated that 21 out of 32 (66 %) of patients with carcinoma of the prostate who received endocrine therapy showed signs of tumour regression within the first 6 months of treatment. Tumour regression was also observed in 44 % of the patients that were treated for a period of 2 years. In 7 out of 32 (22 %), signs of progression were seen in the first 6 months, whilst the remaining four patients did not show evidence of regression or progression and were considered as stable. Some of the patients, who were initially responsive to endocrine therapy, became non-responsive as the treatment continued, while a number of tumours which were initially non-responsive became responsive when the type of hormone therapy was changed. When the mean concentrations of cytoplasmic androgen receptors in responsive and non-responsive tumours were compared, the concentration in the former group was significantly higher at 6 months ($p < 0.05$) but not at 12, 18 or 24 months. However, when the mean nuclear androgen receptor concentration in the hormone responsive tumours was compared to that in non-responsive ones, there were significantly higher receptor concentrations in the hormone responsive group at 6, 12, 18 and 24 months of treatment. This study clearly demonstrated that hormone responsive malignant prostates contain a significantly higher concentration of androgen receptors compared to non-responsive tumours. The non-responsive tumours contained an average of 500 fmol/mg DNA or less of nuclear androgen receptors. In our studies, this value was used as a cut-off point to distinguish between hormone responsive and non-responsive tumours. Analysis of the results showed that 77 % of the tumours with a nuclear androgen receptor concentration of 500 fmol/mg DNA or above responded favourably to endocrine manipulation during the first 6 months of the treatment and the response to endocrine therapy for a similar percentage of patients was maintained for 12, 18 and 24 months. In contrast, only 46 % of the tumours containing less than 500 fmol/mg DNA of nuclear receptors responded to endocrine manipulation during the first 6 months of therapy which was only transient and was not maintained beyond 6 months of treatment. Indeed, none of the tumours containing less than 500 fmol/mg DNA of nuclear receptor responded to endocrine therapy when the period of follow-up was extended to 2 years. The correlation between the cytoplasmic androgen receptor concentration and the response to endocrine therapy was less striking than our finding with the nuclear counterpart. The non-responsive tumours contained approximately 50 fmol/mg protein or less of cytoplasmic androgen receptor. Analysis of the results showed that when this value was used as a cut-off point to discriminate the responsive from non-responsive tumours, 68 % of the prostates with 50 fmol/mg protein or more of this receptor responded to endocrine manipulation within the first 6 months of the treatment. However, at the same time 62 % of tumours which contained a lower concentration of androgen receptors also responded to hormonal therapy. Within a period of 2 years 59–63 % of the tumours at 50 fmol/mg protein or more responded to endocrine therapy, whilst only 18 % with lower concentration (less than 50 fmol/mg protein cytoplasmic androgen receptor) responded to therapy. This finding also demonstrates that the assessment of the tumour response following a short period of 6 months could be misleading. In our experience, five tumours that were judged to be hormone responsive during the first 6 months of therapy became refractory to treatment, when the follow-up was extended to 1 and 2 years. Therefore, a period of at least 1 year for the evaluation of response to endocrine manipulation is more appropriate. As described previously, Jensen's group (Jensen et al., 1976) have employed the terms 'receptor rich' and 'receptor poor' instead of positive and negative with a dividing line which was determined on the basis of clinical experience with breast tumours. A remarkably similar situation is apparent with prostatic tumours. In our study, the concentrations of 50 fmol/mg protein and 500 fmol/mg DNA for cytoplasmic and nuclear androgen receptors are the dividing lines which are obtained on the basis of clinical evaluation. The finding, that the 60 % of the tumours with rich cytoplasmic receptor responded to endocrine therapy whereas only 18 % of those with low receptor level (receptor poor) responded, demonstrates similarities to those studies on the prognostic value of oestrogen receptor measurement in breast tumours. McGuire *et al.* (1975a,b) reported that 55–60% of the breast tumours that were oestrogen receptor positive responded to various forms of endocrine therapy, whilst only 8% of the receptor negative tumours responded to this treatment.

Table 9.1 Correlation between cytoplasmic (fmol/mg protein) and nuclear (fmol/mg DNA) androgen receptor concentrations and response to endocrine therapy in prostatic cancer. Response is expressed as + (regression) or − (progression or stable)

Duration of assessment Months	Response	Cytoplasmic receptors		Nuclear receptors	
		Concentration Mean ± SD	Number and % Responders	Concentrations Mean ± SD	Number and % Responders
6	+	88.5 ± 73.6	13/19 (68%)	1340.6 ± 1342.5	13/17 (77%)
	−	38.2 ± 22.4	8/13 (62%)	519.2 ± 652.2	6/13 (46%)
12	+	94.7 ± 62.7	12/19 (63%)	1874.8 ± 1524.3	12/16 (75%)
	−	55.4 ± 69.0	2/11 (18%)	427.9 ± 521.5	1/12 (8%)
18	+	86.9 ± 64.3	10/17 (59%)	1709.8 ± 1565.1	10/15 (67%)
	−	48.8 ± 45.0	2/11 (18%)	527.5 ± 648.6	1/11 (9%)
24	+	91.7 ± 67.0	9/15 (60%)	1853.8 ± 1571.6	10/13 (77%)
	−	46.9 ± 44.6	2/11 (18%)	476.2 ± 682.2	0/10 (0%)

Data from author's laboratory

A combined measurement of cytoplasmic and nuclear androgen receptors could significantly improve the prognostic value of the receptor and provide a more accurate criteria for the assessment of response of patients with prostatic carcinoma to endocrine manipulation. Prostatic tumours that contained cytoplasmic androgen receptors equal to or more than 50 fmol/mg protein and nuclear androgen receptors of 500 fmol/mg DNA or more revealed a remarkably high response to endocrine therapy. This situation existed in 45% of patients in our study and the response to endocrine manipulation for periods of 6–24 months was 77%–80%. In those tumours that contained 500 fmol/mg DNA or more nuclear androgen receptors but less than 50 fmol/mg protein cytoplasmic androgen receptors, the response to endocrine therapy for the same period ranged between 66% and 75%. The number of tumours in this group was approximately 11%. Another 13% of the tumours that contained high cytoplasmic (over 50 fmol/mg DNA) but low nuclear androgen receptors (less than 500 fmol/mg DNA): the response to endocrine therapy during the first 6 months was 50% but reduced to 25% and 0% after 12 and 24 months respectively. Finally 30% of the tumours in which both cytoplasmic and nuclear androgen receptors were less than their cut-off points: there was 55% response to endocrine therapy within the first 6 months, but no response (0%) after 12 or 24 months. It is quite clear from this data that the initial response within the first 6 months of the treatment is only transient and that the combined cytoplasmic and nuclear receptor measurement could fairly accurately predict the response to hormone manipulation for longer periods.

The importance of the analysis of nuclear androgen receptors is well illustrated in our studies and is in line with the general scheme by which the mechanism of action of androgen has been described. As in the case of breast tumours, a favourable response to endocrine manipulation can only be expected if the tumour has a functional receptor system in which the cytoplasmic receptor is able to translocate to the nucleus and interact with the chromatin components of the prostatic cell nuclei. Indeed, the presence of nuclear receptor could be considered a prerequisite for the tumour to be hormone responsive. If a tumour possesses the cytoplasmic androgen receptor, but lacks the ability to translocate it to the nucleus, then the possibility to respond to endocrine therapy will be significantly reduced, and this has been demonstrated in our study. Following 1 year of treatment 75 % of patients with high nuclear androgen receptor level and only 8 % with low concentration of this receptor responded to endocrine therapy. However, after 2 years treatment the response rate for those with high nuclear androgen receptors was 77 % while none of the tumours containing low levels of this receptor responded to endocrine manipulation. It should be noted that the presence of nuclear receptor does not always guarantee that the tissue is hormone dependent. There may be other mechanisms responsible for the failure of those 23 % tumours with high nuclear androgen receptors that did not respond to endocrine therapy. An explanation for this failure may be the presence of autonomous tumour cells which continue following the destruction of endocrine responsive cells. It is also possible to attribute non-response of receptor rich tumours to endocrine therapy to the heterogeneity of the tumour. Some tumours might be multiclonal in that the patient's tumour possesses both receptor poor and rich clones. This argument could also be applicable for those tumours with low levels of receptor which respond to endocrine manipulation. Finally, another explanation for the failure may be the presence of abnormal receptors, which are incapable of eliciting a physiological response. In this case prostatic tumours may contain two receptor components, one of which does not possess the ability to translocate to the nucleus. If this assumption is correct, those tumours, with high cytoplasmic androgen receptors which failed to respond to endocrine therapy, may have contained more of the non-active receptor. This explanation is consistent with the observation in our study that the number of tumours with high cytoplasmic receptor which did not respond to endocrine therapy following 2 years treatment was 40 % whilst those which failed with high nuclear receptors were 23 %. Fang and Liao (1971) separated two components from rat ventral prostate by the ammonium sulphate precipitation technique. One component (complex I) exhibited low specificity for DHT and could not transfer to the nucleus, whereas the other component (complex II) had a high affinity towards androgens and translocated to the nucleus.

In our study, the histological examination of prostatic tumours revealed a wide variation in the proportion of malignant cells ranging between 2 % and 80 % in between the tissues. Some contained both normal and benign tissues. Correlation between androgen receptor concentration and the proportion of the tumour cells revealed no relationships between these two parameters. This lack of correlation was also apparent when tumours were divided into responsive and non-responsive ones. Similar findings have been reported by Wittliff *et al.* (1980) who examined the relationship between the percentage of the cells of the human mammary carcinoma within the biopsy samples and their concentration of cytoplasmic oestrogen receptor. They concluded that the individual variation between the concentration of oestrogen receptors in different samples of breast tumours is not due to the number of tumour cells but to the differences in the number of binding cells. This conclusion, however, is not totally applicable to prostatic tumours. Feherty *et al.* (1971) suggested that in mammary carcinoma, the malignant epithelium but not the normal is the source of oestrogen receptors. However, there is substantial evidence which suggests that in the human prostate both fibromuscular and epithelial elements contain androgen receptors (Sirett *et al.*, 1980). Therefore, a background receptor level will be present in most prostatic cancer tissues.

There are several other reports on the prognostic value of androgen receptors for predicting the response of patients with prostatic carcinoma to endocrine therapy. de Voogt and Dingjan (1978, 1980) and Wagner (1980) used TUR or biopsy specimens from malignant prostates and measured cytoplasmic androgen receptors using an agar gel electrophoretic technique. These studies suggested a lack of correlation between the concentration of cytoplasmic androgen receptors and the response to endocrine therapy in patients with prostatic carcinoma. This lack of correlation may be explained through the type of method chosen for receptor analysis. They labelled the cytoplasmic androgen receptors by incubation at $0\,^{\circ}C$ for 2 hours with tritiated dihydrotestosterone and then separated the labelled receptor complex from SHBG by agar gel electrophoresis. As discussed in Chapter 8, this procedure could only label the free receptor and not the fraction already bound to steroid. Furthermore, this separation technique is susceptible to contamination by albumin and this point is well illustrated in their reported values which reach 300 fmol/mg cytoplasmic protein for unoccupied binding sites. This is incompatible with other reported values for the unoccupied receptor of the human prostate (Rosen *et al.*, 1975; Ghanadian *et al.*, 1978a, 1980; Mobbs *et al.*, 1978; Kliman *et al.*, 1979). Using the protamine sulphate precipitation technique, Mobbs *et al.* (1978) measured unoccupied (free) cytoplasmic androgen receptors in malignant prostatic tissues. These investigators suggested that in non-treated patients the cytoplasmic receptor level is significantly lower than in tissues obtained from patients who had been orchiectomized or treated with oestrogens. Similar findings have also been reported by Ghanadian *et al.* (1978b, c) and could be due to the decrease in the circulating level of testosterone in treated patients, thus freeing androgen bound to the cytoplasmic receptor and resulting in an increase in the free receptor. Mobbs *et al.* (1980) have also studied the relationship between the free cytoplasmic androgen receptors and the response to endocrine manipulation in patients with prostatic cancer. They found that all patients whose tumours contained a free cytoplasmic androgen receptor concentration of less than 0.4 fmol/mg tissue or 90 fmol/mg DNA were either in relapse at the time of biopsy or did not respond to subsequent endocrine manipulation. They suggested that a certain threshold concentration of this receptor appears to be required for a subsequent response to hormonal manipulation. The most definite response to endocrine therapy occurred in patients whose prostatic cytosol contained free androgen receptor at concentrations of 0.6–3.6 fmol/mg tissue or 80–475 fmol/mg DNA. However, in their study tumours with the highest concentrations of free receptor did not appear to be sensitive to hormonal manipulation. They suggested the possibility that this very high receptor is an abnormal one or is an irrelevant product, not involved in the processes which control androgen sensitivity. Bashirelahi *et al.* (1980) and Ekman (1980) have also studied the relationship between the concentration of cytoplasmic androgen receptors and the response of the patients to endocrine manipulation. Bashirelahi's group reported that the receptor concentration in the seven patients who did not respond to endocrine therapy was approximately double that in the five patients of the hormone responsive group. Ekman (1980) used punch needle biopsies for the assay of androgen receptors and assessed the response to endocrine therapy for a period of 3 months. He found that 18 of the 21 (86%) biopsies with positive androgen receptors had a clear tumour regression. However, three out of eight (37%) patients, in whom the receptor was negative, also showed tumour regression. He found that the non-responsive malignant prostates contained a significantly lower concentration of androgen binding sites than the responsive tumours.

In our studies, when both cytoplasmic and nuclear androgen receptors in 30 prostatic tumours were simultaneously analysed, some degree of exchange between the two androgen receptors was observed. Approximately 13% of those tumours with high cytoplasmic androgen receptors showed low levels of nuclear receptors and the response rates to endocrine therapy in this group were 50%, 25% and 0% following 6, 12 and 24 months of the treatment. A similar proportion of the tissues had high nuclear and low cytoplasmic androgen receptors, but in these tumours the response rate was between 66% and 75%. This data may partially explain the high incidence of false positives (receptor rich tumours that did not respond) and false negatives (receptor poor tumours that responded), when the correlation studies were carried out using the cytoplasmic receptor levels. This observation not only confirms the better prognostic value of nuclear receptors but also emphasizes that the combined measurement of cytoplasmic and nuclear androgen receptors can provide a more reliable criteria for predicting the response to hormone therapy. This is demonstrated by the fact that 80% of those with a high level of both receptors responded to endocrine treatment and the response was maintained for the 2 year period that the patients were investigated. All the patients with low cytoplasmic and nuclear receptors had a very poor prognosis and no response was observed following 1 and 2 years of treatment. In this group, nearly 70% of the patients died of their disease within 2 years.

9.3.2 Oestradiol-17β and progesterone binding proteins

The presence of receptor proteins for oestradiol has been demonstrated in benign and malignant human prostatic tumours and the methodological aspects of the analysis of this receptor have been discussed in Chapter 8. With the introduction of oestrogens for the treatment of patients with prostatic cancer, much attention has been focused on the mechanism by which this class of steroid hormones interacts with prostatic tumours and thereby exerts its suppressive effects. In the course of treatment of patients with prostatic cancer with synthetic oestrogens it has become apparent that some of the prostatic tumours do not respond to this treatment or become refractory to endocrine therapy. As discussed previously, the failure of malignant prostates to respond to endocrine therapy can not always be predicted by the measurement of androgen receptors. Thus it has been suggested that other parameters which might be involved in the development of the tumour should be analysed, in order to provide more information on the control system of prostatic tumours by steroids. Sinha et al. (1977) have compared the ultrastructural features of prostatic cancer cells in both untreated and oestrogen treated responsive and refractory patients. They found that tumours possessed well and poorly differentiated acini and invasive cells. The malignant acini contained numerous columnar (secretory) cells in untreated tumours, whilst few were found in the treated individuals. Two distinct types of basal cells, i.e. type I (light) and type II (dark) cells were observed. These investigators found that prostatic carcinoma, which was non-responsive or subsequently became refractory to oestrogens, showed more abundant type II basal cells than responsive patients. They suggested that the type II basal cells as well as some type I basal cells are endocrine unresponsive from the outset and that the tumour possesses a heterogeneous population of cancer cells. While androgen dependent tumour cells such as columnar cells may be destroyed by endocrine therapy, these endocrine unresponsive cells may continue to proliferate, metastasize and kill the patient.

A number of investigators have measured the cellular receptors for oestradiol in patients with prostatic tumours in order to evaluate the relationship between the content of this tumour and the response to endocrine therapy. Bashirelahi et al. (1980) analysed oestradiol receptor in prostatic tumours in 12 patients with metastatic carcinoma of the prostate and correlated the receptor concentration to subsequent response to endocrine therapy. The receptor concentration was high in 4 out of 5 endocrine responsive tumours, whilst the stable and non-responsive tumours contained low levels of oestradiol receptors. They suggested that patients with absent or low oestradiol receptor content are unlikely to respond to either orchidectomy or diethylstilboestrol therapy. This finding is in contrast with the report by Wagner (1980), who measured the cytoplasmic oestradiol receptor in 11 untreated malignant prostatic tumours and found no correlation between the subsequent response to endocrine therapy and the concentration of oestradiol receptor in the tumour. de Voogt and Dingjan (1978, 1980) reported a positive correlation between the concentration of oestradiol binding protein and the response to endocrine therapy in patients with prostatic tumours. However, this data is open to question as the reported values for oestradiol binding sites in some cases are extremely high, with an upper range of 15 707 fmol/mg protein. This indicates contamination of oestradiol binding protein with other proteins such as albumin during the separation by agar gel electrophoresis.

In a study involving 20 patients with malignant prostate the concentration of cytoplasmic and nuclear oestrogen receptors were measured in our laboratory and the concentration of these receptors in relation to the response of the patients to endocrine therapy was investigated (Auf, 1982). The results of this study demonstrated that 14 out of 20 (70 %) patients showed signs of remission within the first 6 months of therapy and this was evident in 53 % of patients that were followed-up for a 2 year period. In the remaining six patients, three showed signs of tumour regression within the first 6 months and a further three patients were stable. Approximately 47 % of the tumours did not show any signs of regression, when the response to therapy was assessed following 2 years of treatment. There were no significant differences between the mean concentration of cytoplasmic and nuclear oestradiol in the hormone responsive tumours and that of non-responsive. There was also no correlation between the concentration of oestradiol and the response of the patient to endocrine therapy. The available data on oestradiol and progesterone binding components as discriminant markers distinguishing hormone responsive tumours from non-responsive prostatic cancer in inconclusive and requires further investigation.

9.4 CONCLUSIONS

The development of the concept that steroid hormones exert their biological actions in the prostate through a receptor mediated mechanism has significantly contributed to our understanding of the critical events leading to the growth of the prostate and also the mechanism by which the abnormal growth may be controlled. The significance of this in relation to clinical practice lies in the use of steroid receptor measurements in predicting the response of prostatic carcinoma to endocrine therapy. The endocrine manipulation of this tumour is based on the fact that, in general, neoplasms derived from hormone responsive tissues often retain the hormone sensitivity of their parent cells, even though the tumour may be widely dispersed throughout the body. A similar assumption has been made for the growth of the other endocrine dependent tumours such as breast tumours and their relationship to oestrogen receptors. Despite the remarkable advances which have been achieved in the utilization of oestrogen receptors in predicting the response of breast tumours to endocrine therapy, the progress with androgen receptors in prostatic carcinoma has been slow. A number of factors, including the heterogeneity of prostatic tumours, the presence of high levels of endogenous androgens and steroid enzymes and finally the presence of protein binding components with high affinity for androgens, have all been responsible for delaying the development of reliable quantitative assay procedures for androgen receptors in the prostate. However, these problems have now been resolved and reliable techniques for the quantitative analysis of androgen receptors in the cytoplasmic and nuclear fractions of human prostatic tumours have been developed. Furthermore, a more uniform approach for the clinical evaluation of patients following endocrine therapy has been adopted and the subjective and objective criteria of response have been defined.

The current data on the predictive role of androgen receptors in the management of patients with prostatic cancer has been discussed. It is quite apparent that the methodological shortcomings in a number of these reports account for the inconsistencies and often contradictory conclusions. However, in a recent study, the significance of both cytoplasmic and nuclear androgen receptors of malignant prostates in predicting the response to a number of different forms of endocrine therapy for a period of up to 2 years was investigated. The results of this study demonstrate that the hormone responsive malignant prostates contain a significantly higher concentration of androgen receptors than the non-responsive tumours and that about 77 % of the tumours with nuclear receptors' concentration exceeding 500 fmol/mg DNA responded to endocrine therapy during the first 6 months and the response was maintained during the 2 years follow-up period studied. However, the correlation between the cytoplasmic androgen receptor concentration and response was less striking. Combined measurements of cytoplasmic and nuclear androgen receptors appear to improve the prognostic value of androgen receptor analysis and provide a more accurate criteria of the assessment of response to endocrine therapy. In general, these findings are consistent with the prognostic value of oestrogen receptors in breast tumours; that those tumours showing low oestrogen binding or lacking oestrogen receptors, rarely respond to endocrine therapy, whereas most, but not all, patients whose tumours contain significant amounts of receptor benefit from such treatment. Although the measurement of progesterone receptors in breast cancer is complimentary to oestrogen analysis and could improve the prediction rate of response to endocrine therapy, a similar situation has not yet been demonstrated in prostatic cancer and neither oestrogen nor progesterone receptors appear to be of significant values as tumour markers.

9.5 REFERENCES

Auf, G. (1982). The predictive role of androgen and oestrogen receptor proteins in the management of patients with carcinoma of the prostate. *PhD Thesis*, University of London

Bashirelahi, N., Young, Jr., J. D., Sidh, S. M. and Sanefuji, H. (1980). Androgen, oestrogen and progesterone and their distribution in epithelial and stromal cells of human prostate. In Schroder, F. H. and de Voogt, H. J. (eds.) *Steroid Receptors, Metabolism and Prostatic Cancer.* pp. 240–255. (Amsterdam: Excerpta Medica)

Beatson, G. T. (1896). On the treatment of inoperable case of carcinoma of the mamma. Suggestions for a new method of treatment with illustrative cases. *Lancet*, **2,** 1255

Campbell, F. C., Blamey, R. W., Elston, C. W., Morris, A. H., Nicholson, R. I., Griffiths, K. and Haybittle, J. L. (1981). Quantitative oestradiol receptor values in primary breast cancer and response to endocrine therapy. *Lancet*, **2,** 1317

De Sombre, E. R., Carbone, P. P., Jensen, E. V., McGuire, W. L., Wells, Jr., S. A., Whittliff, J. L. and Lipsett, M. B. (1979). Steroid receptors in breast cancer. *N. Engl. J. Med.*, **301,** 1011

De Sombre, E. R., Greene, G. L. and Jensen, E. V. (1978). Estrophlin and endocrine responsiveness of breast cancer. In McGuire, W. L. (ed.) *Hormones, Receptors and Breast Cancer?* pp. 1–14. (New York: Raven Press)

de Voogt, H. J. and Dingjan, P. (1978). Steroid receptors in human prostatic cancer. A preliminary evaluation. *Urol. Res.*, **6**, 151

de Voogt, H. J. and Dingjan, P. G. (1980). Is there a place for the assay of cytoplasmic steroid receptors in the endocrine treatment of prostatic cancer. In Schroder, F. H. and de Voogt, H. J. (eds.) *Steroid Receptors, Metabolism and Prostatic Cancer*. pp. 265–270. (Amsterdam: Excerpta Medica)

Ekman, P. (1980). Clinical significance of steroid receptor assay in the human prostate. In Schroder, F. H. and de Voogt, H. J. (eds.) *Steroid Receptors, Metabolism and Prostatic Cancer*. pp. 208–224. (Amsterdam: Excerpta Medica)

Engelsman, E., Persijn, J. P., Korsten, C. B., Cleton, F. J. (1973). Oestrogen receptors in human breast cancer tissue and response to endocrine therapy. *Br. M. J.*, **2**, 750

Fang, S. and Liao, S. (1971). Androgen receptors: steroid and tissue specific retention of 17-beta-hydroxy-5-alpha-androstan-3-one protein complex by the cell nuclei of ventral prostate. *J. Biol. Chem.*, **246**, 16

Feherty, P., Farrer-Brown, G. and Kellie, A. E. (1971). Oestradiol receptors in carcinoma and benign disease of the breast: an *in vitro* assay. *Br. J. Cancer*, **25**, 697

Folca, P. J., Glascock, R. F. and Irvine, W. T. (1961). Studies with tritium labelled hexoestrol in advanced breast cancer. *Lancet*, **2**, 796

Ghanadian, R. (1976). Endocrine control of the prostate: mechanism of action of androgens. In Williams, D. I. and Chisholm, G. D. (eds.) *Scientific Foundations of Urology*. pp. 138–146. (London: Heinemann)

Ghanadian, R. (1981). Steroid receptors in urologic cancer. In Javadpour, N. (ed.) *Recent Advances in Urologic Cancer*. pp. 67–81. (Baltimore: Williams and Wilkins)

Ghanadian, R. (1982). Mechanism of action of androgens. In Williams, D. I. and Chisholm, G. D. (eds.) *Scientific Foundations of Urology*. 2nd Edn., In Press. (London: Heinemann)

Ghanadian, R. and Auf, G. (1980). Receptor proteins for androgens in benign prostatic hypertrophy and carcinoma of the prostate. In Schroder, F. H. and de Voogt, H. J. (eds.) *Steroid Receptors, Metabolism and Prostatic Cancer*. pp. 110–125. (Amsterdam: Excerpta Medica)

Ghanadian, R., Auf, G., Chaloner, P. J. and Chisholm, G. D. (1978a). The use of methyltrienolone in the measurement of the free and bound cytoplasmic receptors for dihydrotestosterone in benign hypertrophied human prostate. *J. Steroid Biochem.*, **9**, 325

Ghanadian, R., Auf, G. and Chisholm, G. D. (1978b). Androgen receptors in prostatic cancer. In Pavone-Macaluso, M., Smith, P. H. and Edsmyr, F. (eds.) *Bladder Tumours and Other Topics in Urological Oncology*. pp. 453–457 (New York: Plenum Press)

Ghanadian, R., Auf, G., Chisholm, G. D. and O'Donoghue, E. P. N. (1978c). Receptor proteins for androgens in prostatic disease. *Br. J. Urol.*, **50**, 567

Ghanadian, R., Auf, G., Smith, C. B. and Puah, C. M. (1980). Androgen receptors in benign hypertrophied and malignant prostate. In Wittliff, J. L. and Dapunt, O. (eds.) *Steroid Receptors and Hormone-dependent Neoplasia*. pp. 149–150. (New York: Masson Publishing)

Ghanadian, R., Auf, G., Williams, G., Davis A. and Richards, B. (1981). Predicting the response of prostatic carcinoma to endocrine therapy. *Lancet*, **2**, 1418

Glascock, R. F. and Hoekstra, W. G. (1959). Selective accumulation of tritium-labelled hexoestrol by the reproductive organs of immature female goats and sheep. *Biochem. J.*, **72**, 673

Grayhack, J. T. and Wendel, E. F. (1974). Hormone dependent carcinoma of the prostate. In Brans, D. (ed.) *Male Accessory Sex Organs*. p. 425. (New York: Academic Press)

Horwitz, K. B., Costlow, M. E. and McGuire, W. L. (1975). MCF-7: A human breast cancer cell line with oestrogen, androgen, progesterone and glucocorticoid receptors. *Steroids*, **26**, 785

Horwitz, K. B. and McGuire, W. L. (1978). Oestrogen control of progesterone receptor in human breast cancer: correlation with nuclear processing of oestrogen receptor. *J. Biol. Chem.*, **253**, 2223

Huggins, C. and Hodges, C. V. (1941). Studies on prostatic cancer. 1. The effect of castration of oestrogen and of androgen injection on serum phosphatase in metastatic carcinoma of the prostate. *Cancer Res.*, **1**, 293

Jensen, E. V. (1981). Hormone dependency of breast cancer. *Cancer*, **47**, 2319

Jensen, E. V., Block, G. F., Smith, S., Kyser, K. and De Sombre, E. R. (1971). Oestrogen receptors and breast cancer response to adrenalectomy. *Natl. Cancer Inst. Monogr.*, **34**, 55

Jensen, E. V. and Jacobson, H. I. (1962). Basic guides to the mechanism of oestrogen action. In Pincus, G. and Vollmer, E. P. (eds.) *Recent Progress in Hormone Research.* pp. 161, 178. (London: Academic Press)

Jensen, E. V., Polley, T. Z., Smith, S., Block, G. E., Ferguson, D. J. and De Sombre, E. R. (1975). Prediction of hormone dependency in human breast cancer. In McGuire, W. L., Carbone, P. P. and Vollmer, E. P. (eds.) *Oestrogen Receptors in Human Breast Cancer.* pp. 37–56. (New York: Raven Press)

Jensen, E. V., Smith, S. and De Sombre, E. R. (1976). Hormone dependency in breast cancer. *J. Steroid Biochem.*, **7**, 911

King, R. J. B., Hayward, J. L., Masters, J. R. W., Millis, R. R. and Rubens, R. D. (1980). Steroid receptor assays as prognostic aids in the treatment of breast cancer. In Wittliff, J. L. and Dapunt, O. (eds.) *Steroid Receptors and Hormone-dependent Neoplasia.* pp. 249–256. (New York: Masson Publishing)

Kliman, B., MacLoughlin, R. A. and Prout, G. R. (1979). Measurement of androgen receptors in cytosol of human prostatic tissues with a Sepharose-Link antibody system. In Murphy, G. P. and Sandberg, A. A. (eds.) *Prostatic Cancer and Hormone Receptors.* pp. 85–96. *Prog. Clin. Biol. Res.*, (New York: Alan R. Liss)

Knight, W. A., Livingstone, R. B., Gregory, E. J. and McGuire, W. L. (1977). Oestrogen receptor: an independent prognostic factor for early recurrence in breast cancer. *Cancer Res.*, **37**, 4669

Leake, R. E., Laing, L. and Smith, D. C. (1980). Use of nuclear oestrogen receptors in choice of therapy for breast cancer patients. In Wittliff, J. L. and Dapunt, O. (eds.) *Steroid Receptors and Hormone-dependent Neoplasia.* pp. 273–5. (New York: Masson Publishing)

Leung, B. S., Fletcher, W. S., Lindell, T. D., Wood, D. C. and Krippachne, W. W. (1973). Predictability of response to endocrine ablation in advanced breast carcinoma. *Arch. Surg.*, **106**, 515

Maass, H., Engel, B., Hohmeister, H., Lehmann, F. and Trams, G. (1972). Oestrogen receptors in human breast cancer tissue. *Am. J. Obstet. Gynecol.*, **113**, 377

McGuire, W. L. (1978). Hormone receptors: their role in predicting prognosis and response to endocrine therapy. *Semin. Oncol.*, **9**, 428

McGuire, W. L., Carbone, P. P., Sears, M. E. and Esher, G. E. (1975a). Estrogen receptors in human breast cancer. An overview. In McGuire, W. L., Carbone, P. P. and Vollmer, E. P. (eds.) *Estrogen Receptors in Human Breast Cancer.* pp. 1–7. (New York: Academic Press)

McGuire, W. L., Pearson, O. H. and Segaloff, A. (1975b). Predicting hormone responsiveness in human breast cancer. In McGuire, W. L., Carbone, P. P. and Vollmer, E. P. (eds.) *Estrogen Receptors in Human Breast Cancer.* pp. 17–30. (New York: Academic Press)

Mobbs, B. G., Johnson, I. E. and Connolly, J. G. (1980). Androgen receptors and treatment of prostatic cancer. In Schroder, F. H. and de Voogt, H. J. (eds.) *Steroid*

Receptors, Metabolism and Prostatic Cancer. pp. 225–239. (Amsterdam: Excerpta Medica)

Mobbs, B. G., Johnson, I. E., Connolly, J. G. and Clark, A. F. (1978). Androgen receptor assay in human benign and malignant prostatic tumour cytosol using protamine sulphate precipitation. *J. Steroid Biochem.*, **9**, 289

Rosen, V., Jung, I., Baulieu, E. E. and Robel, P. (1975). Androgen binding proteins in human benign prostatic hypertrophy. *J. Clin. Endocrinol. Metab.*, **41**, 761

Savlov, E. D., Wittliff, J. L., Hilf, R. and Hall, T. C. (1974). Correlations between certain biochemical properties of breast cancer and response to therapy: a preliminary report. *Cancer*, **33**, 303

Sinha, A. A., Blackard, C. E. and Seal, U. S. (1977). A critical analysis of tumour morphology and hormone treatments in the untreated and oestrogen treated responsive and refractory human prostatic carcinoma. *Cancer*, **40**, 2836

Sirett, D. A. N., Cowan, S. K., Janeczko, A. E., Grant, J. K. and Glen, E. S. (1980). Prostatic tissue distribution of 17β- hydroxy-5α-androstan-3-one and of androgen receptors in benign hyperplasia. *J. Steroid Biochem.*, **13**, 723

Toft, O. and Gorski, J. (1966). A receptor molecule for oestrogens: isolation from the rat uterus and preliminary characterization. *Proc. Natl. Acad. Sci. USA*, **55**, 1574

Van Rossum, J. M. (1968). Drug receptor theories, In Robson, J. M. and Stacey, R. S. (eds.) *Recent Advances in Pharmacology.* pp. 99–133. (London: J. & A. Churchill)

Wagner, R. K. (1980). Lack of correlation between androgen receptor content and clinical response to treatment with diethylstilboestrol (DES) in human prostate carcinoma. In Schroder, F. H. and de Voogt, H. J. (eds.) *Steroid Receptors, Metabolism and Prostatic Cancer.* pp. 190–7. (Amsterdam: Excerpta Medica)

Wittliff, J. L., Wiehle, S. A., Sandoz, J. P., Fischer, B. and Durant, J. R. (1980). Establishment of uniformity in steroid receptor determination used in clinical studies and drug screening programme. In Raus, J., Martens, H. and Leclercop, G. (eds.) *Cytotoxic Estrogens in Hormone Receptive Tumors.* pp. 147–164. (New York: Academic Press)

10
The response of the malignant prostate to endocrine treatment

G. D. CHISHOLM AND L. L. BEYNON

10.1   NATURAL HISTORY

The need for reviewing the natural history of carcinoma of the prostate becomes apparent whenever the questions arise 'is treatment necessary' or 'should treatment be delayed'. The principle reason for raising these questions is the knowledge that the natural history of the disease, in *some* patients , is such that there are no apparent differences in survival between the treated and untreated groups. These questions are asked more often for two reasons: (1) the methods of staging and grading the tumour are now more precise and (2) the studies by the Veterans Administration Cooperative Urological Group (VACURG) showed that, for early disease and for asymptomatic disease, both morbidity and mortality were worsened by treatment (Byar, 1977).

It might be expected that data from earlier this century, before the advent of endocrine treatment, would give a good idea of the natural history of prostatic cancer but this is not so. Then, as now, most patients presented with symptoms of prostatic obstruction but biopsy techniques were not available, prostatectomy rate was not so high and the need for serial section of prostatic tissue to find a focus of tumour was not appreciated. Thus the disease was diagnosed at a more advanced stage and there are no data for the natural history of early prostatic cancer at that time.

Bumpus, in 1926, recorded the natural history of 485 untreated cases: the average survival from the first symptom to death was approximately 31 months and only four patients in this untreated group lived more than 3 years. When metastases were evident at the initial presentation, 2/3 of these patients died within 9 months. In a group of 125 patients in whom cystostomy was carried out for outflow obstruction, the average survival was 57 months and this represented the best 'treatment' group. A collected series of 795 untreated patients was used by Nesbit and Baum (1950) as the (historical) control group against which they compared their early experience with endocrine treatment. The 5 year survival rate with no metastases at the time of admission was 10 % and 6 % if metastases were present. These data are in striking contrast with current survival rates for patients with non-metastatic disease (irrespective of the primary treatment) which are 40–50 % after 10 years and 20–30 % after 15 years (Chisholm, 1980).

The discussion so far has concerned *clinically* diagnosed prostatic cancer. In 1954, Franks introduced the term *latent* carcinoma for tumours that do not produce signs or symptoms and are found incidentally as with a prostatectomy. He also described a third type – the *occult* tumour which manifested itself by its metastases but the primary tumour remained hidden

(Franks, 1956). There are many reports of an increased incidence of latent cancer with age (Hirst and Bergman, 1954) and a summary of collected data is given in Table 10.1.

Table 10.1 Incidence of latent carcinoma with age (collected data from Gaynor (1938) and Franks (1977))

Age groups (yrs)	Incidence of carcinoma % (postmortem studies)	Number studied
20–29	0	19
30–39	3.0	33
40–49	4.3	140
50–59	12.9	279
60–69	19.2	365
70–79	30.9	307
80–89	43.6	110

The reliability of such data is dependent upon the number of histological sections examined from the prostate. For data obtained from operative specimens there are considerable problems in comparing the study of an enucleated gland with a study of tissue removed by transurethral resection. Thus any study that seeks to determine the incidence of focal tumours is dependent upon the diligence of the pathologist in his examination of the tissues. It is of interest that the proportion of patients with incidental or latent carcinoma diagnosed at prostatectomy appears to have increased in recent years. In 1970, Varkarakis *et al.* reported that 31 of 629 (4.9 %) prostatectomy specimens had incidentally diagnosed carcinoma; other reports up to that time showed an incidence of 9–16 %. More recently the proportion of incidental carcinoma has been reported to be much higher ranging from 37 % (Donohue *et al.*, 1979) to 53 % (McMillen and Wettlaufer, 1976). In the authors' experience 24 of a consecutive series of 100 new cases had incidental carcinoma. Thus this increasing incidence is now close to or even exceeds the incidence reported from postmortem studies (Table 10.1).

An explanation for such a change can be sought from three directions:

(1) Is there an overall increase in the incidence of this disease? Between 1950 and 1970, the reported incidence of prostatic carcinoma in the US did increase from 17 to 21 per 100 000 population (Enstrom and Austin, 1977) while in the same period mortality rates decreased from 7.5 to 7.0 per 100 000. Thus *part* of the increase in incidental tumours can be accounted for.

(2) Is the disease presenting in an earlier age group? There has been no significant change in the number of registrations per decade of age over the period 1968–1977 in Scotland (Fig 10.1).

(3) Are prostatectomies (transurethral resections) being carried out either more frequently or at an earlier age? Although there is a trend towards

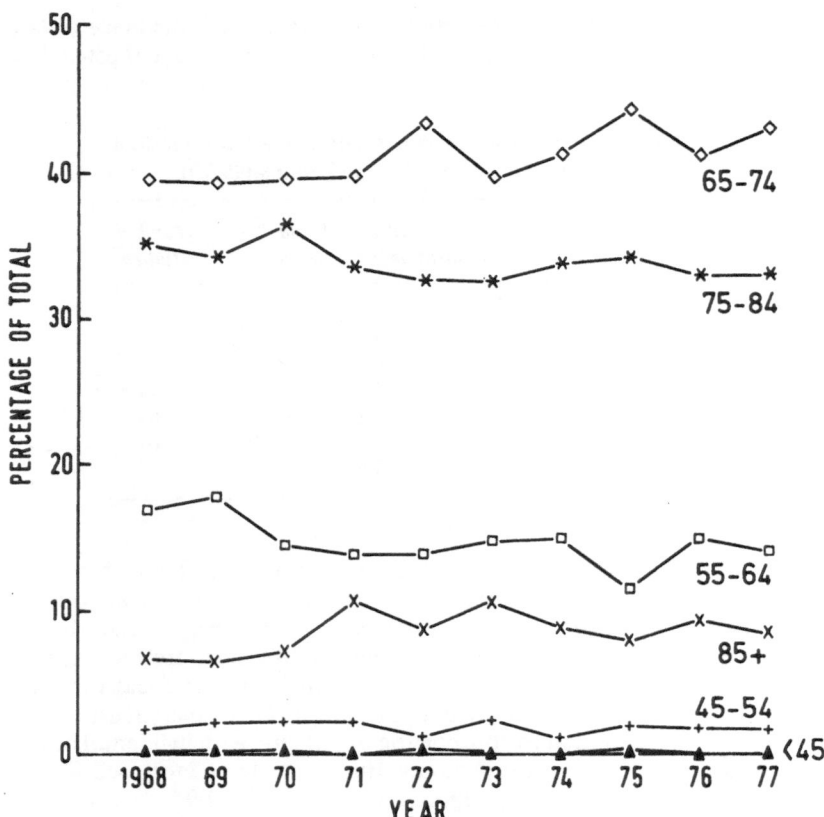

Figure 10.1 Carcinoma of the prostate: number of registrations (percentage of total) by age group and year, Scotland, 1968–77. Source: Cancer Register

an increasing number of 65–74 year olds receiving treatment for obstructive outflow tract symptoms, this has not so far been reflected in reported statistics. If it should prove to be true then this too may add to the trend for an increasing incidence of earlier disease.

The clinical evidence of these trends may be seen from the data just described. With an increasing incidence and decreased mortality rate, the 5 year survival rate has improved from 30 to 59 %. Klein (1979) has stated that 'it is (therefore) erroneous to assume that improved survival is due to improved treatment'. But this is to ignore the fact that for the early, focal, incidental tumour, the prostatectomy was an effective treatment and it could be argued that the data support this.

Of greater concern is whether or not *all* of these incidentally diagnosed tumours have the same favourable natural history. Byar (1973) claimed that survival rates for patients with incidental carcinoma were similar to those of a matched control population. The reliability of this statement is of great practical importance. If it were true that all incidentally diagnosed carcinomas behaved so favourably then there would be no need to consider treatment for these patients. However, as might be suspected, the group is heterogeneous. Some well differentiated tumours will metastasize (Kern, 1978) and those with poor differentiation have a poorer prognosis (Beynon *et al.*, 1981). Other prognostic factors appear to be age (Hanash *et al.*, 1972), tumour bulk (de Vere White *et al.*, 1977) and proximity of tumour to the margin of the resection (Bauer *et al.*, 1960).

Thus the natural history of the incidentally diagnosed or latent tumour remains uncertain. In an attempt to clarify this issue the authors reviewed the histology of 28 untreated cases and used the Gleason method for quantification of these tumours (Gleason *et al.*, 1974). The presence of metastases at diagnosis and the progression to metastases both correlated well with poor histological grade. It was concluded that the natural history of these early tumours was dependent mainly on the histological grade and that a careful grading system is necessary to both classify these patients and to anticipate their prognosis.

It is these changes in our knowledge and in the patterns of natural history of this disease that make it so important to have a proper comparative group in any clinical trial of treatment.

10.2 MONITORING THE RESPONSE

There are four particular points that make the monitoring of response of this tumour difficult.

(1) Although the gland is accessible by rectal examination, it is only so to a limited extent.

(2) The progress of this disease is slow so that serial clinical examinations are generally unreliable and the available tumour markers imprecise.

(3) Carcinoma of the prostate affects the older male (the mean age at presentation in most series is about 70 years) so that these patients are in an age group in which other diseases, especially cardiovascular, are common and will cause problems in monitoring subjective changes.

(4) Some of those patients with incidentally diagnosed untreated prostatic tumours can have a normal life expectancy; thus almost any treatment given to such a patient would give a successful response.

There are therefore considerable difficulties in following the progress of the disease and this has led to definitions of criteria of response most of which are cumbersome to describe and often awkward to apply (see later). Nevertheless, there remains a clear need for such rules in order that the value of any new or different treatment can be reliably evaluated.

Any set of criteria of response must consider both objective and subjective responses. The ability to measure an objective response is a most important aspect of any clinical trial and, indeed, without something to measure there can be no end point to mark response or lack of response to treatment. The expression *evaluable disease** in the context of the prostate refers either to the palpably abnormal primary tumour or to lymph nodes, to bone, to soft tissue metastases or to biochemical tumour markers. A change in any of these is an objective response.

In Phase II clinical trials, which are designed to establish whether a new drug has anti tumour activity worthy of further clinical evaluation, the duration of the trial is usually short (e.g. 3 months) so that the patient must have evaluable disease in order to record objective responses. In Phase III clinical trials, where different drugs or treatment regimes are compared, the need for evaluable disease is less critical and subjective responses, the length of survival and the metastasis-free interval may all be important measures of the response.

10.2.1 Objective criteria of response

10.2.1.1 The primary prostatic tumour

10.2.1.1.1 Size and extent of tumour – The TNM (UICC 1978) description of the primary tumour has six categories:

T   is pre-invasive carcinoma (carcinoma *in situ*).
T0 no palpable tumour (incidental finding at operation or on biopsy).
T1 tumour intracapsular surrounded by palpably normal gland.
T2 tumour confined to the gland. Smooth nodule deforming contour but lateral sulci and seminal vesicles not involved.
T3 tumour extending beyond the capsule with or without involvement of the lateral sulci and/or seminal vesicles.
T4 tumour fixed or infiltrating neighbouring structures.

Reliance upon digital assessment of the primary tumour immediately indicates a serious source of error in the use of this category. Jewett (1975) has reminded us that 50 % of palpably suspicious nodules of the prostate prove to be benign. Thus even the so called educated finger of the urologist is liable to subjective error in describing the size, extent and consistency of the gland. Add to this the well-known variation between observers and also the length of time between assessments and it must be admitted that this is a poor measurement to use in following the progress of the disease (Chisholm, 1981).

Quantification of tumour size has been attempted but generally thought to be too subjective. Byar (1977) has described the VACURG experience. The primary tumour size was drawn on a standard diagram and its surface area estimated in square centimetres. The results showed that there was a good correlation between the size of the primary lesion and probability of death from carcinoma of the prostate.

Recently, the imaging techniques of ultrasound and computerized tomography have been used to judge both tumour size and tumour morphology

---

* The word 'evaluable' is also used for those *patients* in whom the trial protocol has been followed precisely and there are the required data for analysis (Carter *et al.*, 1977).

(Peeling *et al.*, 1979). The use of improved ultrasonic transrectal and transurethral scanning equipment may be of increasing value in monitoring local response of the prostate to treatment (Gammelgaard and Holm, 1980).

10.2.1.1.2 Histological and cytological monitoring of response – The use of serial biopsies to monitor the response of a prostatic tumour to treatment has been advocated but has not proved to be very useful. A transrectal needle biopsy, repeated as an out-patient procedure, at 6 monthly intervals, is feasible whereas a perineal needle biopsy requiring an anaesthetic is not. A more important practical limitation of the repeated biopsy is the problem of interpreting the biopsy. The characteristic effect of endocrine treatment is pyknosis of the cell nuclei and vacuolar degeneration of the cell cytoplasm. These changes may take several months to develop (Esposti, 1971) and even then the precise significance of these findings remains unclear. This problem has been emphasized more recently by the finding that approximately 50 % of those patients treated by primary radiotherapy have, on biopsy at 1 year, malignant cells that show no evidence of treatment (Cox and Stoffel, 1977; Nachtsheim *et al.*, 1978).

Serial cytological studies have proved popular in some centres. Kurth *et al.* (1977) have followed the progress of patients treated by primary radiotherapy, others have used cytological data for monitoring hormone treatment (Spieler *et al.*, 1976) and chemotherapy (Estracyt) (Leistenschneider and Nagel, 1980).

10.2.1.2 Secondary spread from prostatic cancer

10.2.1.2.1 Lymph node metastases – It is now known that lymph node metastases are far more common than is clinically evident and probably antedate metastases to bone (Whitmore *et al.*, 1974; McLaughlin *et al.*, 1976; Chisholm, 1980). The data for this statement have been gathered from a number of studies reporting the relationship between pelvic lymph node biopsies and the primary tumour. Unfortunately pedal lymphography is too unreliable to be of value either in diagnosis or in monitoring the disease so that only palpable nodes, as in the groin or neck, can be used to monitor the course of the disease.

10.2.1.2.2 Bone metastases – In contrast to lymph node metastases, monitoring skeletal metastases by radioisotope bone scans is non-invasive, reproducible and reliable (Fitzpatrick *et al.*, 1978). It is important to emphasize that the technology of bone scanning cannot be assumed to be the same in all centres. The reliability of the bone scan depends not only on high resolution scanning equipment but also upon careful exclusion of other causes of 'hot spots' by appropriate radiography. Careful attention to detail makes this test a most reliable monitor of the progress of bone metastases: in fact it could be regarded as a tumour marker (Stone *et al.*, 1980). In both progression and regression the altered scan may precede changes in serum acid phosphatase and X-ray and in some cases may be the only evidence of response (Chisholm and Habib, 1981).

Quantification of the bone scan has been attempted but no satisfactory methods described. Stone *et al.* (1980) simply counted the number of metastases or the number of involved areas on the scan and found this satisfactory. A method for quantifying X-rays was described by Hovsepian *et al.* (1975) who suggested that the body should be divided into eight sites: shoulders, ribs, lungs, thoracic spine, lumbar-sacral spine, ilia, pubis-ischia and femoral heads/necks. The area of involvement at each site is graded as follows:

Grade 0 – no involvement
Grade 1 – < 25 % of the groin site involved by metastases
Grade 2 – 25–75 % involved
Grade 3 – > 75 % involved

It was found that in untreated carcinoma of the prostate, there was a good correlation between the estimation of the area involved and the survival of the patient.

It has been stated that a favourable response to treatment will render the bone scan insensitive to changes in the course of the disease (Buck *et al.*, 1977). Whether decreased activity represents true regression of the metastasis or simply depression of the osteoblastic response is not known but the scan changes accurately reflect the clinical course and can be used as a reliable clinical monitor.

10.2.1.2.3 Pulmonary metastases – Metastatic involvement of the lung characteristically takes the form of lymphangitic infiltration rather than tumour nodules as in other cancers. These appearances must be distinguished from congestive heart failure or chronic lung disease. Failure to diagnose these latter conditions could easily give a false positive 'improvement' in the lung fields with treatment. Malignant infiltration of the lungs is rare so that this feature is not often available to monitor the progress of a patient.

10.2.1.2.4 Visceral metastases – Liver or cerebral metastases are also relatively uncommon. The accuracy of diagnosis is not very high and these abnormalities can only occasionally be used as objective measures of response.

10.2.1.2.5 Other metastases – Skin metastases or even a metastasis into a corpus cavernosum provide a rare opportunity to monitor progress in that patient but they have no relevance in a clinical trial.

10.2.2 Tumour markers in prostatic cancer

10.2.2.1 Acid phosphatase

Nearly 50 years ago it was observed that normal adult prostatic epithelium had a high acid phosphatase content and that carcinomatous prostatic tissue as well as metastases were also rich in acid phosphatase. Thus the malignant growth appeared to be an overgrowth of adult prostatic epithelium and since this was already known to be influenced by androgens, endocrine manipulation of the gland was studied. In 1941 Huggins and Hodges reported the successful control of this tumour by giving oestrogens or by orchiectomy.

Gutman and Gutman (1938) found that many patients with metastatic cancer had significantly raised serum acid phosphatase and Huggins and Hodges (1941) used the measurement of both acid and alkaline phosphatase as a marker for tumour responsiveness. While the basis of these earlier observations remains correct, considerable controversy has been generated over the reliability of acid phosphatase as a tumour marker.

When the serum acid phosphatase is estimated in a large number of patients, most patients with benign hyperplasia and localized carcinoma have normal levels, whereas half of those with locally invasive tumours and most with distant metastases have elevated levels. A small proportion (< 5%) of patients with benign hyperplasia and some patients with prostatic infarct, myeloma osteogenic sarcoma, thromboembolic disease and thrombocytopaenia can also have raised levels. Thus interpretation of a raised serum acid phosphatase must be made with care; likewise, a normal level does not exclude metastatic disease.

The reason for these variations in patients with proven malignant disease lies mainly in the cellular differentiation of the tumour. Well differentiated cancer cells contain more acid phosphatase than poorly differentiated rapidly progressing tumours but this observation does not correlate well with serum acid phosphatase levels; a poorly differentiated tumour is often not associated with high acid phosphatase levels. However, in the majority of cases, the serum levels of acid and alkaline phosphatase *are* related to prognosis and the response to treatment. The most practical aspect is the use of serial measurement, when the values are raised, to monitor the effect of treatment. There is general agreement that a 50% change in the value is of prognostic significance.

Recent interest has focused on improving the sensitivity of the methods of measuring serum acid phosphatase. Three new techniques are being studied: radioimmunoassay, counter immune electrophoresis and immunofluoroassay. Although preliminary results by Foti *et al.* (1977) were encouraging, both the sensitivity and specificity of the assays require a further evaluation before the so-called standard methods are abandoned.

10.2.2.2 Alkaline phosphatase

Alkaline phosphatases are non-specific for prostatic cancer, but are elevated in patients with bone metastases. Many authors consider that the level of alkaline phosphatase is important when taken in relation to acid phosphatase measurements (Fitzpatrick *et al.*, 1978; Paulson *et al.*, 1979). An initial rise in alkaline phosphatase may represent new reactive bone formation associated with healing of metastases and subsequently, as the bone reaction becomes inactive, it falls to normal levels. Such a sequence was first noted to be accompanied by a good response to treatment by Huggins and Hodges in 1941.

10.2.2.3 Other tumour markers

A range of other tests has been examined in the search for better tumour markers but their practical value is disappointing. Serial CEA levels do not correlate well with clinical changes (Guinan *et al.*, 1974). Tumour associated antigens (Brannen *et al.*, 1975) and polyamines (Cohen, 1977) have not achieved the role of useful markers in carcinoma of the prostate. Urinary hydroxyproline has been shown to be of value in monitoring the patient but its use has not gained wide support (Mundy, 1979). The use of steroid receptors and, in particular, androgen receptors as a marker in prostatic cancer is discussed in Chapter 9.

10.2.3 Length of survival (survival times, time to progression)

The survival time of a patient with cancer is a major index of the response to treatment. Although death provides an end point that can hardly be debated, the cause of death can be varied and this introduces several possibilities for erroneous or misleading conclusions. Death may be due to treatment toxicity or to unrelated other disease. Determining the exact cause of death can be difficult especially if the patient should die at home or in an institution. Even when there is an autopsy there may be some doubt as to whether the tumour was responsible for death. The well-known VACURG studies brought to the attention of the urologist the fact that cardiovascular complications due to oestrogen treatment were important causes of morbidity and mortality (Byar, 1977).

Deaths may be classified:

(1) Due to disease,
(2) Disease related, e.g. renal failure,
(3) Treatment related, e.g. cardiovascular or cytotoxic complications,
(4) Not related to disease or treatment.

Analysis of deaths should first include all causes and then, if possible, the separate causes. Survival time as a criterion of response concerns Phase III clinical trials where substantial numbers of patients are usually entered. Thus the same number of deaths from intercurrent disease can be expected in each treatment arm and the deaths due to or related to prostatic cancer will be apparent. Correction of survival time for age is important in this disease where the mean age at presentation is about 70 years.

Survival time need not necessarily mean survival until death. The 'time' recorded may be the length of response, time to recurrence of disease, time from start of treatment to first response, etc. (Gehan, 1975). Thus in carcinoma of the prostate, in addition to survival time (to death), the time from starting treatment to progression of disease can be recorded and, in those patients with no metastases, the time from diagnosis to the first evidence of metastasis. These are important end points that indicate the failure of the primary treatment but, as with all criteria of response, the reliability of these end points is dependent upon the frequency and detail of the follow-up.

10.2.4 Subjective criteria of response

The use of subjective criteria to monitor the response of prostatic cancer to treatment is debatable. Stoll (1972) has pointed out that palliation is common (66 %) in those whom there is objective evidence of progression.

The problems are that the criteria are difficult to quantify and that changes in the criteria may not necessarily be due to the disease. Such examples are the difficulty in defining the need for analgesics and how to ensure that a fall in weight is due to a tumour effect.

Nevertheless it is these subjective criteria that determine the quality of life for the patient and he is likely to be more impressed with this than the exact number of months he survives.

The criteria usually monitored for a subjective response are:

(1)   activity grading,
(2)   analgesic requirement,
(3)   weight change, and
(4)   other symptoms.

Some studies also include the 'non-specific' criteria of haemoglobulin and erythrocytes sedimentation rate (ESR). Thus, all of these are factors that are influenced not only by the tumour regression or progression while on treatment but also by non-specific effects that can be due to good patient care, e.g. analgesia, treatment of anaemia and diet.

Analysis of these non-specific criteria by both Byar (1977) and Kvols et al. (1977) demonstrate different approaches to providing a guide to tumour response. Byar used 11 factors for his multivarate risk factor model. Kvols used six – pain, performance status, weight, haemoglobulin and total acid and alkaline phosphatases (Table 10.2).

Table 10.2 Ancillary Score System (Kvols et al., 1977) for quantifying patient response in prostatic cancer

Ancillary factors	Score and changes*			
	0	1	2	4
Pain	none	improved	stable	worse
Performance status	asymptomatic	improved	stable	worse
Weight (%)	normal	increased >5	stable	decreased >5
Haemoglobin (g/100 ml)	normal (13 g/100 ml)	increased >1	stable	decreased >1
Total acid & alkaline phosphatases	normal	decreased >25	stable	increased >25

* Overall score of 9 or less considered a response; overall score of 10–14 considered stable; overall score >15 considered progression

10.2.5 Rules for criteria of response

There are no universally accepted rules for defining the criteria of response and, as a result, each group involved in assessing such responses has produced its own set of rules. Thus the British Prostate Group (BPG), National Prostatic Cancer Project (NPCP), Eastern Cooperative Oncological Groups (ECOG) and the European Organization for Research and Treatment of Cancer (EORTC) all have their own specific rules for criteria of response. It has to be admitted that efforts to simplify the rules invariably fail for competent clinicians can easily see alternative interpretations unless the rules are detailed and almost laborious.

All sets of rules have four divisions for objective response and one subjective response.

(1) Complete objective response,
(2) partial objective response,
(3) no change or stable state,
(4) progressive response, and
(5) subjective response.

The details of the criteria for response recommended by the British Prostate Group are shown in Tables 10.3 and 10.4.

10.3 PRIMARY TREATMENT

The selection of primary treatment for a patient with carcinoma of prostate is based on the clinician's assessment of tumour stage and grade and the prognostic significance of this assessment based on a knowledge of the patient's age and general health. Radical therapy, be it surgical or radiotherapeutic, should be reserved for those most likely to benefit, allowing for the inadequacies of clinical staging.

10.3.1 Surgery

The relief of bladder outlet obstruction by transurethral resection of the prostate allows the patient rapid symptomatic benefit and the clinician adequate histological material. The option of prolonged catheterization while awaiting hormone induced local tumour regression carries a significant morbidity and is tiresome for the patient. The possibility remains, however, that partial resection of the tumour may encourage dissemination of tumour cells into the circulation and increase the incidence of later metastases (McGowan, 1980).

Radical prostatectomy by either the retropubic or perineal route has gained favour mainly in North America. Applied to patients with clinically localized tumours, 33 % 15 year tumour-free survival has been reported (Jewett, 1975). The incidence of urinary continence problems and impotence is high with this form of surgery and the clinical results reported suggest that it should be used only in patients with palpable disease confined within the prostatic capsule.

10.3.2 Deferred treatment

The use of radiotherapy or hormonal therapy can be delayed until patients develop signs or symptoms of local or metastatic disease progression. Byar

Table 10.3 Criteria for *objective* responses in carcinoma of the prostate

Complete objective regression
No tumour palpable (TO) and
No evidence of distant metastases (MO)
(Note: lymph nodes not assessed = NX)

Partial objective regression Any of the following
Reduction in primary tumour by one or more T category
Reduction in primary tumour area by 50%
Return to normal serum acid phosphatase, if elevated
Reduction in size of soft tissue metastases by 50%
Recalcification of any osteolytic metastases, if present
(Note: regression in primary tumour but other evidence of progression = objective progression)

Stable response
No changes in T and M categories
(Note: there must be documented progression of disease prior to this response)

Objective progression Any of the following
Increase in primary tumour by one or more T category
Increase in primary tumour area by 50%
Increase in serum acid phosphatase on 2 or more occasions (state levels)
Increase in size of soft tissue metastases by 50%
New bony lesions on scans/X-ray

Table 10.4 Criteria for *subjective* responses in carcinoma of the prostate

At least a 2 point reduction in the overall subjective score:
(Note: a score system is recommended (see also Table 10.2))

(1) *Activity grade*	0	Normal activity, no symptoms
	1	Restricted activity but ambulatory
	2	Confined to bed <50% of time
	3	Confined to bed >50% of time
	4	Bedridden 100% of time (Reference: Karnofsky, 1961)
(2) *Pain*	0	No analgesia
	1	Occasional non-narcotics
	2	Frequent non-narcotics
	3	Occasional oral narcotics
	4	Frequent oral narcotics
	5	Parenteral narcotics
(3) *Weight*	0	No change or weight gain
	1	>10% weight loss
(4) *Other symptoms*	0	None
	1	Mild
	2	Moderate
	3	Severe

(1977) claimed that survival figures for patients with incidentally diagnosed carcinoma of prostate were similar to those of a matched control population. Despite this report there seems little doubt that patients with locally unsuspected tumours do not form a homogenous group since those with diffuse or multifocal involvement of the gland have a poorer prognosis than those with tumour localized in one lobe (de Vere White *et al.*, 1977). This finding may reflect the poorer histological grade of these more extensive tumours (Bauer *et al.*, 1960).

The Veterans Administration studies have revealed the importance of cardiovascular deaths in patients treated with oestrogen and have identified as high risk groups those with a previous history of cardiovascular disease and those over the age of 75. This raises the question of whether deferred treatment is justified in patients with advanced prostatic cancer who are, at the time of diagnosis, symptom free. Measurement of not only survival time but subjective factors such as performance and pain makes this a difficult study but there was no evidence in the Veterans studies that initial treatment with placebo, delaying oestrogen treatment until it was required for control of symptoms, adversely affected the patients in any way (Byar, 1977).

10.3.3 Radiotherapy

Although radiation therapy for prostatic carcinoma has been used since the 1920s it is only in the past 15 years that results to match those of other forms of treatment have been achieved. This change has been due to improvements in both staging of the disease and treatment techniques.

Whether megavoltage external beam irradiation or interstitial implantation with ^{198}Au or ^{125}I is used, the aim of treatment is a cure and so this form of therapy is restricted to patients without evidence of distant metastases. The inaccuracy of pedal lymphography makes assessment of pelvic lymph node involvement difficult, and so many external beam treatments cover the whole pelvis with additional therapy to the prostate. The advantage of open isotope implantation is that it allows pelvic lymph node biopsy, but the theoretical advantages of improved local dosimetry are not easy to achieve in practice (Shipley *et al.*, 1980).

Complication rates following radiation therapy vary in different series but a large percentage will develop troublesome proctitis and in about 5 % this will persist for a year or longer. A similar percentage will suffer significant urinary symptoms with urethral stricture formation in some. Potency is retained in 50–60 % of patients (Bagshaw *et al.*, 1975).

Reference has already been made to the difficulties in assessing the response to treatment. Digital examination of the prostate is unreliable after radiotherapy because of the changes in periprostatic as well as prostatic tissues. The result of prostatic biopsy is also difficult to interpret (Kiesling *et al.*, 1980; Cox and Stoffel, 1977) because of the following reasons:

(1) Possible slow tumour regression over at least the first year.
(2) The possibility of false negative biopsies.
(3) The difficulty in attributing viability to residual tumour tissue.

Although not a universal finding, a highly significant association is reported between tumour grade and both patient survival and disease free interval (Cupps *et al.*, 1980). This may in part be a reflection of undetected micrometastases from poorly differentiated tumours rather than a difference in radio sensitivity.

The results of treatment are difficult to compare between centres because of rapid improvements and variation in technique but for tumours with no extra capsular spread a 5 year survival of 80 % can be expected with a corresponding figure around 50 % for locally advanced disease (Cupps *et al.*, 1980). There is no evidence that radiotherapy alters the response to later oestrogen therapy should it be required.

10.3.4 Endocrine treatment

When Huggins and Hodges (1941) first described the symptomatic and biochemical changes in patients with advanced prostatic carcinoma treated by orchiectomy or with oestrogen, the benefits were so dramatic that there seemed little question that the same treatment would produce improved survival in all patients shown to have hormone sensitive tumours. The first Veterans Administration Cooperative Urological Research Group (VACURG) study (1967) not only dispelled this illusion, but demonstrated that those patients receiving oestrogen in the dose of stilboestrol 5 mg daily had a poorer survival than those treated with placebo. This difference was due to increased deaths from cardiovascular causes, tended to occur in the first year of therapy and was found to occur predominantly in patients with a previous history of cardiovascular problems and in those over 75 years of age. The results of this study have profoundly influenced later work on hormone therapy (Byar, 1973) but the timing and precise indications for endocrine manipulation remain a subject of controversy. Although survival is not altered by immediate treatment and palliation is no worse if treatment is withheld until the onset of symptomatic progression (Byar, 1977) it is still the practice in many centres to use hormone therapy in all cases of metastatic disease from the time of diagnosis. Once the decision to treat has been made, the choice of regimes available is a wide one.

10.3.4.1 Stilboestrol

The widely used synthetic oestrogen, stilboestrol is generally used in a dose of 1 mg t.d.s., although no clinical data on the incidence of cardiovascular side effects at this dosage are available. The lower dose of 1 mg daily does not produce consistent suppression of plasma testosterone (Shearer *et al.*, 1973) although it may not be valid to equate antitumour effect with testosterone levels (Resnick and Grayhack, 1975). Certainly the 1 mg dose was found to be as effective as the 5 mg dose in controlling cancer in both locally advanced and metastatic groups in the second VACURG study. Gynaecomastia and impotence are significant side-effects of stilboestrol therapy.

10.3.4.2 Orchiectomy

Although it was concluded from the VACURG study I (1967) that oestrogen was more effective than orchiectomy in preventing cancer deaths (Byar, 1977), orchiectomy does have advantages to the patient. The need for continuous medication is avoided, there are no cardiovascular complications, gynae-comastia does not occur and impotence is not invariable. Some patients do however suffer 'hot flushes'. The operation of subcapsular orchiectomy is aesthetically and psychologically more acceptable to many patients than simple castration and when carefully performed produces effective androgen suppression (Clark and Houghton, 1977). The combination of oestrogen and orchiectomy has not been shown to have any therapeutic advantage over either treatment alone (Byar, 1977).

It has been suggested that orchiectomy is more effective than oestrogen or antiandrogen therapy in patients with ureteric obstruction (Michigan and Catalona, 1977) but the hormone treatment group in this study was too small to be conclusive.

10.3.4.3 Other drugs

Stilboestrol diphosphate (Honvan) can be given by mouth or intravenously. By the latter route high blood levels of stilboestrol are achieved and it is suggested that the high acid phosphatase concentration in the prostate results in increased dephosphorylation at the site, thus maximizing the cytotoxic effect of stilboestrol on the malignant cells. These high levels are almost certainly transient but a regime of 300–600 mg daily i.v for 2–4 weeks followed by an oral dose of 120–600 mg daily finds favour in many centres.

Chlortrianisene (TACE) is a synthetic compound developed from stilboes-trol. Claimed to have fewer side effects than other oestrogens, it directly inhibits testicular androgen production without depressing gonadotrophin levels. It may be of value in cases of gastrointestinal intolerance to stilboestrol.

Dienoestrol in a dose of 0.15–1 mg daily has been widely used for many years but manufacturing health hazards have now made it less readily available in the UK.

Polyoestradiol phosphate (Estradurin) is a polymerized oestrogen which by slow dephosphorylation provides a long acting preparation. Monthly i.m. injection of 80–160 mg provides a constant oestrogenic effect.

Attempts to localize a chemotherapeutic effect in the prostate have led to the development of estramustine phosphate (Estracyt), a combination of oestradiol and nitrogen mustard gas. There have been favourable reports of its use as primary treatment in advanced cases (Jönsson and Hogberg, 1971) of metastatic cancer.

Some progestogens have the ability to suppress gonadotrophin production, to inhibit testicular steroid production and to directly inhibit the intracellular prostatic effects of testosterone. In addition they have the advantage of avoiding feminization and the cardiovascular side effects of oestrogen therapy. Medroxyprogesterone (Provera) has been included in the VA Study III with no advantage recorded to date over 1 mg stilboestrol daily. Cyproterone acetate (Cyprostat) has a direct antiandrogen effect but is expensive. It is currently being evaluated in patients with metastatic disease in several clinical trials; early reports indicate fewer side effects and complications when compared with oestrogens. 'The British Prostate Group trial of stilboestrol (1 mg tds), cyproterone acetate (100 mg bd) and orchiectomy show no differences in the uncorrected survival data but other details are not yet available.'

10.4 SECONDARY OR FAILED PRIMARY TREATMENT

It has long been known that approximately 20 % of prostatic tumours show little or no response to hormone treatment. Identification of these non-responders prior to treatment is at present impossible but in clinical terms they can usually be identified in cases of metastatic disease within 3 months of starting treatment.

In those cases where primary hormone therapy is successful in producing stabilization or regression of disease, later resistance to treatment or 'oestrogen escape' may occur. Although clinically this may appear to be a fairly sudden event, the emergence of these androgen independent cells, whether by selective cell population growth or dedifferentiation and consequent metabolic adaptation, is probably a gradual process. Thus, the endpoint at which secondary treatment is indicated may be difficult to define. Average survival time following relapse after endocrine therapy is 6 months (Scott *et al.*, 1975).

10.4.1 Hormone treatment

As the different physiological mechanisms for hormone control of prostatic cancer have become more accurately defined, the rationale for changing the drug or dose in the 'oestrogen-escaped' patient has been if anything more compelling. Nesbit and Baum (1950) claimed significant benefit when relapse followed orchiectomy by adding oestrogen, and additional benefit when relapse occurred in oestrogen therapy from carrying out castration, but the criteria of response were inadequate. The VA Study I did not demonstrate any benefit from the combination of orchiectomy and oestrogen when compared with either treatment alone and in 'oestrogen-escaped' patients Stone *et al.* (1980) found no objective evidence of a response to secondary orchiectomy and only a 20 % subjective response.

Adrenalectomy to remove extragonadal sources of androgen has produced disappointing results (Brendler, 1973) and attempts at a similar effect pharmacologically using aminoglutethamide have produced little benefit.

10.4.2 Hypophysectomy

The mechanism of action of hypophysectomy in relieving metastatic bone pain is not understood. While it does not improve survival, it does provide dramatic symptomatic benefit in up to 80 % of cases of those with metastatic pain and long pain-free survivals can occur after successful ablation of the pituitary (Fitzpatrick *et al.*, 1980). The results of this procedure do not appear to relate to prior hormone responsiveness or the length of hormone remission.

10.4.3 Chemotherapy

The difficulty in assessing response in these patients has made the investigation of chemotherapy for prostatic cancer a slow and often unrewarding task. Several agents have demonstrated antitumour activity, 5-fluorouracil, cyclophosphamide, nitrogen mustard, razoxane, adriamycin, hydroxyurea and cisplatinum being some of the more promising. Others, such as streptozotocin, melphalan, vincristine, methyl CCNU and hexamethylmelamine have proved to be either ineffective or toxic or both and often incompletely assessed. Further investigation of the active drugs either singly or in combination regimes will be required in collaborative controlled studies with tightly defined response criteria (Schmidt, 1980).

Combination drugs such as Estracyt and Prednimustine (an ester of chlorambucil plus prednisone) have also been studied in patients with 'oestrogen-escaped' tumours. In this patient group Estracyt produces a subjective response rate of 20–30 % and an objective response rate of approximately 15 % (Chisholm et al., 1977).

10.4.4 Radiotherapy

Localized bone metastases pain can often be quickly alleviated by a short course of palliative radiotherapy. This treatment can be repeated at several sites if required.

10.4.5 Analgesia

When other treatment modalities have failed it is important to achieve adequate pain control during terminal care. The non-steroidal anti-inflammatory drug Froben has been found of great benefit in ambulatory patients and the administration of glucocorticoids may enhance the patient's feeling of well-being. Local analgesia by nerve 'blocks' is helpful in some patients. Opiates when required should be given regularly and the patient's family given adequate nursing support with home, hospital or hospice care.

10.5 CONCLUSIONS

Carcinoma of the prostate is a common tumour, second only to carcinoma of the lung in the male. Thus it might be expected that its management would, by now, have become established along certain standard lines. This is not so and because of the variations in the choice of treatment, only a consensus opinion of management has been given in this chapter.

There is no debate that the malignant prostate *does* respond to endocrine treatment in most cases. However, because the treatment is palliative there remains a strong desire to treat the localized tumour by something that will be curative. Surgery or radiotherapy appear to offer such a choice but unfortunately there are no data that adequately support the claims for either treatment, compared to so-called standard endocrine treatment.

Clinical trials in an elderly population are difficult to carry out for any condition, but carcinoma of the prostate is especially difficult because of the limitations in monitoring the course of the disease and its response to treatment. An approach to the problems of monitoring response is given in detail in this chapter to emphasize and illustrate the present 'state of the art'. It will be evident that most of the present methods are unsatisfactory and it will also be evident that, even applying these criteria carefully, it is possible to produce data that are quite misleading. Nowhere is this better illustrated than in the many unhelpful reports of 'encouraging results' with various chemotherapeutic agents.

Despite these negative comments there has in fact been very substantial progress in understanding many aspects of this tumour. Even the appreciation that the diagnosis of carcinoma of the prostate does not automatically indicate hormone treatment, is important. Greater care in staging now enables the clinician to select the most appropriate management plan.

A major challenge for the future is to find an effective method for treatment for those who no longer respond to endocrine treatment. At present the choice is very limited and only chemotherapy offers any reasonable prospect. The fact that this is a hormone responsive tumour should not be overlooked and some combination of endocrine treatment and chemotherapy still appears the most logical approach for the future.

10.6 REFERENCES

Bagshaw, M. A., Ray, G. R., Pistenma, D. A., Castellino, R. A. and Meares, E. M., Jr. (1975). External beam radiation therapy of primary carcinoma of the prostate. *Cancer*, **36**, 723

Bauer, W. C., McGavran, M. H. and Carlin, M. R. (1960). Unsuspected carcinoma of prostate in suprapubic prostatectomy specimens: a clinicopathological study of 55 consecutive cases. *Cancer*, **13**, 370

Beynon, L. L., Busuttil, A. and Chisholm, G. D. (1981). Pathological characteristics and prognosis of patients with category TO carcinoma of the prostate. (Abstract). *Clin. Oncol.*, **7**, 259

Brannen, G., Gomolka, D. and Coffey, D. (1975). Specificity of cell membrane antigens in prostatic cancer. *Cancer Chemother. Rep.*, **59**, 127

Brendler, H. (1973). Adrenalectomy and hypophysectomy for prostatic cancer. *Urology*, **2**, 99

Buck, A. C., Chisholm, G. D. and Merrick, M. V. (1977). Follow-up of prostate carcinoma with serial bone scanning using cyclotron-produced 18-fluorine. *Recent Results Cancer Res.*, **60**, 91

Bumpus, H. C. (1926). Carcinoma of the prostate: a clinical study of 1000 cases. *Surg. Gynecol. Obstet.*, **43**, 150

Byar, D. P. (1973). The Veterans Administration Co-operative Urological Research Group's studies of cancer of the prostate. *Cancer*, **32**, 1126

Byar, D. P. (1977). VACURG studies on prostatic cancer and its treatment. In Tannenbaum, M. (ed.) *Urologic Pathology: the Prostate*. pp. 241–267. (New York: Lea and Febiger)

Carter, S. K., Bakowski, M. T. and Hellman, K. (1977). *Chemotherapy of Cancer*. (New York: Wiley)

Chisholm, G. D., O'Donoghue, E. P. N. and Kennedy, C. L. (1977). The treatment of oestrogen-escaped carcinoma of the prostate with estramustine phosphate. *Br. J. Urol.*, **49**, 717

Chisholm, G. D. (1980). Urological malignancy: prostate. In Chisholm, G. D. (ed.) *Tutorials in Postgraduate Medicine: Urology*. pp. 223–246. (London: Heinemann)

Chisholm, G. D. (1981). The TNM classification of prostatic cancer and activities of British Prostate Group. In Jacobi, G. H. and Hohenfellner, R. F. (eds.) *International Perspectives in Urology: Prostatic Cancer*. In press

Chisholm, G. D. and Habib, F. K. (1981). Prostatic cancer: experimental and clinical advances. In Hendry, W. F. (ed.) *Recent Advances in Urology/Andrology 3*. pp. 211–213. (London: Churchill Livingstone)

Clark, P. and Houghton, L. (1977). Subcapsular orchidectomy for carcinoma of the prostate. *Br. J. Urol.*, **49**, 419

Cohen, S. (1977). Conference on polyamines in cancer. *Cancer Res.*, **37**, 939

Cox, J. D. and Stoffel, T. J. (1977). The significance of needle biopsy after irradiation for stage C adenocarcinoma of the prostate. *Cancer*, **40**, 156

Cupps, R. E., Utz, D. C., Fleming. T. R., Carson, C. C., Zincke, H. and Myers, R. P. (1980). Definitive radiation therapy for prostatic carcinoma: Mayo Clinic experience. *J. Urol.*, **124**, 855

de Vere White, R., Paulson, D. F. and Glenn, J. F. (1977). The clinical spectrum of prostate cancer. *J. Urol.*, **117**, 323

Donohue, R. E., Fauver, H. E., Whitesel, J. A. and Pfister, R. R. (1979). Staging prostatic cancer: a different distribution. *J. Urol.*, **122**, 327

Enstrom, J. E. and Austin, D. F. (1977). Interpreting cancer survival rates. *Science*, **195**, 847

Esposti, P. L. (1971). Cytological malignancy grading of prostatic carcinoma by transrectal aspiration biopsy. *Scand. J. Urol. Nephrol.*, **5**, 199

Fitzpatrick, J. M., Constable, A. R., Sherwood, T., Stephenson, J. J., Chisholm, G. D. and O'Donoghue, E. P. N. (1978). Serial bone scanning: the assessment of treatment response in carcinoma of the prostate. *Br. J. Urol.*, **50**, 555

Fitzpatrick, J. M., Gardiner, R. A., Williams, J. P., Riddle, P. R. and O'Donoghue, E. P. N. (1980). Pituitary ablation in the relief of pain in advanced prostatic carcinoma. *Br. J. Urol.*, **52**, 301

Foti, A. G., Cooper, J. F., Herschman, H. and Malvaez, R. R. (1977). Detection of prostatic cancer by solid phase radioimmunoassay of serum prostatic acid phosphatase. *N. Engl. J. Med.*, **297**, 1357

Franks, L. M. (1954). Latent carcinoma of the prostate. *J. Pathol. Bac.*, **68**, 603

Franks, L. M. (1956). The natural history of prostatic cancer. *Lancet*, **2**, 1037

Franks, L. M. (1977). Etiology and epidemiology of human prostatic disorders. In Tannenbaum, M. (ed.) *Urologic Pathology: the Prostate*. pp. 23–29. (Philadelphia: Lea and Febiger)

Gammelgaard, J. and Holm, H. H. (1980). Transurethral and transrectal ultrasonic scanning in urology. *J. Urol.*, **124**, 863.

Gaynor, E. P. (1938). Zur Frage des Prostatakrebses. *Virchows Arch. Pathol. Anat. Physiol. Klin. Med.*, **301**, 602

Gehan, E. A. (1975). Statistical methods for survival time studies. In Staquet, M. J. (ed.) *Cancer Therapy: Prognostic Factors and Criteria of Response*. pp. 7–35. (New York: Raven Press)

Gleason, D. F., Mellinger, G. T. and The Veterans Administration Cooperative Urological Research Group (1974). Prediction of prognosis for prostatic adenocarcinoma by combined histological grading and clinical staging. *J. Urol.*, **111**, 58

Guinan, P., Sadoughi, N., John, T., Ablin, R. J. and Bush, I. M. (1974). The prognostic value of carcinoembryonic antigen in carcinoma of the prostate. *Urol. Res.*, **2**, 79

Gutman, A. B. and Gutman, E. B. (1938). An 'acid' phosphatase occurring in the serum of patients with metastasizing carcinoma of the prostate gland. *J. Clin. Invest.*, **17**, 473

Hanash, K. A., Utz, D. C., Cook, E. N., Taylor, W. F. and Titus, J. L. (1972). Carcinoma of the prostate: a 15-year follow up. *J. Urol.*, **107**, 450

Hirst, A. E., Jr. and Bergman, R. T. (1954). Carcinoma of the prostate in men 80 or more years old. *Cancer*, **7**, 136

Hovsepian, J. A., Byar, D. P. and VACURG. (1975). Carcinoma of prostate. *Urology*, **6**, 11

Huggins, C. and Hodges, C. V. (1941). Studies on prostatic cancer. I. The effect of castration, of estrogen and of androgen injection on serum phosphatases in metastatic carcinoma of the prostate. *Cancer Res.*, **1**, 293

Jewett, H. J. (1975). The present status of radical prostatectomy for stages A and B prostatic cancer. *Urol. Clin. N. Am.*, **2**, 105

Jönsson, G. and Hogberg, B. (1971). Treatment of advanced prostatic carcinoma with Estracyt. *Scand. J. Urol. Nephrol.*, **5**, 103

Karnofsky, X. X. (1961).

Kern, W. H. (1978). Well differentiated adenocarcinoma of the prostate. *Cancer*, **41**, 2046

Kiesling, V. J., McAninch, J. W., Goebel, J. L. and Agee, R. E. (1980). External beam radiotherapy for adenocarcinoma of the prostate: a clinical follow up. *J. Urol.*, **124**, 851

Klein, L. A. (1979). Prostatic carcinoma. *N. Engl. J. Med.*, **300**, 824

Kurth, K. H., Altwein, J. E., Skoluda, D. and Hohenfellner, R. (1977). Follow-up of irradiated prostatic carcinoma by aspiration biopsy. *J. Urol.*, **117**, 615

Kvols, L. K., Eagan, R. T. and Myers, R. P. (1977). Evaluation of Melphalan, ICRF-159, and Hydroxyurea in metastatic prostate cancer: a preliminary report. *Cancer Treat. Rep.*, **61**, 311

Leistenschneider, W. and Nagel, R. (1980). Estracyt therapy of advanced prostatic cancer with special reference to control of therapy with cytology and DNA cytophotometry. *Eur. Urol.*, **6**, 111

McGowan, D. G. (1980). The adverse influence of prior transurethral resection on prognosis in carcinoma of prostate treated by radiation therapy. *Int. J. Radiat. Oncol. Biol. Phys.*, **6**, 1121

McLaughlin, A. P., Saltzstein, S. L., McCullough, D. L. and Gittes, R. G. (1976). Prostatic carcinoma: incidence and location of unsuspected lymphatic metastases. *J. Urol.*, **115**, 89

McMillen, S. M. and Wettlaufer, J. N. (1976). The role of repeat transurethral biopsy in Stage A carcinoma of the prostate. *J. Urol.*, **116**, 759

Michigan, S. and Catalona, W. J. (1977). Urethral obstruction from prostatic carcinoma: Response to endocrine and radiation therapy. *J. Urol.*, **118**, 733

Mundy, A. R. (1979). Urinary hydroxyproline excretion in carcinoma of the prostate. A comparison of 4 different modes of assessment and its role as a marker. *Br. J. Urol.*, **51**, 570

Nachtsheim, D. A., Jr., McAninch, J. W., Stutsman, R. E. and Goebel, J. L. (1978). Latent residual tumour following external radiotherapy for prostatic adenocarcinoma. *J. Urol.*, **120**, 312

Nesbit, R. M. and Baum, W. C. (1950). Endocrine control of prostatic carcinoma: clinical and statistical survey of 1818 cases. *J. Am. Med. Assoc.*, **143**, 1317

Paulson, D. F. and Uro-oncology Research Group. (1979). The impact of current staging procedures in assessing disease extent of prostatic adenocarcinoma. *J. Urol.*, **121,** 300

Peeling, W. B., Griffiths, G. J., Evans, K. T. and Roberts, E. E. (1979). Diagnosis and staging of prostatic cancer by transrectal ultrasonography. A preliminary study. *Br. J. Urol.*, **51,** 565

Resnick, M. I. and Grayhack, J. T. (1975). Treatment of stage IV carcinoma of the prostate. *Urol. Clin. N. Am.*, **2,** 141

Schmidt, J. D. (1980). Chemotherapy of hormone-resistant stage D prostatic cancer. *J. Urol.*, **123,** 797

Scott, W. W., Johnson, D. E., Schmidt, J. D., Gibbons, R. P., Prout, G. R., Jomer, J. R., Saroff, J. and Murphy, G. P. (1975). Chemotherapy of advanced prostatic carcinoma with cyclophosphamide or 5-fluorouracil: results of first national randomized study. *J. Urol.*, **114,** 909

Shearer, R. J., Hendry, W. F., Sommerville, I. F. and Fergusson J. D. (1973). Plasma testosterone: an accurate monitor of hormone treatment in prostatic cancer. *Br. J. Urol.*, **45,** 668

Shipley, W. U., Kopelson, G., Novack, D. H., Ling, C. C., Dretter, S. P. and Prout, G. R., Jr. (1980). Pre-operative irradiation, lymphadenectomy and [125]Iodine implant for patients with localised prostatic carcinoma: a correlation of implant dosimetry with clinical results. *J. Urol.*, **124,** 639

Spieler, P., Gloor, F., Egle, N. and Bandhauer, K. (1976). Cytological findings in transrectal aspiration biopsy on hormone- and radio-treated carcinoma of the prostate. *Virchows Arch. Pathol. Anat. Hist.*, **372,** 149

Stoll, B. A. (1972). Assessment of tumour-host relationship. In Stoll, B. A. (ed.) *Endocrine Therapy in Malignant Disease.* pp. 85–108. (London, Philadelphia, Toronto: Saunders)

Stone, A. R., Hargreave, T. B. and Chisholm, G. D. (1980). The diagnosis of oestrogen escape in prostatic cancer. *Br. J. Urol.*, **52,** 535

UICC. Union Internationale contre le Cancer (1978). *TNM Classification of Malignant Tumours.* 3rd Edn. (Geneva: International Union against Cancer)

Varkarakis, M., Castro, J. E. and Azzopardi, J. G. (1970). Prognosis of stage I carcinoma of the prostate. *Proc. R. Soc. Med.*, **63,** 91

Veterans Administration Cooperative Urological Research Group (1967). Treatment and survival of patients with cancer of the prostate. *Surg. Gynecol. Obstet.*, **124,** 1011

Whitmore, W. F., Jr., Hilaris, B. and Grabstald, H. (1974). Implantation of ^{125}I in prostatic cancer. *Surg. Clin. N. Am.*, **54,** 887

11

The response of the benign hypertrophied prostate to endocrine therapy

GORDON WILLIAMS

Histological evidence of benign prostatic hypertrophy (BPH) can be found in the prostates of almost all men as they exceed the age of 40. The true incidence is difficult to determine as most available data relate to selected groups of patients. BPH, the most common neoplasm in man, results in clinical symptoms in 65 % of men over the age of 60 years (Flocks, 1964) and it is estimated that one in ten men will require an operation (Lytton *et al.*, 1968).

With improved medical care and surgical technique the overall mortality following a surgical prostatectomy is between 1–2 % (Chilton *et al.*, 1978; Smith and O'Flynn, 1979). When carried out in a specialist urological unit the operation should have a high degree of success in relieving symptoms of urinary outflow obstruction and carry a low morbidity. As a result, double blind controlled clinical trials of endocrine therapy for the treatment of BPH have been limited and at present most symptomatic patients referred to a urological unit are advised to undergo a surgical prostatectomy. The frequency of the disease creates certain problems with over 33 000 men admitted to hospital in England and Wales in 1978 with prostatic hyperplasia as the primary diagnosis. With an ageing population the number of new referrals can be expected to increase and, depending on the type of operation, the mean time in hospital in a specialist unit, including time wasted before surgery, will vary from 7 days for a transurethral resection and up to 19 days for a retropubic prostatectomy (Argyrou *et al.*, 1974). The morbidity following surgery is increased in patients not treated in a specialist unit (Lytton, 1980). It is unlikely that further improvements in surgical technique or pre- and postoperative management will be sufficiently great to allow surgical treatment to be recommended to all patients irrespective of their age or medical condition. Furthermore, it is unlikely that medical facilities will be expanded to an extent whereby all patients with urinary outflow obstruction will be offered surgical treatment before significant complications of this condition arise. Prophylaxis aimed at preventing the disease or treatment in the symptomatic patient, obviating the need for surgery with its attendant risks, would be highly desirable. The clinical features of the disease BPH are a consequence of its anatomical site and the variations in biological behaviour of the epithelial and stromal elements of which it is comprised. This chapter reviews the endocrine dependence of the prostate and attempts which have been made to treat BPH with endocrine therapy.

11.1 THE ENDOCRINE DEPENDENCE OF BPH

Many theories have been proposed to explain the occurrence of benign prostatic hypertrophy, ranging from an absolute excess of androgens to a relative excess of oestrogens. The two essential factors for the initiation of the disease are the presence of the testes and ageing. Evidence for the permissive role of testicular hormones and the initiation of BPH is considerable. John Hunter in 1786 discovered that the prostate of animals is dependent on testicular function. He noted that the prostates of castrated animals were 'small, flabby, tough, ligamentous and had little secretion'. BPH does not occur in men who are castrated before puberty. Moore (1944) carried out serial sections of the prostate of 28 patients who had all lived beyond the age of 45 years and were either eunuchs, eunuchoid or had pituitary infantilism and had lost their secondary sexual characteristics before the age of 40. In none of this group was there any evidence of benign prostatic hypertrophy. A Russian sect, the Skoptzys, were castrated at approximately 35 years of age. These men were reported to have small prostates and lacked symptoms attributable to BPH (Zuckerman, 1936).

11.1.1 Regression of BPH after castration

In 1895 White reported the effect of castration carried out on 200 men for the treatment of urinary obstruction secondary to BPH. The operation carried a mortality of 20 % but in his summary of 111 cases he reported a rapid atrophy of the prostatic enlargement in 87 %, return of vesical contractility, measured by observed rate of urine flow and reduction in residual volume in 66 %, reduction or improvement in long standing cystitis in 52 % and a return of local conditions not far removed from normal in 46 %. Cabot (1896) reported longer follow-up of 61 orchidectomized patients. Five showed no improvement, one improved initially then relapsed and four still required a catheter but this entered more easily. In 27 cases of retention of urine all improved. Seven of these were acute, that is, of less than 1 month's duration and 20 chronic ranging from 1 month to 18 years. In percentage terms his cases showed a 9.8 % failure, 6.6 % moderate improvement and 83.6 % substantial or very good improvement. Cabot felt able to tell his 'enquiring patients' that they had eight chances in ten of getting through the operation and, if successful in this 8 chances in 10, or a little better, of getting very substantial relief from their urinary difficulties. These studies were carried out without controls and in the light of more recent studies are difficult to interpret. In some of White's patients who died, the prostate was examined histologically. A substantial number showed an almost complete disappearance of all glandular elements. Cabot, however, felt that these changes were also seen in men who had not been castrated as a result of degeneration of the prostate. Huggins and Stevens (1940) obtained prostatic biopsies for histological study from three patients prior to castration. Two had BPH and one BPH and carcinoma. Repeat biopsies of the prostate 29, 86 and 91 days after castration were also obtained. Those at 86 and 91 days showed smaller prostatic acini with loss of cell height and layering of the epithelium compared to the precastration biopsy. Wendel *et al.* (1972) studied autopsy specimens of three groups of patients, those with carcinoma of the prostate treated by orchidectomy or oestrogens, a similar age-matched group with no premortem evidence of carcinoma of the prostate and a group of patients with untreated carcinoma of the prostate. It was found that the BPH present in patients with treated carcinoma was of a lower grade than in untreated patients. Infolding of the acinar epithelium and the secretory phase were virtually absent in the treated group compared to the non-treatment group. These differences correlated with the orchidectomy and oestrogen but not with the presence of prostatic cancer.

These observed changes in the epithelium of the prostate in patients who have undergone an orchidectomy support the concept that it is subjected to continuing stimulation by the testis.

11.1.2   Changes in circulating and tissue steroids in BPH

These subjects are fully covered in Chapters 3 and 4 and are briefly summarized in this section.

11.1.2.1   Alterations in plasma androgens with age in normal men and those with BPH

In spite of a marked individual variation, considerable evidence has been presented to show the circulating levels of bound and free testosterone (Vermeulen, 1976; Lewis *et al.*, 1976), 5α-dihydrostestosterone (DHT) (Lewis *et al.*, 1976) and 5α-androstane-3α,17β-diol (Ghanadian and Puah, 1981a) decrease with age in normal men, i.e. those without clinical evidence of benign prostatic hyperplasia, such decreases being most marked in the 60–80y age group. In symptomatic patients with BPH the level of testosterone does not differ significantly from age-matched asymptomatic controls (Chisholm and Ghanadian, 1976; Harper *et al.*, 1976; Hammond *et al.*, 1978). In contrast, levels of DHT in patients with benign prostatic hypertrophy are elevated compared to normal subjects (Ghanadian *et al.*, 1977a; Hammond *et al.*, 1978). Others, however, have not confirmed this finding (Bartsch *et al.*, 1979). A significant increase in the level of circulating 5α-androstane-3α,17β-diol in patients with BPH compared to their age-matched controls has been reported by Ghanadian *et al.* (1981). These changes in circulating androgens may represent a permissive rather than a causative role in the production of BPH as they are most marked many years after the earliest histological changes of prostatic hyperplasia can be detected.

11.1.2.2   Alterations in plasma oestrogens in normal men and men with BPH

In normal men there is an increase in the plasma level of oestradiol-17β with age (Pirke and Doerr, 1975; Skoldefors *et al.*, 1978). However, there does not appear to be a difference in plasma oestrogens in men with prostatic hyperplasia as compared with age-matched control subjects (Harper *et al.*, 1976; Hammond *et al.*, 1978; Bartsch *et al.*, 1979).

11.1.2.3 Steroid changes in normal prostates and BPH tissues

Siiteri and Wilson (1970) demonstrated a marked increase in DHT concentration in hyperplastic prostatic tissue but more significantly the concentration of DHT in areas of early periurethral hyperplasia was higher than that in normal tissue of the same gland. However, the main metabolite of DHT, 5α-androstane-3α,17β-diol has been found to be significantly lower in benign hypertrophied tissue than in normal tissue (Geller *et al.*, 1976).

Although the level of oestradiol-17β in benign prostatic tissues has been reported (Ghanadian and Puah, 1981b), no measurement of endogenous oestradiol-17β has been reported for normal prostatic tissue. Similarly, the presence of oestrogen receptors has been reported in benign hypertrophied prostatic tissues (Bashirelahi *et al.*, 1976; Auf and Ghanadian, 1982) though their concentration has not been compared with levels in the normal prostate.

11.2 THE EFFECT OF ENDOCRINE MANIPULATION ON THE PROSTATE OF ANIMALS

The administration of testosterone to a variety of animals produces a larger than normal growth of the prostate. In several species there is correlation between the animal's ability to produce dihydrotestosterone in the prostate and the ability of the prostate to grow (Gloyna and Wilson, 1969). Histologically, however, these changes are dissimilar to the human disease.

The administration of oestrogens to many different species, including mouse, rat, guinea-pig, Rhesus monkey and dog, produces primarily an increase in the fibromuscular stroma and metaplastic changes in the epithelium (Geller, 1974). The concomitant administration of androgens prevents some of these histological changes giving support to the theory that benign prostatic hypertrophy might be the result of excess stimulation of an oestrogenic substance.

11.2.1 Prostatic hyperplasia in the dog

Man and dog are the two species which commonly develop spontaneous prostatic hyperplasia. There are many similarities between the prostatic hypertrophy of man and that of the dog. The disease occurs most frequently in the ageing male. The presence of the testes are necessary in both species and prepubertal castration prevents its onset. The size of the gland is similar (30–100 g) and regression of the established disease following castration or treatment with antiandrogens occurs routinely in the dog (Huggins and Clark, 1940; Neri and Monahan, 1972) and has been reported in humans (White, 1895; Geller *et al.*, 1969). In both the concentration of DHT is increased compared to the normal gland (Siiteri and Wilson, 1970; Gloyna *et al.*, 1970).

There are also considerable differences. The human disease is a multifocal process arising as a periurethral nodule which is secondarily invaded by glandular elements (Moore, 1943; Pradhan and Chandra, 1975). In contrast, in the dog two types of hyperplasia may occur – glandular hyperplasia and cystic hyperplasia due to cystic degeneration of the glandular acinar. These types may occur concomitantly, are diffuse and may involve the whole gland.

De Klerk et al. (1979) induced prostatic hyperplasia in young beagles with intact testes using either DHT or 5α-androstane-3α,17β-diol alone or with either of these steroids in conjunction with oestradiol-17β. Furthermore, this group were able to induce BPH in the castrated animal using DHT or 5α-androstane-3α,17β-diol in combination with oestradiol-17β. This experimentally induced hyperplasia is identical to the naturally occurring glandular hyperplasia of the ageing dog. 5α-androstane-3α,17β-diol appears to exert its effects through its metabolism to 5α DHT. Moore et al. (1979a) reported that exogenous 5α-androstane-3α,17β-diol is a better precursor of prostatic DHT than exogenous DHT itself. It causes the level of DHT in the prostate to increase to a level equal to that of the naturally occurring disorder. Because the administration of DHT induces prostatic hyperplasia and because 5α-androstane-3α,17β-diol induces hyperplasia by its conversion to DHT, it is suggested that the accumulation of DHT in spontaneous prostatic hypertrophy is the intracellular mediator of this condition (Wilson, 1980). The accumulation of DHT in the prostate may be due in part to the decreased metabolism of DHT to 5α-androstane-3α,17β-diol and to androsterone and an increased back-conversion of 5α-androstane-3α, 17β-diol to DHT. In addition to this, an increased concentration of DHT cytosol receptor may be brought about by the action of oestradiol-17β (Moore et al., 1979b). The role for oestrogens in the pathogenesis of prostatic hyperplasia was first suggested by Zuckerman and Groom (1937). Their demonstration that oestradiol-17β exerts a synergistic effect with androgens in promoting prostatic growth in the dog is of considerable importance and may explain why the hyperplastic process continues with ageing which in itself is associated with a lowered serum testosterone level.

It is impossible to carry out in man the studies that are being carried out in the dog and to accept that the canine disorder is a valid model for the human disease would necessitate that the underlying endocrine changes are the same and that the species difference accounts for the difference in the site of initiation of the glandular rather than mesenchymal proliferation (Wilson, 1980). If the pathogenesis of prostatic hyperplasia in the dog is, as has been suggested, similar to that of man, a considerable possibility exists for the development of medical treatment for this condition which, provided that it was safe and free from side-effects, could be used as prophylactic treatment before surgery was necessary. In symptomatic patients, the treatment would have to be safer and more effective than the well-tried surgical removal of the adenoma. Attempts at medical treatment of benign prostatic hypertrophy in man have been aimed at medical castration. These treatments are all associated with side-effects, and, in particular, impotence. Specific therapy based on the suggested pathogenesis would be aimed at either reducing DHT formation or blocking the synthesis or action of oestradiol-17β. This might inhibit prostatic growth and prevent the onset of symptoms or induce regression of the prostate and relieve the symptoms of outflow obstruction.

11.2.2 The effect of various antiandrogens in animals

Cyproterone acetate, a 17α-hydroxy progesterone derivative, and other antiandrogens caused the prostate to atrophy in both intact animals and those which had been castrated and substituted with androgens (Neumann and Steinbeck, 1974). The dog is reported to react more sensitively than rodents, the epithelium almost disappearing with a relative increase in the stroma (Neumann *et al.*, 1976). In the canine model for the development of prostatic hyperplasia using 5α-androstane-3α,17β-diol and oestradiol-17β, the concomitant addition of cyproterone acetate abolished the epithelial or metaplastic proliferation and induced atrophy of the glandular epithelium (Tunn *et al.*, 1980). The non-steroidal antiandrogen, flutamide, is also effective in the treatment of canine prostatic hypertrophy. Oral administration of flutamide to 12 intact dogs for 6 weeks reduced the hyperplastic gland size by an average of 80 %. When the antiandrogen therapy was withdrawn the prostate reverted to the original hyperplastic condition with respect to size, epithelial cell height and histology (Neri and Monahan, 1972).

11.3 EVALUATION OF CRITERIA FOR RESPONSE TO TREATMENT OF BPH

The purpose of treatment of BPH is the alleviation of urinary outflow obstruction. The indications are still based in most units almost entirely on a subjective assessment except when there is retention of urine. Without objective measurements or knowledge of the natural history of the disease it is too easy to attribute the favourable response to a new pill or operation.

11.3.1 Subjective symptoms

Clarke (1937) showed that improvement in clinical symptoms of prostatism lasting approximately 3 years occurred in 60 % of patients with mild or moderate prostatism who were followed without specific therapy. Even in advanced BPH transient remissions in clinical symptoms occurred in 60 % of patients followed for 1 year. Castro *et al.* (1971) in a double blind study found improvement of symptoms of frequency and nocturia in almost 70 % of placebo treated patients over 6 months. The only measurements which did not respond to the placebo were the maximum urine flow rate and the catheter measured residual urine. If subjective clinical symptoms of frequency, nocturia, hesitancy, urgency, dribbling or change in urinary stream are to be used then the study must have adequate placebo treated controls and a double blind technique must be used. Alternatively, the study should continue for at least 3 years. A symptomatic study of multiple parameters and the correlation with prostatic obstruction was reported by Castro *et al.* (1969) and

Lacassagne (1933) who found that the maximum urine flow rate could be correlated best with a cross-sectional diameter of the urethra (R = 0.96, this being the expression of outflow obstruction).

11.3.2 Objective measurements

If objective measurements for the relief of outflow obstruction are to be preferred and when the patient acts as his own control, the following criteria should be used:

(1) Changes in maximum urine flow rate.
(2) Changes in catheterized residual urine.
(3) The ability to void in patients with retention.

The great majority of studies on the endocrine response of benign prostatic hypertrophy in man do not fulfil these criteria. As such the results are often uninterpretable.

11.4 HORMONAL THERAPY OF BPH

Following studies on the effect of various hormones on the accessory sex organs of animals (Lacassagne, 1933; Korenchevsky and Dennison, 1934) a large number of clinical trials using androgens, oestrogens or a combination of both were commenced in the 1930s. These studies are only mentioned briefly as they invariably lack randomization of patients, rigid controls, the use of placebos, adequate follow-up and objective reproducable data. This subject has been reviewed by Geller (1974) and Scott and de Klerk (1976).

11.4.1 Androgen therapy

The idea that patients with BPH might be androgen deficient came from both animal experiments and clinical observations. Lacassagne (1933) reported that the abnormalities in the prostate caused by oestrogens could be prevented by androgens. In man, the onset of the disease occurs around the time of the so-called 'male menopause'. Many attempts to treat BPH using androgens were made but without any control studies or objective evidence of reduction in prostatic size or histological change. Lesser *et al.* (1955) compared the incidence of BPH in 100 men over the age of 45 who had received testosterone for either angina pectoris or the male climacteric with the incidence of BPH in 100 age-matched controls. Testosterone had been given in doses of 25–75 mg per week for periods ranging from 3 months to 4 years. Twenty-seven treated patients and 34 controls had benign prostatic hypertrophy. Within the limitations of this study, testosterone administration did not appear to affect the incidence of BPH. Testicular extracts have also been used by Lower *et al.* (1935). They suggested that a lack of inhibin would stimulate gonadotrophin release leading to an excess androgen production. They reported subjective improvement in their patients.

11.4.2 Oestrogen therapy

Oestrogen therapy for BPH is based on the fact that oestrogens in sufficient dosage will reduce the levels of circulating testosterone. Most studies using oestrogens for the treatment of BPH lack controls and are without objective evidence of improvement.

11.4.3 Combined androgen and oestrogen therapy

A trial based on the combined use of androgens and oestrogen was reported by Kaufman and Goodwin (1969). Forty-four patients were treated for 6 months and followed for 6–24 months after completion of therapy. Their uncontrolled study showed 'an appreciable amelioration of symptoms in the majority of patients. There was improved voiding velocity in most subjects and several patients showed a reduction in residual urine. Approximately half the patients showed histological changes in the prostate and in approximately one third there seemed to be reduction in the size of the prostate.' However, these authors felt that these features were too inconstant and unpredictable to warrant absolute conclusions.

11.4.4 Antiandrogens

With a greater understanding of the mechanism and action of androgens within the prostate a search has been made for drugs which inhibit the biological activity of testosterone metabolites. A variety of compounds have been synthesized and are known as antiandrogens. There are three main groups:

(1) Those derived from 17α-hydroxy-progesterone.
(2) Those derived from 19 nor-testosterone.
(3) Synthetic non-steroidal antiandrogens.

There are a number of identifiable sites where antiandrogens exert their effects. They inhibit the action of 5α-reductase and steroid dehydrogenase, and also lower plasma testosterone levels (Ghanadian et al., 1979). They competitively inhibit the binding of DHT to cytoplasmic and nuclear receptors at the target cell (Ghanadian et al., 1977b; Smith et al., 1978). They also reduce oestrogen production rates in the male to castrate levels (Fishman and Geller, 1970). It has been shown in animal studies and in clinical practice that this group of drugs has a considerable effect both in benign hyperplasia and carcinoma of the prostate. Because of their many sites of action they are associated with side-effects which detract from their usefulness. The most commonly reported effects are breast enlargement, nipple tenderness, loss of libido, impotence and acne.

11.4.4.1 17α-Hydroxy-progesterone caproate

The first report of the use of these derivatives was in an uncontrolled study by Geller et al. (1965). In a later report (Geller et al., 1969), 20 patients with urine retention requiring a catheter were studied. Ten were treated, seven with hydroxy-progesterone caproate and three with chlormadinone acetate. The other 10 acted as controls. Seven of the ten treated patients were able to void spontaneously with residual urines of less than 50 ml after 5 months treatment. In the control group only two voided spontaneously after 3 months of catheter or cystotomy tube drainage. Suprapubic prostatectomy was carried out in three of the patients who received hydroxy-progesterone caproate for 2 months. Histology of the removed glands showed the epithelial cells were more cuboidal than columnar, there was a reduction in acinar size and less intra-acinar papillation. No pretreatment tissue was available for comparison.

Following cessation of treatment with hydroxy-progesterone caproate four of the five patients remained stable for an average period of 13 months. In a more recent study, 17 patients suffering from benign prostatic hypertrophy were treated using this drug with urine flow and residual urine measured pre- and post-therapy. No statistically significant trend could be shown despite subjective improvement in almost 50% of the patients (Brooks and Braf, 1981).

11.4.4.2 17α-Hydroxy-19-nor-progesterone caproate (SH582) gestronol hexanoate

In a double blind cross-over trial involving 24 patients, Aubrey and Khosla (1971) reported that 'in most subjects there was subjective and objective evidence that SH582 had a beneficial effect which exceeded that of the placebo. Only two subjects emerged from the trial without improvement.' Their objective evidence for improvement was in reduction of residual urine and decrease in prostatic weight. Using a similar protocol, Gingell et al. (1972) were unable to show any significant alteration in residual urine or peak urinary flow rate during their 3 months trial period, though beneficial effect on residual urine carried over into the placebo period suggesting that the effects of treatment require a longer time interval to become manifest.

11.4.4.3 Nor-progesterone caproate

Treatment with 12 weekly intramuscular injections significantly reduced residual urine in ten of 15 patients with prostatism. It was of no value in a further ten patients with retention (Ibrahim and Elnur, 1978).

11.4.4.4 Cyproterone acetate

Vahlensieck and Gödde (1968) reported on 12 patients who were treated with cyproterone acetate 100 mg daily for up to 4 months. Their objective criteria was residual urine and this decreased in all cases. In a study devoid of adequate controls but with objective assessment of urine flow rate and residual volume, Scott and Wade (1969) treated 13 patients for periods of up to 15 months with 50 mg of cyproterone acetate per day. Urine flow rates improved in nine patients and measured residual urine in eight. Pretreatment biopsies were obtained and compared to tissue removed while the patients were on treatment. In eight of the 11 patients a decrease in epithelial cell height was noted.

11.4.4.5 Megestrol acetate

Lebech and Nordentoft (1967), without a parallel control group but using objective measurements of residual urine and urine flow, studied the effects of megestrol acetate in 15 randomly selected patients with benign prostatic hypertrophy. They were followed for 10 months. The mean residual urine prior to treatment was 200 ml and after 6 months had decreased to 30 ml. The mean urine flow rate had increased from 3 ml/sec to 7 ml/sec. Geller *et al.* (1979) in a double blind control study randomly assigned 61 patients with benign prostatic hypertrophy to placebo or megestrol 120 mg daily for 5 months. Patients on megestrol had significant increases in maximum and mean urine flow rates from the sixth to the twentieth week compared to their own control baseline values. The placebo treated patients showed no significant change at any time in their 20 week period in their mean flow rate but their maximum flow rate did demonstrate statistically significant increases above their own baseline value at 8, 12, 18 and 20 weeks. Megestrol-treated patients in comparison to the placebo group showed statistically significant increases in mean flow rate compared to the placebo group at 14, 16 and 20 weeks of therapy and in the maximum flow rate at 10, 12, 14 and 20 weeks. Loss of libido was noted in 70 % of the treated patients.

11.4.4.6 Medrogestone

In a randomized double blind study Rangno *et al.* (1971) assessed the effects of medrogestone in a dose of 50 mg b.d. in 24 patients. They reported very favourable results for the test drug in both subjective and objective parameters. Constant histological changes were observed after treatment. The epithelium was flat, broken and lytic fragments filled the lumen. There was an absence of acinar fronds and there was a complete reversal of the changes at the end of the placebo period which followed. In another study, no effect of medrogestone in a dose of 15 or 30 mg per day was found (Paulson and Kane, 1975).

11.4.5 19-Nor-testosterone derivatives

Studies on the effect of this group of synthetic steroids on benign prostatic hypertrophy have been limited to only two compounds:

(1) 17-ethyl-19-nor-testosterone (Norlutate),
(2) 17α (2-methallyl)-19 nor testosterone (SC9022).

The effects of these two steroids and a placebo have been studied by Wolff and Madsen (1968). Forty patients were treated for 6 months. The results showed no difference between the treated and control groups. These authors emphasized that the absence of response could be entirely due to the dose used.

11.4.6   Non-steroidal antiandrogens (flutamide)

In a study of 30 patients randomized to a placebo or flutamide 100 mg three times a day for 12 weeks, the only objective in the treatment group was improvement in urine flow rate. No difference was found in residual urine or prostatic size or any histological change in prostatic biopsies (Caine *et al.*, 1975a).

11.4.7   Other drugs with certain antiandrogenic effects

11.4.7.1   Spironolactone

Some aldosterone antagonists are known to be progestogens. In a double blind controlled clinical trial, Castro *et al.* (1971) showed that spironolactone was better than a placebo for short term treatment of benign prostatic hypertrophy, but this advantage was not maintained over a longer period. Their patients also showed a considerable response to the placebo.

11.4.7.2   Cimetidine

Some antiandrogenic effects of cimetidine have been reported recently in both animal and human studies (Van Thiel *et al.*, 1979; Winters *et al.*, 1979). Despite its widespread use there are no reports of its effects on the male with prostatic outflow obstruction.

11.5   NON-HORMONAL MEDICAL TREATMENT

A number of other drugs have been used to attempt to relieve the outflow obstruction caused by the prostate. Phyto drugs and vitamins can be considered along with placebos. Castro *et al.* (1971) showed a 70 % subjective improvement in a placebo-treated group.

11.5.1   Polyene macrolides

Gordon and Schaffner (1968) showed that polyene macrolides reduce the size of the prostate gland of older dogs. In the only reported controlled double blind study using nystatin 500 000 units 8-hourly for 6 weeks, no benefit was seen compared to the control group (Bourke *et al.*, 1974).

11.5.2   Bromocriptine

The anterior pituitary hormone, prolactin, has been shown to have an effect on prostatic size. When given to hypophysectomized rats it resulted in increase in prostatic weight (Grayhack and Lebowitz, 1967) and when prolactin antisera is administered to rabbits there is a marked decrease in prostatic size (Asano *et al.*, 1971). Bromocriptine (2-bromo-α-ergocriptine) is a specific central prolactin antagonist. Furthermore, *in vitro* isometric studies of the effects of bromocriptine on the human prostatic capsule and prostatic adenoma revealed transient direct stimulant actions, α-adrenergic blocking actions and anticholinergic actions (Shapiro *et al.*, 1980). In a double blind cross-over study in 14 patients (Farrar and Pryor, 1976), only nine patients completed the trial, five withdrawing because of side-effects. Six patients had subjective improvement and three had objective evidence of improvement with an increased urinary flow rate. This may be due to a combination of its effect on smooth muscle and on its endocrine effects.

11.5.3 Phenoxybenzamine

As a result of the finding of a high α-adrenergic activity both in the prostatic capsule and in the adenoma itself (Caine *et al.*, 1975b) a number of studies have been carried out using phenoxybenzamine in the medical management of patients with BPH. In a placebo controlled double blind study of 49 patients, Caine *et al.* (1978) found a significant improvement in peak and mean flow rate and reduction in frequency but no decrease in residual urine. Though side-effects occurred in 11 patients receiving phenoxybenzamine, they were insufficient to cause the patients to stop treatment. However, this trial only lasted 2 weeks and may account for the failure to reduce residual urine. If the treatment is given for longer periods, the side-effects may be more trouble-some. This treatment is not aimed at reducing the size of the basic mechanical obstruction but depends on the basal activity of α-adrenergic stimulation of the prostatic muscle. Abrams *et al.* (1982) in a study of 61 patients noted an overall symptomatic improvement in patients treated with phenoxybenz-amine. The symptoms of slow stream and hesitancy were significantly improved. The urethral pressure profile features of prostatic plateau height and prostatic plateau area were significantly decreased and they felt that the effect of phenoxybenzamine on bladder outflow obstruction was by reducing the pressure in the proximal urethra. They again reported a high incidence of dizziness in patients in their studies, which may preclude its long-term use in those patients who are unfit for surgery.

11.6 CONCLUSIONS

It is quite apparent that there is a potential role for medical treatment of benign prostatic hypertrophy. However, more clinical trials are required with drugs which can be tested initially on experimental models such as the canine prostatic model. New drugs should be specific in their action on dihydrotes-tosterone or oestradiol-17β production within the prostatic cell and free of other side-effects. The trials reported in this chapter are only a selection of those which have been carried out to assess the value of endocrine manipulation in patients with BPH. One fundamental question arising from these studies is how should the relative merits of these drugs or new drugs be assessed when they become available. Properly constructed clinical trials are a considerable undertaking and very few have been carried out in assessing these various agents. In the clinical studies reported here, the effects of these treatments may vary with the proportion of stroma and epithelium within the prostate gland or on the dose and duration of treatment. Evaluation of histological changes occurring within the glands was often superficial or not carried out. Of all the treatments so far tried, the side-effects have been considerable, particularly in the development of impotence.

The mortality and morbidity in patients undergoing surgical treatment is low. However, patients, who are poor surgical risks or those having to face months or years on a waiting list, should receive benefit from medical treatment and perhaps make surgery unnecessary.

11.7 REFERENCES

Abrams, P. M., Shah, P. J. R., Stone, R. and Choa, R. G. (1982). Bladder outflow obstruction treated with phenoxybenzamine. *Br. J. Urol.* (In Press)

Argyrou, F., Blandy, J. P., Gow, J. G., Singh, M., Tresidder, G. C. and Vinnicombe, J. (1974). The price of prostatectomy. *Br. Med. J.*, **2**, 511

Asano, M., Kanzaki, S., Sekiguchi, E. and Tasaka, T. (1971). Inhibition of prostatic growth in rabbits with anti-ovine prolactin serum. *J. Urol.*, **106**, 248

Aubrey, D. A. and Khosla, T. (1971). The effect of 17α-hydroxy-19-nor progesterone caproate (SH582) on benign prostatic hypertrophy. *Br. J. Surg.*, **58**, 648

Auf, G. and Ghanadian, R. (1982). Characterisation and measurement of cytoplasmic and nuclear oestradiol-17β receptor proteins in benign hypertrophied human prostate. *J. Endocrinol.*, **93**, 305

Bartsch, W., Becker, H., Pinkenburg, F. A. and Krieg, M. (1979). Hormone blood levels and their inter-relationships in normal men and men with benign prostatic hyperplasia (BPH). *Acta Endocrinol.*, **90**, 727

Bashirelahi, N., O'Toole, J. N. and Young, J. D. (1976). A specific 17β-oestradiol receptor in human benign hyperplastic prostate. *Biochem. Med.*, **15**, 254

Bourke, J. B., Griffin, J. P. and Theoorides, P. (1974). A double-blind trial of a polyene macrolide – Nystatin – in the treatment of benign prostatic hyperplasia in man. *Br. J. Urol.*, **46**, 463

Brooks, M. E. and Braf, Z. F. (1981). Effect of 17α-hydroxy progresterone 17-n-caproate on urine flow. *Urology*, **17**, 488

Cabot, A. T. (1896). The question of castration for enlarged prostate. *Ann. Surg.*, **24**, 266

Caine, M., Perlberg, S. and Gordon, R. (1975a). The treatment of benign prostatic hypertrophy with Flutamide (SCH13521): a placebo controlled study. *J. Urol.*, **114**, 564

Caine, M., Perlberg, S. and Meretyk, S. (1978). A placebo controlled double-blind study of the effect of phenoxybenzamine in benign prostatic obstruction. *Br. J. Urol.*, **50**, 551

Caine, M., Raz, S. and Zeigler, M. (1975b). Adrenergic and cholinergic receptors in the human prostate, prostatic capsule and bladder neck. *Br. J. Urol.*, **47**, 193

Castro, J. E., Griffiths, H. J. L. and Edwards, D. E. (1971). A double-blind controlled clinical trial of spironolactone for benign prostatic hypertrophy. *Br. J. Surg.*, **58**, 485

Castro, J. E., Griffiths, H. J. L. and Shackman, R. (1969). Significance of signs and symptoms in benign prostatic hypertrophy. *Br. Med. J.*, **2**, 598

Chilton, C. P., Morgan, R. J., England, H. R., Paris, A. M. I. and Blandy, J. P. (1978). A critical evaluation of the results of transurethral resection. *Br. J. Urol.*, **50**, 542

Chisholm, G. D. and Ghanadian, R. (1976). Comparison between changes in serum 5α-dihydrotestosterone and testosterone in normal men and patients with benign prostatic hypertrophy. Presented at the *5th International Congress of Endocrinology*, July 18–24, Hamburg

Clark, R. (1937). The prostate and the endocrines: a controlled series. *Br. J. Urol.*, **96**, 479

De Klerk, D. P., Coffey, D. S., Ewing, L. L., McDermott, I. R., Reiner, W. G., Robinson, C. H., Scott, W. W., Strandberg, J. D., Talalay, P., Walsh, P. C., Wheaton, L. G. and Zirkin, B. R. (1979). Comparison of spontaneous and experimentally induced canine prostatic hyperplasia. *J. Clin. Invest.*, **64**, 842

Farrar, D. J. and Pryor, J. S. (1976). The effect of bromocriptine in patients with benign prostatic hypertrophy. *Br. J. Urol.*, **9**, 254

Fishman, J. and Geller, J. (1970). The effect of the anti-androgen cyproterone acetate on oestradiol production and metabolism in man. *Steroids*, **16**, 531

Flocks, R. H. (1964). Benign prostatic hypertrophy: its diagnosis and management. *Med. Times*, **92**, 519

Geller, J. (1974). Medical treatment of benign hypertrophy. In Castro, J. E. (ed.) *The Treatment of Prostatic Hypertrophy and Neoplasia*. pp. 27–58. (Lancaster: MTP Press)

Geller, J., Albert, J., Lopez, D., Geller, S. and Niwayama, G. (1976). Comparison of androgen metabolites in benign prostatic hypertrophy (BPH) and normal prostate. *J. Clin. Endocrinol. Metab.*, **43**, 686

Geller, J., Angrist, A., Nakao, K. and Newman, H. (1969). Therapy with progestational agents in advanced benign prostatic hypertrophy. *J. Am. Med. Assoc.*, **210**, 1421

Geller, J., Nelson, C. G., Albert, T. D. and Pratt, C. (1979). The effect of megestrol acetate on uroflow rates in patients with prostatic hypertrophy. *Urology*, **14**, 467

Geller, J., Roberts, T., Newman, H., Lin, A. and Silva, R. (1965). Treatment of benign prostatic hypertrophy with hydroxy progesterone caproate: the effect on clinical symptoms, morphology and endocrine function. *J. Am. Med. Assoc.*, **193**, 121

Ghanadian, R., Lewis, J. G., Chisholm, G. D. and O'Donoghue, E. P. N. (1977a). Serum dihydrotestosterone in patients with benign prostatic hypertrophy. *Br. J. Urol.*, **49**, 541

Ghanadian, R., O'Donoghue, E. P. N. and Puah, C. M. (1979). Changes in dihydrotestosterone and testosterone following endocrine manipulation in carcinoma of the prostate. *Cancer Treat. Rep.* **63**, 1192

Ghanadian, R. and Puah, C. M. (1981a). Age related changes of serum 5α-androstane-3α, 17β-diol in normal men. *Gerontology*, **27**, 281

Ghanadian, R. and Puah, C. M. (1981b). Relationships between oestradiol-17β, testosterone, dihydrotestosterone and 5α-androstane-3α,17β-diol in human benign hypertrophy and carcinoma of the prostate. *J. Endocrinol.*, **88**, 255

Ghanadian, R., Puah, C. M. and Williams, G. (1981). Serum androstane 5α,17β-diol in patients with prostatic tumours. *Br. J. Cancer*, **44**, 308

Ghanadian, R., Smith, C. B., Williams, G. and Chisholm, G. D. (1977b). The effect of anti-androgens and stilboestrol on the cytosol receptor in rat prostate. *Br. J. Urol.*, **49**, 695

Gingell, J. C., Miller, I. N. and Roberts, J. B. N. (1972). A clinical trial of gestronol hexanoate (SH582) in benign prostatic hypertrophy. (Preliminary report: *Proc. R. Soc. Med.*, **65**, 130)

Gloyna, R. E., Siiteri, P. K. and Wilson, J. D. (1970). Dihydrotestosterone in prostatic hypertrophy. II. The formation and content of dihydrotestosterone in the hypertrophic canine prostate and the effect of dihydrotestosterone on prostate growth in the dog. *J. Clin. Invest.*, **49**, 1746

Gloyna, R. E. and Wilson, J. D. (1969). A comparative study of the conversion of testosterone to 17β-hydroxy 5α-androstan-3-one (dihydrotestosterone) by prostate and epididymis. *J. Clin. Endocrinol.*, **29**, 970

Gordon, H. W. and Schaffner, C. P. (1968). The effect of polyene macrolides on the prostate gland and canine hyperplasia. *Proc. Natl. Acad. Sci. (Washington)*, **60**, 1201

Grayhack, J. T. and Lebowitz (1967). The effect of prolactin on citric acid of lateral lobe of prostate of Sprague-Dawley rat. *Invest. Urol.*, **5**, 87

Hammond, G. L., Kontturi, M., Vihko, P. and Vihko, R. (1978). Serum steroids in normal males and patients with prostatic diseases. *Clin. Endocrinol.*, **9**, 113

Harper, M. E., Peeling, W. B., Cowley, T., Brownsey, B. G., Phillips, M. E. A., Groom, G., Fahmy, D. R. and Griffiths, K. (1976). Plasma steroid and protein hormone concentrations in patients with prostatic carcinoma before and during oestrogen therapy. *Acta Endocrinol.*, **81**, 409

Huggins, C. and Clark, P. J. (1940). Quantitative studies of prostatic secretion. II. The effect of castration and of oestrogen injection on the normal and on the hyperplastic prostate glands of dogs. *J. Exp. Med.*, **72**, 747

Huggins, C. and Stevens, R. A. (1940). The effect of castration on benign hypertrophy of prostate in man. *J. Urol.*, **43**, 705

Hunter, J. (1786). Observations on the glands situated between the rectum and the bladder called the vesiculae seminales. In Palmer, J. F. (ed.) *Collected Works*. p. 31. (New York: AMS Press)

Ibrahim, A. and Elnur, S. H. (1978). A clinical trial with nor progesterone caproate (Primostat) in benign prostatic hyperplasia. *E. Afr. Med. J.*, **55**, 429

Kaufman, J. J. and Goodwin, W. E. (1969). Hormonal management of the benign obstructing prostate – the use of combined androgen oestrogen therapy. *J. Urol.*, **81**, 165

Korenchevsky, V. and Dennison, M. (1934). The effect of oestrone on normal and castrated male rats. *Biochem. J.*, **28**, 1474

Lacassagne, A. (1933). Metaplasie epidermoide de la prostate provoquée chez la souris par des injections répétées des fortes doses de follicutine. *C.R. Soc. Biol. (Paris)*, **113**, 590

Lebech, P. E. and Nordentoft, E. L. (1967). A study of endocrine function in the treatment of BPH with megestrol acetate. *Acta Obstet. Gynaecol. Scand.*, **46** (Suppl. 9), 25

Lesser, M. A., Vose, S. N. and Dixey, G. M. (1955). The effect of testosterone propionate on the prostate gland of patients over 45. *J. Clin. Endocrinol. Metab.*, **15**, 297

Lewis, J. G., Ghanadian, R. and Chisholm, G. D. (1976). Serum 5α-dihydrotestosterone and testosterone changes with age in man. *Acta Endocrinol.*, **82**, 444

Lower, W. E., Engle, W. J. and McCullagh, D. R. (1935). A summary of the experimental research on the control of benign prostatic hypertrophy and a preliminary clinical report. *J. Urol.*, **34**, 670

Lytton, B. (1980). Prostatectomy at a district general hospital. *Ann. R. Coll. Surg. (Engl.)*, **62**, 306

Lytton, B., Emery, J. M. and Harvard, B. M. (1968). The incidence of benign prostatic obstruction. *J. Urol.*, **99**, 639

Moore, R. A. (1943). Benign hypertrophy of the prostate: a morphological study. *J. Urol.*, **50**, 680

Moore, R. A. (1944). Benign hypertrophy and carcinoma of the prostate – occurrence and experimental production in animals. *Surgery*, **16**, 152

Moore, R. J., Gazak, J. N., Quebbeman, J. F. and Wilson, J. D. (1979a). The concentration of dihydrotestosterone 3α-androstane diol in naturally occurring and androgen induced prostatic hyperplasia in the dog. *J. Clin. Invest.*, **46,** 1003

Moore, R. J., Gazak, J. N. and Wilson, J. D. (1979b). The regulation of cytoplasmic dihydrotestosterone binding in dog prostate by 17β-oestradiol. *J. Clin. Invest.*, **63,** 351

Neri, R. O. and Monahan, M. (1972). The effects of a novel non-steroidal anti-androgen on canine prostatic hyperplasia. *Invest. Urol.*, **10,** 123

Neumann, F., Schenck, B., Senge, T. H. and Richter, K. D. (1976). Anti-androgens and prostatic tumours (experimental base and clinical use). In Marberger, H. (ed.) *Prostatic Disease.* p. 169. (New York: Alan R. Liss)

Neumann, F. and Steinbeck, H. (1974). Anti-androgens. In Eichler, O., Farah, A., Herken, H. and Welch, A. D. (eds.) *Handbook of Experimental Pharmacology.* pp. 235–45. (Berlin, Heidelberg, New York: Springer)

Paulson, D. F. and Kane, R. D. (1975). Medrogestone: a prospective study in the pharmaceutical management of benign prostatic hyperplasia. *J. Urol.*, **113,** 811

Pirke, K. M. and Doerr, P. (1975). Age related changes in free plasma testosterone, dihydrotestosterone and oestradiol. *Acta Endocrinol.*, **80,** 171

Pradhan, B. H. and Chandra, K. (1975). Morphogenesis of nodular hyperplasia of the prostate. *J. Urol.*, **113,** 210

Rangno, R. E., McLeod, P. J., Ruedy, J. and Ogilvy, R. I. (1971). Treatment of benign prostatic hypertrophy with Medrogestone. *Clin. Pharmacol. Ther.*, **12,** 658

Scott, W. W. and de Klerk, D. P. (1976). Benign prostatic hyperplasia: the current status of medical treatment. In Grayhack, J. T., Wilson, J. D. and Scherbenske, M. J. (eds.) *Benign Prostatic Hyperplasia.* pp. 135—151. (Washington DC: US Department of Health, Education and Welfare. Publication number NIH76/1113)

Scott, W. W. and Wade, J. C. (1969). Medical treatment of benign prostatic hyperplasia with cyproterone acetate. *J. Urol.*, **101,** 81

Shapiro, A., Ron, M., Caine, M. and Kramer, J. (1980). The pharmacological effect of bromocriptine on the human prostate. *Urol. Res.*, **8,** 25

Siiteri, P. K. and Wilson, J. D. (1970). Dihydrotestosterone in prostatic hypertrophy. I. The formation and content of dihydrotestosterone in the hypertrophic prostate of man. *J. Clin. Invest.*, **49,** 1737

Skoldefors, H., Bolmstedt, B. and Carlstrom, K. (1978). Serum hormone levels in benign prostatic hyperplasia. *Scand. J. Urol. Nephrol.*, **12,** 111

Smith, C. B., Ghanadian, R. and Chisholm, G. D. (1978). Inhibitor of the nuclear dihydrotestosterone receptor complex from rat ventral prostate by anti-androgens and stilboestrol. *Mol. Cell. Endocrinol.*, **10,** 13

Smith, J. M. and O'Flynn, J. D. (1979). Prostatectomy mortality. Observations based on 7454 cases. *J. Ir. Med. Soc.*, **72,** 296

Tunn, U., Senge, T., Schenck, B. and Neumann, F. (1980). The effects of cyproterone acetate on experimentally induced canine prostatic hyperplasia. *Urol. Int.*, **35,** 125

Vahlensieck, W. and Gödde, S. (1968). Behandlung der prostatahypertrophie mit gestagenen. *München Med. Wochenschr.*, **110,** 1573

Van Thiel, D. H., Gavaler, J. S., Smith, W. I. and Paul, G. (1979). Hypothalamic pituitary gonadal disfunction in men using cimetidine. *N. Engl. J. Med.*, **300,** 1012

Vermeulen, A. (1976). Testicular hormonal secretion and ageing of males. In Grayhack, J. T., Wilson, J. D. and Scherbenske, M. (eds.) *Benign Prostatic Hyperplasia.* (Washington DC: US Department of Health, Education and Welfare. Publication number NIH76/1113)

Wendel, E. F., Brannen, G. E., Pu Tong, P. B. and Grayhack, J. T. (1972). The effect of orchidectomy and oestrogens on benign prostatic hypertrophy. *J. Urol.*, **108,** 116

White, J. W. (1895). The results of double castration in hypertrophy of the prostate. *Ann. Surg.*, **22,** 1

Wilson, J. D. (1980). The pathogenesis of benign prostatic hyperplasia. *Am. J. Med.*, **68,** 745

Winters, S. J., Banks, J. L. and Loriaux, D. L. (1979). The histamine H_2 antagonist Cimetidine is an anti-androgen. *Gastroenterology*, **76,** 504

Wolff, H. and Madsen, P. O. (1968). Treatment of benign prostatic hypertrophy with progestational agents: a preliminary report. *J. Urol.*, **99,** 780

Zuckerman, S. (1936). The endocrine control of the prostate. *Proc. R. Soc. Med.*, **29,** 1557

Zuckerman, S. and Groom, J. R. (1937). The aetiology of benign enlargement of the prostate in the dog. *J. Pathol. Bact.*, **44,** 113

12
Experimental models for prostatic tumours

R. GHANADIAN

12.1 ANIMAL MODELS

The search for experimental animal models, to study the biology of the prostate, to induce benign or malignant tumours of the gland and to investigate the usefulness of therapeutic agents, constitutes an important aspect of prostate research. Despite limitations in extrapolating data obtained from animal experiments to human conditions, animal models offer certain advantages, although ultimate evaluation of any biological or clinical concepts or therapeutic agent should be in the human. However, progress in these investigations will be seriously hampered if all these studies are to be carried out in man. Thus the need for other experimental models and, in particular, those related to animals becomes apparent. A number of factors

281

have influenced the choice of experimental animals. In most cases, the experimental practicality, together with availability and financial considerations, have been determining factors in the choice of an animal model. An example has been the use of rodents, especially rats, in this field of research. A great majority of the experiments concerning the biochemistry and endocrinology of the prostate have been carried out in this species, despite substantial differences to the human prostate. The prostate of the rat is composed of a discrete paired ventral lobe, located at the neck of the bladder, a dorsolateral group of prostatic acini and ducts surrounding the urethra and base of the bladder, and a paired coagulating gland (Price, 1963). These lobes possess different biochemical properties, e.g. the ventral lobe is rich in citric acid, but lacks fructose, whilst the dorsolateral group produce both fructose and citric acid. The ventral lobes are larger and have been widely used in prostatic research, despite their dissimilarities from the human prostate.

The availability, uniformity of genetic strains and ability to control both age and experimental conditions have thus made the rat an attractive animal for prostate research. The mouse prostate has also been used for research purposes. The mouse has dorsal and ventral prostatic lobes as well as paired coagulating glands. However, the ventral lobes are relatively less well developed than in the rat. Lateral lobes are absent or only slightly developed. In addition to the rat and mouse, the prostate of mastomys is considered to be suitable for prostatic research. The females of this species possesses a well developed prostate which responds to steroid hormones (Holland, 1970). The prostate of the female mastomys consists of two lobes lying posterior to and on each side of the bladder neck. Dorsally, these lobes are separated by the urethra and vagina and this anatomical arrangement resembles the ventral lobes of the male mastomys (Fig. 12.1). Hormonal studies on this female prostate (Ghanadian et al., 1975b, 1977b, c, 1978) have shown remarkable similarity with that of the male prostate from this species (Ghanadian et al., 1976; Smith, C. B. et al., 1978, 1979). The ultrastructure of the male and female prostate in this species has also been investigated (Smith, A. K. et al., 1978). The advantage of the female prostate of mastomys as an experimental model lies in the low androgen environment in which this prostate functions (Ghanadian et al., 1977b) which can be utilized for the studies of the hormone action, drug effects and other variables affecting the prostate. Although there are considerable advantages in the use of rodent prostates for a number of research purposes, only certain strains of rodents are suitable for investigations into the development of prostatic tumours. This aspect will be discussed in this chapter.

The dog prostate has also been useful in the study of benign prostatic hyperplasia. The dog possesses a large prostate which constitutes 0.01–0.07 % of its body weight (Fig. 12.1). De Klerk et al. (1979) reported the average weight in animals aged 1–3 years to be 14.7 ± 6.4 g increasing to 23.65 ± 10.45 g for those 5–10 years old. The body weight in these dogs ranged from 7.0 to 18.6 kg (11.3 ± 2.2, mean ± SD). The large size of the prostate gland as well as the occurrence of benign hyperplasia in the old dog has made this animal suitable for a number of prostatic research projects.

The prostates of primates and, in particular those of the Rhesus monkey

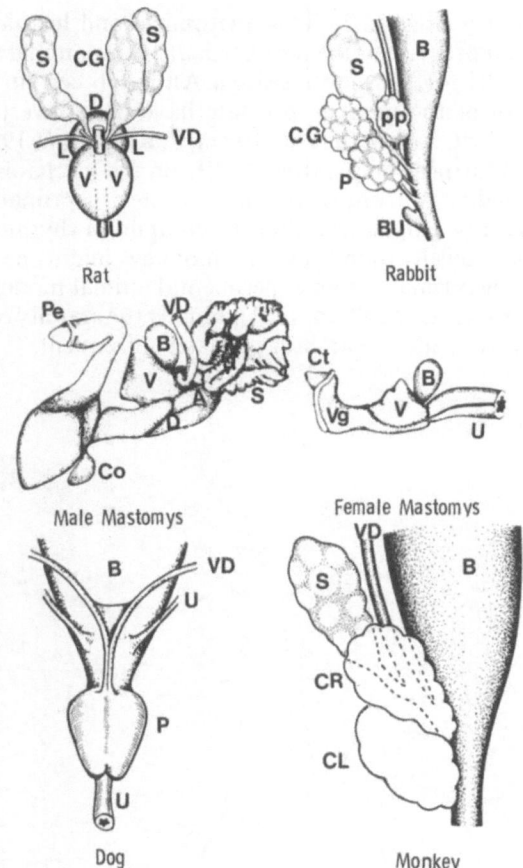

Figure 12.1 Diagrams of prostate glands in rat, rabbit, male and female mastomys, dog and Rhesus monkey. Key words: Prostate (P), Dorsal prostate (D), Ventral prostate (V), Lateral prostate (L), Anterior prostate (A), Para prostate (PP), Coagulating glands (CG), Cranial lobe (CR), Caudal lobe (CL), Bladder (B), Urethra (U), Penis (Pe), Clitoris (Ct), Vagina (Vg). Drawings were kindly supplied by Professor N. J. Blacklock (Rat, rabbit and monkey), Ghanadian *et al*, (1975) (Male and female mastomys) and J. Barr (dog).

and the baboon, are reported to be suitable for a number of research purposes. Comparative studies of the monkey and human prostates have shown remarkable similarities between the two glands. The prostate in the monkey is composed of two distinct lobes, a cranial and a caudal. The surface of the cranial lobe is deeply furrowed and resembles the seminal vesicles in external appearance, but is easily separable from them. The caudal lobe is closely associated with the urethra and has a smooth surface (Fig. 12.1). Blacklock (1977) has suggested that the cranial and the caudal lobes of the monkey prostate are analogous with the central and peripheral zones of the human

prostate respectively (Fig. 12.2). This anatomical and histological resembl-
ance of the human prostate to the monkey makes this animal an appropriate
experimental model for prostate research. Although certain aspects of the
endocrine control of the monkey prostate have been investigated (Arora-
Dinakar *et al.*, 1977; Ghanadian *et al.*, 1977a, d; Karr *et al.*, 1978; Ghanadian
and Smith, 1981) further comparative studies on the mechanism of action of
hormones and endocrine control of the prostates in primates and man is
required. It should be emphasized that the compound rhythmic variation of
plasma androgen levels found in the monkey might be considered a
disadvantage in the primate as an experimental animal model for endocrine
studies of the prostate (Ghanadian, 1981). Finally the scarcity of these animals
and their cost have made research in primates infrequent.

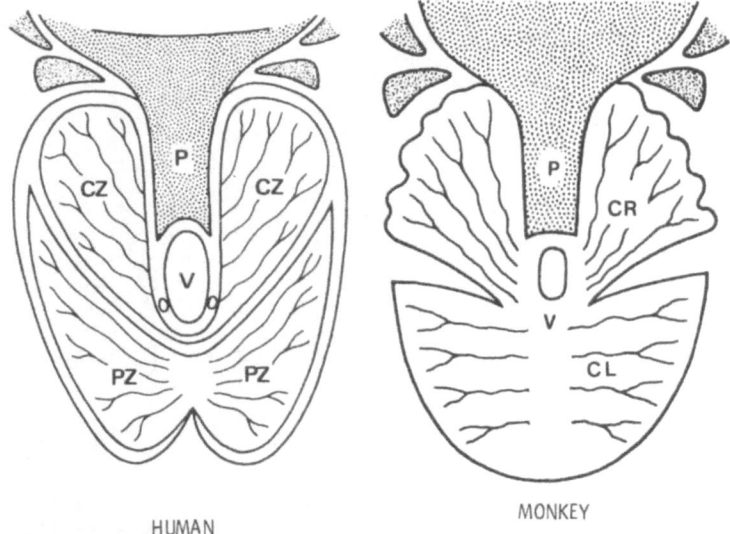

HUMAN

MONKEY

Figure 12.2   Coronal sections of the prostates of human and monkey. Key words:
Central zone (CZ), Peripheral zone (PZ), Preprostatic sphincter (P), Verumontanum
(V), Cranial lobe (CR), Caudal lobe (CL). Drawings were kindly supplied by
Professor N. J. Blacklock.

12.1.1   Animal models for benign prostatic hypertrophy

12.1.1.1   *Spontaneous and experimentally induced tumours*

In rodents, the occurrence of spontaneous hyperplasia is rare. However, there
are a number of reports of experimentally induced hyperplasia. Studies with
mice have shown that certain glandular and stromal changes similar to benign
prostatic hypertrophy can be induced. Fingerhurt and Veenema (1966, 1967)
have induced BPH in mice which has similarities to the human condition

including urinary retention. Both intact and castrated animals received subcutaneous implantation of stilboestrol which induced nodules of connective tissue and smooth muscle as well as an increase in the weight of the pituitary and adrenal glands. In these studies, subsequent adrenalectomy relieved urinary retention and caused gradual atrophy of the prostate. Prostatic hyperplasia has also been induced in the prostate of female mastomys. As discussed before, all females of this species possess a well-developed prostate gland which responds to androgens. It is reported that the treatment of this animal with testosterone causes hyperplasia and substantial increase in prostatic size. It has also been noted that certain strains of golden hamster, e.g. B10 87.2, develop spontaneous tumours of the prostate (Finney et al., 1978).

Of the experimental animals, the dog has been considered to be the most appropriate model for the study of prostatic hyperplasia, as both the ageing dog and man spontaneously develop benign prostatic hyperplasia (Moore, 1944; Huggins, 1945, 1947). The frequency of the tumour is high in dogs over 5 years of age. The benign tumour of the dog has certain differences from that in man (Ofner, 1968). Whilst canine prostatic hyperplasia is a diffuse epithelial or glandular process, involving the entire gland, the human tumour is a multinodular process. The development of both tumours requires functioning testes, but whilst the incidence of the tumour is different in human races, it is not breed dependent in the dog. Benign prostatic hyperplasia can be induced experimentally in the dog. Huggins (1963, Vollmer and Kauffman, p. 27) originally reported that the combined administration of testosterone and stilboestrol to the castrated dog for a period of 30 days caused prostatic enlargement. Walsh and Wilson (1976) were the first to demonstrate that the long-term administration of 5α-androstane-3α,17β-diol can induce prostatic hyperplasia in castrated dogs. In their study the administration of DHT did not induce the tumour. However, subsequent studies by others have revealed that DHT is capable of inducing this tumour in the intact animal. De Klerk et al. (1979) have extensively investigated the experimental conditions for the induction of canine prostatic hyperplasia by hormone manipulation. These investigators have compared the experimentally induced tumour with that of the spontaneous one. The tumour was induced in young dogs with intact testes, when treated with either DHT or 5α-androstane-3α,17β-diol alone or with either of these steroids in combination with oestradiol-17β. In contrast, the induction of the tumour in young castrated dogs, in which the gland had been allowed to involute for one month, required both oestradiol-17β and either 5α-androstane-3α,17β-diol or DHT. Neither testosterone nor oestradiol-17β alone or in combination could produce the tumour. De Klerk et al. (1979) have also studied spontaneous prostatic hyperplasia in the beagle and confirmed the two types of the tumour, i.e. glandular and cystic hyperplasia, in this animal. These authors have emphasized that the experimentally induced glandular hyperplasia could not be distinguished from spontaneous glandular hyperplasia. However, cystic hyperplasia was not produced by any of the hormonal manipulations. This study provided support for the dog prostate as an experimental model. Despite some dissimilarities with that of the human, this model produces useful information for the understanding of hormonal factors which influence the development of this tumour in man.

The development of benign prostatic hyperplasia has also been reported in the lion (Huggins, 1943) and the rate of DHT formation in this species has been found to be similar to the dog (Gloyna and Wilson, 1969). However, this animal has obviously not been considered a suitable model for experimentation.

There is a paucity of information on the incidence of benign prostatic hyperplasia in aged primates. A major reason has been the cost of maintaining sufficient numbers of primates and permitting them to get old enough to develop this tumour.

12.1.2   Animal models for carcinoma of the prostate

The occurrence of malignant tumours of the prostate in experimental animals is not common. Nevertheless, there are several reports of this tumour in experimental animals. A difficulty in this field is the variability of human prostatic cancer, its cell type, differentiation growth rate and the variation in response to hormonal manipulation or other treatment. Thus it is quite apparent that a single animal model is incapable of providing the necessary criteria for all types of human prostatic cancer. A more realistic approach would be to search for a model which could meet the characteristics of a more typical human prostatic cancer with high incidence. Most of the necessary requirements for an animal model for this tumour have been described by Coffey *et al.* (1979). The tumours should be spontaneous in origin from prostatic tissue and develop in the aged animal. The adenocarcinoma's slow growing nature, its malignant and metastatic pattern and its histological and biochemical similarities to human prostatic cancer are important factors in experimental animal tumours. Further requirements are a hormone sensitivity and a response to castration and oestrogen therapy which is similar to that in man. Finally, the similarities in immunology and in the therapeutic response to human prostatic cancer are relevant when selecting animal models.

12.1.2.1   *Spontaneous carcinoma of the prostate*

The incidence of spontaneous carcinoma in rodents has been relatively small. Fortner *et al.* (1963) reported a transplantable spontaneous adenocarcinoma in one Syrian (golden) hamster. Dunning (1963) also reported a spontaneous tumour of the prostate in a Copenhagen rat. This tumour was identified in 1961 in a 22-month-old retired breeder from the 54th brother × sister generation of line 2337. The tumour occupied a large part of the lower abdominal cavity and appeared to involve primarily the dorsal prostate gland. This primary tumour was classified as a papillary adenocarcinoma. No metastases were identified. Subsequently ten rats, four of the same inbred line as the host of the primary tumour and 6 F_1 hybrids from a Copenhagen × Fisher cross were inoculated on the right side with 10 mg grafts of the soft tumour tissue and on the left side with somewhat larger quantities of the gelatinous material. The transplanted tumours grew very slowly and became palpable on the 60th day on the right side of each of the inoculated rats, whereas no tumour appeared at the site of injection of the gelatinous material on the left side of the rat. Dunning in addition reported glandular formation with a great deal of cellular material corresponding to the normal dorsal-type gland of the rat prostate. The tumour remained histologically a well-differentiated adenocarcinoma. Voigt and Dunning (1974) studied the hormone dependency of this transplantable tumour and found that the tumour grew well only in intact males, but did not grow in castrates. They also found that the major metabolites of testosterone in the tumour are 5α-dihydrotestosterone in the androgen sensitive R-3327 but not in the androgen insensitive R-3327A. This androgen insensitive squamous cell carcinoma of the prostate is derived from an established line (R-3327). They also noted R-3327A tumours have a growth rate of approximately ten times that of R-3327 (Voigt et al., 1975). Further characterization of Dunning R-3327 tumour was carried out by Smolev et al. (1977) who used the term R-3327H for their tumour which was a relatively pure, well-differentiated adenocarcinoma. Histologically this tumour was similar to a well-differentiated human prostatic cancer and the biochemical profile of the tumour indicates its origin from the rat dorsolateral prostate. The cell kinetics and growth rate of this tumour following a variety of hormonal manipulations have established that 70–90% of this tumour require androgens for their growth. However, 10–30% of the cells are capable of growth in the absence of androgens. After the tumour was well established in an intact animal, subsequent oestrogen therapy or castration resulted in a marked diminution in tumour volume. This was followed by a subsequent relapse. Based on the characterization of the tumour at the morphological, biochemical and therapeutic levels these investigators concluded that R-3327H prostatic adenocarcinoma fulfils the criteria of an animal model for carcinoma of the prostate. The original tumour arose spontaneously in the aged animal, grew slowly and demonstrated malignant cellular characteristics and metastases. Smolev et al. (1977) also suggested that the androgen dependence of most of the cells within this tumour mimics the human situation, as does the occurrence of a non-hormonally dependent phase of tumour growth. Further investigations into the hormonal control and suitability of this experimental model were carried out by Isaacs et al. (1978, 1979). Apart from the R-3327 and R-3327H which is a well-differentiated slow growing androgen-insensitive tumour, they established two other sub-lines: a well-differentiated slow growing insensitive tumour (R-3327HI) and a fast growing androgen-insensitive, anaplastic tumour (R-3327AT). The latter was very distinct in all parameters examined except the tissue protein electrophoretic patterns, which contained a uniform pattern in all tumours. The significant differences between R-3327H and HI sub-lines were the inability of testosterone to stimulate DNA synthesis in the R-3327HI tumour and certain differences in enzymes of these sub-lines. The specific activity of these enzymes (3α-hydroxy steroid dehydrogenase, leucine aminopeptidase and lactic-dehydrogenase) increased, while the activity of another three enzymes (6α, 7α-hydroxylase, 5α-reductase and alkaline phosphatase) decreased in the sub-lines which are androgen insensitive and less differentiated (Isaacs et al., 1979). Lopez and Voigt (1977) and Lubaroff et al.

(1977) have studied the immunological aspects of R-3327 tumours and have suggested that this tumour line appears to be suitable for immunological and possible immunotherapeutic studies of this type of neoplasia.

Spontaneous prostate adenocarcinomas have also been reported in aged germ-free random bred Lobund Wistar rats. Pollard (1973) reported four spontaneous adenocarcinomas, three with metastases and leukemoid reactions. This animal develops spontaneous tumour in increasing frequency from the age of 24 months. Most tumours involved endocrine organs or their target organs. The malignant characteristics were noted in individual animals over 30 months. Pollard and Luckert (1975) examined 52 male germ-free Wistar rats older than 30 months. Seven (13 %) had adenocarcinoma in the prostate gland. One exception was a younger rat (age 22 months) which had a prostate tumour plus lung metastases. Among 17 over 35 months old, six (35 %) had prostate carcinoma. Thus, as in man, the incidence of autochthonous prostate carcinomas appears to increase with age. The germ-free status of the Wistar rats was thought unlikely to have influenced the development of tumours, but merely to have allowed the rats to live long enough for tumours to develop. Pollard and Luckert (1975) transplanted three prostate carcinomas and propagated them in a series of conventional random bred Lobund Wistar rats, which, in addition to subcutaneous implanted tumour, developed lymph node and pulmonary metastases Pollard and Luckert (1976) subjected germ-free and conventional rats with metastasizing prostate carcinoma cell to chemotherapy schedules of cyclophosphamide (NSC-26271) which modified the pattern of established and metastatic lesions. The germ-free mice and rats tolerated larger subtoxic doses of cyclophosphamide over longer periods than conventional animals.

Iglesias et al. (1966) reported the occurrence of a spontaneous adenocarcinoma of the prostate in a 39-month-old male AXC rat, when investigating more than 807 intact male rats of which 207 had different tumours. The tumour was an undifferentiated infiltrating adenocarcinoma without metastases. They transplanted the tumour in 16 intact and castrated AXC rats and the tumour grew in all except one female. Metastases were found in the lung of three castrated males. Shain et al. (1975) also found spontaneous adenocarcinoma of the ventral prostate in seven of 41 aged (34–37 months old) virgin untreated male AXC rats. The detected frequency of prostatic adenocarcinoma in this group was 17 %. However, these investigators suggested that because a visible lesion was present in only one of the seven rats, the reported detected frequency rate may be a significant underestimate of the actual frequency as microscopic neoplasm unassociated with haemorrhage would go undetected, when visually examined. In this study the principal intraglandular neoplasm was composed of marked anaplastic epithelial cells which retained a moderate propensity to form glandular patterns. Interglandular connective tissue was invasive in one rat, but metastases were not demonstrated. Shain et al. (1975) concluded that the high frequency of spontaneous prostate adenocarcinoma in the aged rat and its absence in the young individual suggest a positive correlation between frequency and age, as is true for man. Shain et al. (1977) reported that the incidence of adenocarcinoma of the prostate in old virgin AXC male rat increased to 70 % when animals were treated with testosterone. The principle morphologic features which distinguish neoplasia in rats receiving exogenous testosterone from those in untreated rats were (1) more extensive glandular enlargement due to neoplastic growth, (2) more numerous mitotic figures, (3) an increased frequency of invasion and (4) neoplastic cells that were more anaplastic. Testosterone metabolism by spontaneous and transplantable ventral prostate adenocarcinoma in this animal demonstrated increased Δ^4-androstenedione and diminished 5α-dihydrotestosterone synthetic capacity relative to lesion-free ventral prostate of senescent AXC rats. Shain *et al.* (1977) suggested that senescent changes in regulation of ventral prostate cell function, indicated by diminished cytoplasmic androgen receptors and altered testosterone metabolism, may be pathogenic in prostatic neoplasia and indicate that the rat represents an appropriate model for the study of prostate carcinogenesis. Medel *et al.* (1980) have studied the characteristics of androgen receptors in prostatic adenocarcinoma of AXC rats and compared them with those of the normal prostate in this strain. In their studies an originally spontaneous adenocarcinoma of the prostate, which was identified by Iglesias *et al.* (1966), was transplanted subsequently into the neck of 2-month-old AXC rat for several generations over 12 years. The comparison of the physical parameters of the normal and malignant tissues showed identical molecular weight (280 000 daltons), sedimentation coefficient (8s), Stokes radius (87 Å) and isoelectric point (5.8 pH units). There was a slight difference at the level of migration in polyacrylamide gel electrophoresis between DHT receptor complexes. Furthermore, the dissociation constant of the DHT receptor complex from adenocarcinoma was significantly lower than that from normal prostate. These investigators suggested that, probably due to the presence of malignancy, there are changes at the level of cytoplasmic DHT receptor, which facilitate their association with the steroid. These changes appear to be subtle enough to maintain the properties of the receptor complex with the exception of its electrophorectic mobility.

The occurrence of adenocarcinoma of the prostate in the prostate of one untreated virgin female *Praomys* (*Mastomys*) *natalensis* has been reported by Snell and Stewart (1965). They examined the prostate of 55 female mastomys and found 4 cases of proliferative hyperplasia and one adenocarcinoma. Holland (1970) has also found proliferative changes of the prostate with increasing age in untreated female mastomys over 24 months old. This papillary hyperplasia was seen often with granulosa cell proliferation of the ovary and proliferative changes of breast and endometrium. Treatment of the animal with testosterone caused enlargement of the prostate. Long-term treatment caused marked papillary hyperplasia which led to the suspicion of malignancy. However, he did not observe all the cellular criteria of malignancy or metastases.

Spontaneous adenocarcinoma of the prostate has been found in the dog. However, it is a much rarer condition than benign hyperplasia in this species. Adenocarcinoma of the canine prostate is often difficult to differentiate clinically from prostatic hyperplasia. Most of the prostates which harbour adenocarcinoma contain hyperplastic foci, which further confuse the differential diagnosis. Leav and Ling (1968) have studied 20 cases of adenocarcinoma of the canine prostate, using clinical and autopsy materials. Similarities of this neoplasm to the one in man were observed. These included morphological similarities, a frequency of the tumour in older animals, skeletal metastases, histochemical demonstration of acid phosphatase and lipids in neoplastic cells and routes of metastasis similar to those thought to exist in man. The main differences between the two species are reported to be the lower incidence of the tumour in the dog, as well as the unspecific anatomical region and the absence of latent carcinoma in this species.

In addition to dog, spontaneous primary carcinoma of the prostate has been reported in one monkey, *Macaca mulatta* (Engle and Stout, 1940). Lack of evidence for spontaneous carcinoma of the prostate in other domestic animals may be more apparent than real, because of the widespread practice of castrating the immature animal (Ofner, 1968).

12.1.2.2 Experimentally induced malignant tumours of the prostate

Carcinoma of the prostate has been induced in several species of rodents including rats, mice and mastomys by direct inoculation of carcinogenic compounds such as 20-methyl cholanthrene (Moore and Melchionna, 1937; Dunning *et al.*, 1946; Horning and Demochovski, 1947; Holland, 1970). However, most of the induced tumours are reported to be squamous cell carcinomas and fibrosarcomas which are different to that observed in man. Ishibe *et al.* (1975) have extensively investigated the influence of a number of hormones on the induction of prostatic tumour by 20-methylcholanthrene. When the compound was administered alone, there was an initial period of 90 days before the appearance of neoplasms, and by 200 days 57.3% of the animals exhibited neoplasm. Oestradiol benzoate enhanced the carcinogenic properties of 20-methylcholanthrene, whereas when combined with triiodothyronin the carcinogenic effect was reduced. Testosterone propionate, castration, hydrocortisone, human chorionic gonadotrophin and prolactin do not appear to produce any significant changes. These authors concluded that endocrine manipulation may be a major environmental factor in the formation and biochemical activities of 20-methylcholanthrene induced neoplasm in rat prostate. Fingerhurt and Veenema (1977) have developed tumours consistent with prostatic adenocarcinoma following the injection of the potent carcinogen, 9, 10-dimethyl-1,2-benzanthracene (DMBA) into small rats (Fisher/Furth), mice (Strong A/J) and golden hamsters. The animals were previously castrated and the prostate had become histologically atrophic. Three to 4 months following the injection of DMBA, evidence of prostatic adenocarcinoma was consistently found in each of the groups of castrated animals which survived the experiment. The prostates were found to be enlarged and urethral obstructions were also noted. Metastases to the lung were observed in five mice, three rats and one hamster.

The induction of malignant tumours of the prostate with endocrine manipulation has not been successful (Brendler, 1963). However, Noble (1977) found that the low spontaneous incidence of grossly recognizable adenocarcinoma of the dorsal lobe of the prostate in Nb rats over 13 months old (0.45 %) could be increased to 18.38 % by prolonged treatment of animal with testosterone propionate and oestrone. The tumours tended to metastasize, transplanted readily and were mostly autonomous.

12.2 IN VIVO MODELS FOR GROWING HUMAN PROSTATIC TUMOURS

12.2.1 Immunosuppressed mice

Fragments of human tumours and tissues have been maintained in mice made deficient in cell mediated immunity by thymectomy, lethal irradiation and reconstitution with syngeneic bone marrow, which is a graft between individuals of identical genetic constitution such as identical twins and mice of the same pure line strain (Davies et al., 1969; Castro, 1972). Both benign and malignant human prostates have been maintained in this system (Castro, 1973; Castro and Cass, 1974; Williams et al., 1978a). In these studies, CBA male mice were thymectomized at 4 weeks of age by sternal approach (Miller, 1961) and 2 weeks later they were given 900 rad whole body irradiation from a cobalt source. Within 24 hours they received an intravenous injection of 5×10^6 cells of syngeneic (CBA mice) bone marrow which were obtained by irrigating donor femurs and tibias with tissue culture medium TC199. Three weeks to 3 months later fragments of $2-5$ mm^3 human prostatic tumours were implanted beneath the snout skin of the anaesthetized mice and 1 month later animals were killed and the viability of the implants assessed and compared with the original tumour. The criteria for the assessment in these studies were changes in the size of the tumour, histological appearance of the tumour and histochemical demonstration of the presence or absence of acid phosphatase. The implants were also transplanted into a second series of immunosuppressed mice which showed they could grow. The hormonal environment and the ability of prostatic explants to take up and retain testosterone in this system have been investigated in our laboratory (Williams et al., 1978a, b). This in vivo experimental model is suitable for maintenance and growth of prostatic tumours and might be useful for the assessment of therapeutic agents and their effects on prostatic tumours. However, it should be noted that there are considerable differences between the serum hormone concentrations of immunodeficient mice and of man (Williams et al., 1978b).

12.2.2 Nude mice

The mouse mutant 'nude' was first described by Flanagan (1966) and is a genetic variant of the BALB/C mouse which is characterized by being hairless. The homozygotes 'nu nu' are hairless and their growth is retarded. Pantelouris (1968) found that the thymus is absent in the homozygotes while in all normal phenotypes (homozygote wild type or heterozygotes) the organ is normally developed. The absence of the thymus was confirmed for both sexes and all ages. Okada et al. (1976) have transplanted human benign and malignant prostatic tissues as well as cells from permanent cell lines originating from prostatic tumours into the subcutaneous space of the nude mice. In this study transplantation of single pieces of 50 mg of benign and malignant tissues provided the best results. These investigators found that carcinoma was present in seven out of 25 nude mice that were castrated and treated with testosterone, but only in one of 21 transplantations into castrates without testosterone substitution, suggesting that heterotransplants of human prostatic carcinoma tissue can be established more easily in androgenized animals. The histological appearance of the benign tumours was found to be strikingly similar to the original tumours. However, heterotransplantation of cells from permanent cell lines resulted in a fast growing carcinoma not similar to the original tumours.

12.2.3 Neonatal rats

Neonatal rats have also been used for maintaining human benign hypertrophied prostate (Senge *et al.*, 1972). The required immunosuppression has been achieved by subcutaneous application of antilymphocyte serum which was obtained by immunization of rabbits with lymphocytes from mesenteric lymph nodes of the rat. Benign prostatic tissues have been transplanted into the femoral musculature and 3 weeks later the implanted tissue samples have been examined and found to be similar to the original tissue. These workers have found metaplastic alterations characterized by a decrease in enzymic activity. The treatment of animals with testosterone resulted in stimulation of the implant, whereas oestrogen produced marked vacuolar degeneration of the epithelium. These workers did not investigate the suitability of this model for malignant tissues.

12.3 IN VITRO MODELS

Despite certain advantages in the growth and maintenance of prostatic tumours by *in vivo* methods using experimental animals, the influence of many systemic factors complicate the interpretation of the results in these investigations. Thus, for a number of purposes, the use of *in vitro* systems alone or in parallel with the *in vivo* models for a comparative study is most desirable. In the *in vitro* systems, the experimental conditions can be more strictly controlled and the exposure of the cells to chemical or therapeutic agents can easily be manipulated. The most commonly used technique for the *in vitro* growth of the prostatic tumours has been tissue culture which consists of the two main categories of cell and organ culture. In cell culture, cells are grown as colonies in monolayer or suspension or more rarely now as cells migrating and surrounding explant cultures. Fraley *et al.* (1970) have developed a cell line from tissue cultures of a human benign prostatic adenoma. These workers explanted a small fragment of the tumour which became surrounded by fibroblast-like as well as epithelial cells, but the epithelial type finally dominated. The cells were designated MA160 and have been carried through numerous passages. The long survival of MA160 *in vitro* is thought to be an indication that the cells have undergone spontaneous transformation, as normally human adult cells have a finite life span in culture. However, the cells may become transformed and acquire the ability to survive indefinitely *in vitro* (Lasnitzki, 1976). It has been reported that the MA160 cell line has been contaminated with He La cells (Nelson-Rees *et al.*, 1974). Lasnitzki (1976) suggested that even if the risk of contamination with other cells is excluded, it is doubtful whether the transformed cell line is still comparable to the fresh tumours. Therefore short-term culture would be preferable for relating hormonal response *in vitro* to that of the patients. Brehmer *et al.* (1972) also established cell culture from benign hyperplasia and adenocarcinoma which remained viable for 2–3 months. These cell lines were developed from explant cultures or by repeated trypsinization of the tumour.

Schröder *et al.* (1971) developed primary and subculture of prostatic carcinoma and Okada and Schröder (1974) reported the characterization of the prostatic carcinoma epithelial cell line, ED33. It has been suggested that this cell line may also have been contaminated with He La cells (Webber, 1981). Other human cell lines are HPC-36, DU-145 and PC-3 (Lubaroff, 1977, Stone *et al.*, 1978; Kaighn *et al.*, 1979).

The cell line PC-3 has been derived from a poorly differentiated adenocarcinoma of the prostate, whilst the line DU-145 was derived from a metastatic lesion in the brain with widespread metastatic carcinoma of the prostate. An important consideration in prostatic cell culture is that there is a 2–3 week elapse between the removal of the tumour and the establishment of the isolated cell in monolayer. Even during this short period, a selection of cells which are best adapted to *in vitro* conditions will take place and it is not certain whether these are still closely comparable to the more heterogenous cell population of the tumour (Lasnitzki, 1976). This is most important, as according to Franks *et al.* (1970) epithelium and stroma form a functional unit and the expression of hormonal action depends on an intact epithelial-stromal relationship. In organ culture, the two components and their anatomical relationships are well preserved. A number of research groups have grown benign hypertrophied and malignant prostates for short periods in organ culture. Schrodt and Foreman (1971) explanted prostatic adenoma for a period of up to 9 days. The morphology of epithelium and stroma were well preserved for the first 3 days and in some explants up to 9 days. McRae *et al.* (1973) and Ghanadian *et al.* (1975a) have cultured explants of benign hypertrophied prostate for 8 days and have investigated the morphology, DNA content, and glucose utilization in the presence and absence of testosterone and dihydrotestosterone. McMahon *et al.* (1972) and McMahon and Thomas (1973) also grew prostatic adenoma and carcinoma in organ culture for periods up to 7 days. It is quite apparent that both cell and organ cultures of the prostatic tumours have several advantages in that satisfactory growth or maintenance of prostatic tumours can be achieved by these techniques, despite their limitations.

12.4 CONCLUSIONS

In this chapter the significance of experimental animal models in relation to research and development in human prostatic tumours is discussed. A comparative study of the prostates of the most commonly used animals has been made and emphasis is given to the advantages of these animals in research. Studies of the spontaneous and experimentally induced benign prostatic hyperplasia in animals suggest that the dog is a suitable experimental model for this tumour, and despite differences between the tumour in this species and in man, this model provides valuable information on the aetiology and pathogenesis of this tumour. The search for experimental animal models for carcinoma of the prostate has been mainly focused on the rodent. The incidence of spontaneous carcinoma of the prostate in Syrian hamster, Copenhagen rat, germ-free random bred Lobund Wistar rat, AXC rat and female mastomys is reported. The current information on these animal tumours as models for human prostatic carcinoma has been discussed. These studies suggest that a single animal model is often incapable of providing the necessary criteria for all types of human prostatic cancer. Therefore, the search for a comprehensive model which could meet the essential requirements of a more typical human prostatic cancer should continue.

The *in vivo* and *in vitro* models for the growth and maintenance of human prostatic tumours have also been reviewed. A number of *in vivo* models including immunosuppressed mice, nude mice and neonatal rats are presented. For the *in vitro* systems cell and organ cultures of human prostatic tumours have been discussed.

12.5 REFERENCES

Arora-Dinakar, R., Dinakar, N. and Prasad, M. R. N. (1977). Metabolism *in vitro* of ^{3}H-testosterone in testis, epididymis and sex accessories of the Rhesus monkey, *Macaca mulatta*: effects of cyproterone acetate on androgen metabolism. *Indian J. Exp. Biol.*, **15**, 953

Blacklock, N. J. (1977). The morphology of the parenchyma of the prostate. *Urol. Res.*, **5**, 163

Brendler, H. (1963). Experimental prostatic cancer. Background of the problem. *Natl. Cancer. Inst. Monogr.*, **12**, 343

Brehmer, B., Marquardt, H. and Madsen, P. O. (1972). Growth and hormonal response of cells derived from carcinoma and hyperplasia of the prostate in monolayer cell culture. A possible *in vitro* model for clinical chemotherapy. *J. Urol.*, **108**, 890

Castro, J. E. (1972). Human tumours grown in mice. *Nature New Biol.*, **239**, 83

Castro, J. E. (1973). A method of *in vivo* maintenance of human prostatic tissue in immunosuppressed mice. *Br. J. Urol.*, **45**, 163

Castro, J. E. and Cass, W. (1974). Maintenance of human tumours and tissues in immunosuppressed mice. *Br. J. Surg.*, **61**, 421

Coffey, D. S., Isaacs, J. T. and Weisman, R. M. (1979). Animal models for the study of prostatic cancer. In Morphy, G. P. (ed.) *Prostatic Cancer*. pp. 89–109. (Littleton: PSG Publishing)

Davies, A. J., Carter, R. L., Leuchars, E., Wallis, V. and Koller, P. C. (1969). The morphology of immune-reaction in normal thymectomised and reconstituted mice. The response to sheep erythrocytes. *Immunology*, **16**, 57

De Klerk, D. P., Coffey, D. S., Ewing, L. L., McDermott, I. R., Reiner, W. G., Robinson, C. H., Scott, W. W., Strandberg, J. D., Talalay, P., Walsh, P. C., Wheaton,

L. G. and Zirkin, B. R. (1979). Comparison of spontaneous and experimentally induced canine prostatic hyperplasia. *J. Clin. Invest.*, **64**, 842

Dunning, W. F. (1963). Prostatic cancer in the rat. *Natl. Cancer Inst. Monogr.*, **12**, 369

Dunning, W. F., Curtis, M. R. and Segaloff, A. (1946) Methylcholanthrene squamous cell carcinoma of the rat prostate with skeletal metastases and failure of the rat liver to respond to the same carcinogen. *Cancer Res.*, **6**, 256

Engle, E. T. and Stout, A. P. (1940). Spontaneous primary carcinoma of the prostate in a monkey (*Macaca mulatta*). *Am. J. Cancer.*, **39**, 334

Fingerhurt, B. and Veenema, R. J. (1966). Histology and radiocultography of induced benign enlargement of the mouse prostate. *Invest. Urol.*, **4**, 112

Fingerhurt, B. and Veenema, R. J. (1967). The effect of bilateral adrenalectomy on induced benign prostatic hyperplasia in mice. *J. Urol.*, **97**, 508

Fingerhurt, B. and Veenema, R. J. (1977). An animal model for the study of prostatic adenocarcinoma. *Invest. Urol.*, **15**, 42

Finney, R. W., Harper, M. E., Gaskell, S. J., and Griffiths, K. (1978). Endogenous androgen concentrations in the dorsal and ventral prostate gland of golden hamsters with benign prostatic tumours. *J. Endocrinol.*, **79**, 53

Flanagan, S. P. (1966). 'Nude' a new hairless gene with pleiotrophic effects in the mouse. *Genet. Res.*, **8**, 295

Fortner, J. G., Funkhauser, J. W. and Cullen, M. R. (1963). A transplantable spontaneous adenocarcinoma of the prostate in the syrian (golden) hamster. *Natl. Cancer Inst. Monogr.*, **12**, 371

Fraley, E. E., Ecker, S. and Vincent, M. M. (1970). Spontaneous *in vitro* transformation of adult human prostatic epithelium. *Science*, **170**, 540

Franks, L. M., Riddle, P. N., Carbonell, A. W. and Gey, G. D. (1970). A comparative study of the ultra-structure and lack of growth capacity of adult human prostatic epithelium mechanically separated from its stroma. *J. Pathol.*, **100**, 113

Ghanadian, R. (1981). Androgen regulation in the prostate of Rhesus monkey (*Macaca mulatta*). In Hafez, E. S. E. and Spring-Mills, E. (eds.) *Clinics in Andrology. Vol. 6: Prostatic Carcinoma, Biology and Diagnosis.* pp. 160–164. (The Hague: Martinus Nijhoff)

Ghanadian, R., Auf, G., Smith, C. B., Chisholm, G. D. and Blacklock, N. J. (1977a). Androgen receptors in the prostate of Rhesus monkey. *Urol. Res.*, **5**, 169

Ghanadian, R., Chisholm, G. D. and Ansell, I. D. (1975a). 5α-dihydrotestosterone stimulation of human prostate in organ culture. *J. Endocrinol.*, **65**, 253

Ghanadian, R., Holland, J. M. and Chisholm, G. D. (1975b). Identification of a prostate in female *Praomys (Mastomys) natalensis* using ^{3}H steroids. *Br. J. Urol.*, **47**, 77

Ghanadian, R., Holland, J. M. and Chisholm, G. D. (1976). Uptake and distribution of ^{3}H testosterone in tissues of male *Praomys (Mastomys) natalensis*: an *in vivo* and *in vitro* study on the prostate. *Urol. Res.*, **4**, 77

Ghanadian, R., Lewis, J. G. and Chisholm, G. D. (1977b). Androgen concentrations in prostate and serum of the male and female *Praomys (Mastomys) natalensis*. *Invest. Urol.*., **15**, 212

Ghanadian, R. and Smith, C. B. (1981). Androgen metabolism within the lobes of Rhesus monkey prostate. *Eur. Urol.*, **7**, 89

Ghanadian, R., Smith, C. B. and Chisholm, G. D. (1977c). Identification of an androgen receptor in the cytosol of the female Mastomys prostate. *Mol. Cell. Endocrinol.*, **8**, 147

Ghanadian, R., Smith, C. B. and Chisholm, G. D. (1978). Receptor protein for dihydrotestosterone in nuclei of the female prostate of *Praomys (Mastomys) natalensis. Invest. Urol.*, **16**, 119

Ghanadian, R., Smith, C. B., Chisholm, G. D. and Blacklock, N. J. (1977d).

Differential androgen uptake by the lobes of the Rhesus monkey prostate. *Br. J. Urol.*, **49**, 701

Gloyna, R. E. and Wilson, J. D. (1969). A comparative study of the conversion of testosterone to 17β-hydroxy-5α-androstan-3-one (dihydrotestosterone) by prostate and epididymes. *J. Clin. Endocrinol.*, **29**, 879

Holland, J. M. (1970). Prostatic hyperplasia and neoplasia in female *Praomys (Mastomys) natalensis*. *J. Natl. Cancer Inst.*, **45**, 1229

Horning, E. S. and Demochovski, L. (1947). Induction of prostate tumours in mice. *Br. J. Cancer*, **1**, 59

Huggins, C. (1943). Endocrine control of prostatic cancer. *Science*, **97**, 541

Huggins, C. (1945). The physiology of the prostate gland. *Physiol Rev.*, **25**, 281

Huggins, C. (1947). The aetiology of benign prostatic hypertrophy. *Bull. NY Acad. Med.*, **23**, 697

Iglesias, R., Vukusic, P., Panasevich, V. and Salinas, S. (1966). Spontaneous, transplantable adenocarcinoma of the prostate of the AXC rat. *Proc. Am. Assoc. Cancer Res.*, **7**, 33

Isaacs, J. T., Heston, W. D. W., Weissman, R. M. and Coffey, D. S. (1978). Animal models of the hormone-sensitive and insensitive prostatic adenocarcinoma, Dunning R3327-H, R3327-HI and R3327-AT. *Cancer Res.*, **38**, 4353

Isaacs, J. T., Isaacs, W. B. and Coffey, D. S. (1979). Model for development of non-receptor methods for distinguishing androgen-sensitive and insensitive prostatic tumours. *Cancer Res.*, **39**, 2652

Ishibe, T., Takenaka, I. and Kazuta, M. (1975). Prostate and 20-methylcholanthrene. In Goland, M. (ed.) *Normal and Abnormal Growth of the Prostate*. pp. 759–787. (Springfield: Charles C. Thomas)

Kaighn, M. E., Narayan, S., Ohnuki, Y. and Lechner, J. F. (1979). Establishment and characterization of a human prostatic carcinoma cell line (PC-3). *Invest. Urol.*, **17**, 16

Karr, J. P., Sufrin, G., Kirdoni, R. Y., Murphy, G. P. and Sandberg, A. A. (1978). Prostatic binding of oestradiol-17β in the baboon. *J. Steroid Biochem.*, **9**, 87

Lasnitzki, I. (1976). Action of hormones on the normal prostate and prostatic tumours grown *in vitro*. In Williams, D. I. and Chisholm, G. D. (eds.) *Scientific Foundation of Urology*. pp. 365–370. (London: Heinemann)

Leav, I. and Ling, G. V. (1968). Adenocarcinoma of the canine prostate. *Cancer*, **22**, 1329

Lopez, D. M. and Voigt, W. (1977). Adenocarcinoma R-3327 of the Copenhagen rat as a suitable model for immunological studies of prostate cancer. *Cancer Res.*, **37**, 2057

Lubaroff, D. M. (1977). Development of an epithelial tissue culture line from human prostatic adenocarcinoma. *J. Urol.*, **118**, 612

Lubaroff, D. M., Canfield, L., Feldbush, T. L. and Bonney, W. W. (1977). R3327 Adenocarcinoma of the Copenhagen rat as a model for the study of the immunologic aspects of prostate cancer. *J. Natl. Cancer Inst.*, **58**, 1677

McMahon, M. J., Butler, A. J. V. and Thomas, G. H. (1972). Morphological response of prostatic carcinoma to testosterone in culture. *Br. J. Cancer.*, **26**, 388

McMahon, M. J. and Thomas, G. H. (1973). Morphological changes of benign prostatic hyperplasia in culture. *Br. J. Cancer*, **27**, 323

McRae, C. U., Ghanadian, R., Fotherby, K. and Chisholm, G. D. (1973). The effect of testosterone on the human prostate in organ culture. *Br. J. Urol.*, **45**, 156

Medel, M. R., Pino, Z. A. M. and Sierralta, L. W. (1980). Comparison of the characteristics of androgen receptors from normal prostate and prostatic adenocarcinoma of AXC rats. *J. Steroid Biochem.*, **13**, 653

Miller, J. F. (1961). Immunological function of the thymus. *Lancet*, **2**, 748

Moore, R. A. (1944). Benign hypertrophy and carcinoma of the prostate. Occurrance and experimental production in animals. *Surgery (St. Louis)*, **16**, 152

Moore, C. A. and Melchionna, R. H. (1937). Production of tumours of the prostate of the white rat with 1:2 benzpyrene. *Am. J. Cancer*, **30**, 731

Nelson-Rees, W. A., Flandermeyer, R. R. and Hawthorne, P. K. (1974). Banded marker chromosomes as indicators of intra-species cellular contamination. *Science*, **184**, 1093

Noble, R. L. (1977). The development of prostatic adenocarcinoma in Nb rats following sex hormone administration. *Cancer Res.*, **37**, 1929

Ofner, P. (1968). Effects and metabolism of hormones in normal and neoplastic prostate tissue. *Vit. Horm.*, **26**, 237

Okada, K. and Schröder, F. H. (1974). Human prostatic carcinoma in cell culture: preliminary reports on the development and characterization of an epithelial cell line (E. B. 33). *Urol. Res.*, **2**, 111

Okada, K., Schroder, F. H., Jellinghaus, W., Wullstein, H. K. and Heinemeyer, H. H. (1976). Human prostatic adenocarcinoma and carcinoma: transplantation of cultured cells and primary tissue fragments in 'nude' mice. *Invest. Urol.*, **13**, 395

Pantelouris, E. M. (1968). Absence of thymus in a mouse mutant. *Nature (London)*, **217**, 370

Pollard, M. (1973). Spontaneous prostatic adenocarcinoma in aged germfree Wistar rats. *J. Natl. Cancer Inst.*, **51**, 1235

Pollard, M. and Luckert, P. H. (1975). Transplantable metastasizing prostate adenocarcinoma in rats. *J. Natl. Cancer Inst.*, **54**, 643

Pollard, M. and Luckert, P. H. (1976). Chemotherapy of metastatic prostate adenocarcinoma in germfree rats. I. Effects of cyclophosphamide (NSC-26271). *Cancer Treat. Rep.*, **60**, 619

Price, D. (1963). Comparative aspects of development and structure in the prostate. In Vollmer, E. P. and Kauffman, G. (eds.) *Biology of the Prostate and Related Tissue. Natl. Cancer Inst. Monogr.*, **12**, pp. 1–25. (Bethesda: US Dept. Health Education and Welfare)

Schrodt, G. R. and Foreman, C. D. (1971). *In vitro* maintenance of human hyperplastic prostate tissue. *Invest. Urol.*, **9**, 85

Schröder, F. H., Sato, G. and Gitters, R. F. (1971). Human prostatic adenocarcinoma: growth in monolayer tissue culture. *J. Urol.*, **106**, 734

Senge, T. H., Richter, K. D. and Lunglmayr, G. (1972). Vitality of human adenomatous prostatic tissue grafted into neonatal rats. *Invest. Urol.*, **10**, 115

Shain, S., McCullough, B., Nitchuk, M. and Boesel, R. W. (1977). Prostatic carcinogenesis in the AXU rat. *Oncology*, **34**, 114

Shain, S. A., McCullough, B. and Segaloff, A. (1975). Spontaneous adenocarcinomas of aged AXC rats. *J. Natl. Cancer Inst.*, **55**, 177

Smith, A. K., Landon, G. V., Ghanadian, R. and Chisholm, G. D. (1978). The ultrastructure of the male and female prostate of *Praomys (Mastomys) natalensis*. *Cell Tissue Res.*, **190**, 539

Smith, C. B., Ghanadian, R. and Chisholm, G. D. (1978). A soluble androgen receptor in the cytoplasm of the mastomys prostate. *Urol. Res.*, **6**, 29

Smith, C. B., Ghanadian, R. and Chisholm, G. D. (1979a). Nuclear androgen receptors in the prostate of male *Praomys (Mastomys) natalensis*. *Urol. Res.*, **7**, 243

Smolev, J. K., Heston, W. D. W., Scott, W. W. and Coffey, D. S. (1977). Characterization of the Dunning R3327H prostatic adenocarcinoma. An appropriate animal model for prostatic cancer. *Cancer Treat. Rep.*, **61**, 273

Snell, K. C. and Stewart, H. L. (1965). Adenocarcinoma and proliferative hyperplasia of the prostate gland in female *Rattus (Mastomys) natalensis. J. Natl. Cancer Inst.*, **35**, 7

Stone, K. R., Mickey, D. D., Wunderli, H., Mickey, G. H. and Paulson, D. F. (1978). Isolation of a human prostate carcinoma cell line. *Int. J. Cancer.*, **21**, 274

Voigt, W. and Dunning, W. F. (1974). *In vivo* metabolism of testosterone ^{3}H in R-3327, an androgen sensitive rat prostatic adenocarcinoma. *Cancer Res.*, **34**, 1447

Voigt, W., Feldman, M. and Dunning, W. F. (1975). 5α-dihydrotestosterone-binding proteins and androgen sensitivity in prostatic cancers of Copenhagen rats. *Cancer Res.*, **35**, 1840

Vollmer, E. P. and Kauffman, G. (1963). Biology of the prostate. *Natl. Cancer Inst. Monogr.*, **12**, 27

Walsh, P. C. and Wilson, J. D. (1976). The induction of prostatic hypertrophy in the dog with androstanediol. *J. Clin. Invest.*, **57**, 1093

Webber, M. M. (1981). *In vitro* models. In Hafez, E. S. E. and Spring-Mills, E. (eds.) *Prostatic Carcinoma: Biology and Diagnosis.* pp. 145–159. (The Hague: Martinus Nijhoff)

Williams, G., Ghanadian, R. and Castro, J. E. (1978a). The growth and viability of human prostatic tissue maintained in immunosuppressed mice. *Clin. Oncol.*, **4**, 347

Williams, G., Ghanadian, R., Papadopoulos, A. S. and Castro, J. E. (1978b). Hormonal environment of immunosuppressed mice. *Br. J. Cancer*, **37**, 123

Index

acid phosphatase 4, 26, 89
  assessment methods 249
  in BPH, epithelial and stromal 90
  in carcinoma 24
  tumour marker 248, 249
acini 19
  composition in BPH 96
  dormant in tumours 20
  function 105
actinomycin D, steroid action 159
adenocarcinoma 21, 24
  sites of origin 25, 26
  spontaneous in rats 287, 288
adenoid cystic carcinoma 26
adenosarcoma 26
adrenalectomy 38, 257
  and hormone levels 71
  survival 71
affinity chromatography
  steroid receptor analysis 182, 183
  uses 182
AFP *see alpha*-fetoprotein
agarose 178, 180
  cyanogen bromide activated 181
age
  androgen changes 42, 43, 46, 266
  and atrophy 9
  and carcinoma of the prostate 18, 19, 243, 244
  and dihydrotestosterone in BPH 61, 62
  oestrogen changes 45, 46
albumin, hormone binding 41
alkaline phosphatase, tumour marker 249
alpha-amanitin 157
ammonium sulphate *see* precipitation
analgesia 258
Ancillary Score System 251
androgen metabolism 64, 113–33
  and BPH in humans 123–7
  clearance rate 40
  cofactor requirement in BPH 126
  malignant prostate 127, 128
  normal, benign and malignant comparison 128–32, 135
  normal human prostate 122, 123
  organ culture 128
  pathways in human prostate 124, 125

  pathway in rat 116, 118
  steroid effects 132
  and tissue preparation 123, 124, 130
androgens *see also* individual androgens, receptor
  adrenal 38, 39
  age-related changes 42, 43, 266
  BPH therapy 270
  changes with age and BPH 266
  circulating in normal man 40–3
  DNA unmasking 154
  guanylate cyclase stimulation 160
  mechanism of action in prostate 143–62
  mesenchyme mediation 160
  nongenomic responses 159, 160
  plasma concentrations 41
  prostate, mechanism of action 223, 224
  protein bound 41
  rat prostate protein synthesis 153
  -receptor model 161, 162
  RNA and protein synthesis effects 152–4
  specific protein induction 155–7
  suppression in prostate 70, 72
  testicular 36–8
5*alpha*-androstane-3*alpha*, 17*beta*-diol
  BPH induction 285
  in BPH and removal technique 100
  changes in BPH 61–3, 68, 78, 285
  changes in carcinoma of the prostate 65, 66
  clearance rate 40
  experimental tumours 106
  human prostate 124, 125
  metabolic pathways 118
  metabolism in dog prostate 121
  metabolism in rat prostate 119
  normal prostate concentration 48–50
  plasma concentration 41
  prostate in BPH 73–5
  prostate in carcinoma 73–5
  secretion and age 42
androstanetriol 118, 123
androstenediol
  formula 37
  plasma concentration 41
androstenedione
  adrenal origin 38
  changes in BPH 61–3

299